Transition mechanisms in child development

Transition mechanisms in child development:
The longitudinal perspective

Edited by
ANIK DE RIBAUPIERRE
Faculté de Psychologie et des Sciences de l'Education
Université de Genève

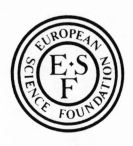

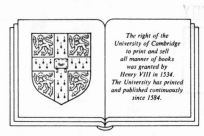

The right of the
University of Cambridge
to print and sell
all manner of books
was granted by
Henry VIII in 1534.
The University has printed
and published continuously
since 1584.

CAMBRIDGE UNIVERSITY PRESS
Cambridge
New York   New Rochelle   Melbourne   Sydney

Published by the Press Syndicate of the University of Cambridge
The Pitt Building, Trumpington Street, Cambridge CB2 1RP
32 East 57th Street, New York, NY 10022, USA
10 Stamford Road, Oakleigh, Melbourne 3166, Australia

First published 1989

Printed in Canada

Library of Congress Cataloging-in-Publication Data
Transition mechanisms in child development.
Includes index.
1. Child psychology – Longitudinal studies – Congresses
I. Ribaupierre, Anik de.
BF721.T69   1989   155.4   88–30512
ISBN 0-521-37138-4 hard covers

British Library Cataloging-in-Publication applied for

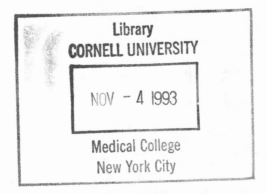

Contents

Foreword

A main characteristic of traditional research on individual development, whether it is performed in education, medicine, psychology, or any other discipline, is its reliance on cross-sectional studies. Thus, the studies that have dominated the scene are those in which the relationship among variables has been investigated using data collected at a certain point in time for a sample of individuals. Although this type of research is important and highly valuable, it has definite and serious limitations. For research to contribute to understanding and explaining individual development in all its psychological and biological facets, it is necessary to complement the cross-sectional approach with research planned and conducted in a longitudinal perspective – by studying individuals over time in relation to relevant variables.

Longitudinal research on individual development has a long history. The necessity for and benefits of such a perspective have become increasingly apparent during the past decades in all disciplines concerned with understanding and explaining the biological, psychological, and social structures and processes involved in individual life courses. The manifestation of the importance of longitudinal research in many fields, both in basic research and in application, and the need for stimulation and support of such research were determining factors for the European Science Foundation's decision to give this type of research high priority and to establish in 1985 the ESF Network on Longitudinal Research on Individual Development (ENLS).

Effective longitudinal research on individual development must deal with far-reaching, substantive, methodological and research strategy problems. Of crucial importance for successful scientific progress is the need to handle methodological problems appropriately. Few areas in research are so full of traps as developmental research. However, a relevant discussion of appropriate methodologies must be founded in appropriate substantive models and theories for the developmental phenomena that we try to understand and explain. Therefore, as a first step in its endeavors to contribute effectively to longitudinal developmental research, the coordination committee of ENLS has taken the initiative in the publication of a series of books focusing on central substantive issues. The main topic of the present volume – transition mechanisms in cognitive, emotional, and social development – is concerned with a substantive area of great importance for developmental research. It is my conviction, and that of my colleagues responsible for directing the ENLS, that the essays presented here will enhance the effectiveness of theoretical and empirical analyses related to important topics of individual development.

David Magnusson
Chairman
The ESF Network on Longitudinal Research
on Individual Development

Preface

This book is the outcome of a joint effort by the participants in the second workshop organized by the European Science Foundation Network on Longitudinal Studies on Individual Development (ENLS), held in Grächen, Switzerland, in March 1987. The current chapters represent the main papers presented at the workshop and a selection of the discussants' contributions. The final versions incorporate many of the ideas and comments discussed during the workshop. Although the book will fail to communicate to the reader the atmosphere of the workshop – whether the intellectual and personal relations among the participants or the pleasant blend of hard work and sportive between-session skiing effort – I hope it will convey the many good ideas and interesting directions that were discussed.

The workshop was organized around the six following themes, each consisting of a main presentation paper and two discussants' papers: cognition, memory, language, and social, emotional, and motor development. Each contributor, dealing with one of these areas, addressed the issues of developmental transitions, transition mechanisms, and the role of longitudinal research in clarifying these issues. In the present volume, the six themes are retained but reorganized in four sections, due to an unequal number of contributions in each theme. In an introductory chapter, Siegfried Hoppe-Graff deals with the delicate task of defining some of the core concepts used throughout this book – such as transition and transition laws and mechanisms – and pleads for the necessity of longitudinal research in developmental psychology. The first content section is devoted to cognitive and memory development, with one chapter by Kurt Fischer and Susie Lamborn and the other by Wolfgang Schneider and Franz Weinert. In the second section, which deals with language development, Luigia Camaioni discusses the transition to oral language and Peter Bryant and Jesus Alegria the transition to written language. The third section includes three chapters on social and emotional development, contributed by Håkan Stattin and David Magnusson, Paul Harris, and Grazia Attili. The fourth section includes three essays concerned with motor development by Claes von Hofsten, Henriette Bloch, and George Butterworth. Finally, in an epilogue, Anik de Ribaupierre attempts a summary of these different theoretical perspectives along three directions, by focusing on definitions of transition mechanisms given in the four sections, and on the role assigned to longitudinal research and to individual differences; she also discusses the lack of longitudinal studies in developmental psychology.

It is a pleasure to thank the many colleagues who participated in the workshop, especially the European Science Foundation, for endorsing a series of such interesting workshops and resolutely attempting to advance longitudinal research; and the Network Committee Members, particularly Chairman David Magnusson, who are so enthusiastic and efficient in organizing the Network's activities. Pierre Mounoud and Klaus Scherer helped to plan the workshop and select many of the participants. Isabelle Neirynck and Ana Sancho were of great assistance in attending to the many organizational details that such a workshop necessarily entails. The participants at the workshop and authors of this book are to be thanked for having met, most of the time, the stringent deadlines that were given. Finally, I would like to express my gratitude to the many people who contributed, by their comments and reviews, to the look of this book: Paul Baltes, Johan Brandtstatter, Michael Chapman, Willem Doise, Klaus Grossmann, Pierre Mounoud, Laurence Rieben, Chirstiane Robert-Tissot, Ana Sancho, Klaus Scherer, Dan Stern, Martti Takala, and Alexander von Eye. Thanks are also due to the Cambridge University Press editors for their patience in waiting for long overdue manuscripts and for their efficiency.

Anik de Ribaupierre
February 1989

Contributors

Jesus Alegria
Laboratoire de Psychologie
  Expérimentale
Université Libre de Bruxelles
Av. Ad-Buyl 117
B-1050 Bruxelles
Belgium

Grazia Attili
CNR
Istituto di Psicologia
Viale Marx 15
I-00156 Roma
Italy

Henriette Bloch
Laboratoire de Psycho-Biologie
  de l'Enfant
Ecole Pratique des Hautes
  Etudes
41, rue Gay-Lussac
F-75005 Paris
France

Peter Bryant
Department of Experimental
  Psychology
University of Oxford
South Parks Road
UK-OX1 3UD Oxford
England

George Butterworth
Department of Psychology
University of Stirling
UK-FK9 4LA Stirling
Scotland

Luigia Camaioni
Department di Psicologia dei
  Processi di Sviluppo
Universita degli Studi di Roma
Via degli Apuli 8
I-00185 Roma
Italy

Kurt W. Fischer
Department of Human
  Development
Larsen Hall
Harvard University
Cambridge, Massachusetts 02138
United States

Paul L. Harris
Department of Experimental
  Psychology
University of Oxford
South Parks Road
UK-OX1 3UD Oxford
England

Claes von Hofsten
Department of Psychology
University of Umeå
S-901 87 Umeå
Sweden

Siegfried Hoppe-Graff
Psychologisches Institut
Universität Heidelberg
Haupstrasse 47–51
D-6900 Heidelberg
Germany

Susie D. Lamborn
National Center on Effective
    Secondary Schools
School of Education
1025 W. Johnson #685
University of Wisconsin
Madison, Wisconsin 53706
United States

David Magnusson
Department of Psychology
University of Stockholm
S-106 91 Stockholm
Sweden

Anik de Ribaupierre
Faculté de Psychologie et des
    Sciences de l'Education
Université de Genève
av. Général Dufour 24
CH-1211 Genève 4
Switzerland

Wolfgang Schneider
Max-Planck Institut für
    Psychologische Forschung
Léopoldstrasse 24
D-8000 München 40
Germany

Håkan Stattin
Department of Psychology
University of Stockholm
S-106 91 Stockholm
Sweden

Franz E. Weinert
Max-Planck Institut für
    Psychologische Forschung
Leopoldstrasse 24
D-8000 München 40
Germany

1 The study of transitions in development: potentialities of the longitudinal approach

SIEGFRIED HOPPE-GRAFF

In longitudinal research "the entity under investigation is observed repeatedly as it exists and evolves over time" (Baltes & Nesselroade, 1979, p. 4). Since Wohlwill's (1973) well-known pleading there seems to be agreement among developmentalists that we can resolve our main problems only by this type of observational strategy. It is the aim of this article to relate the longitudinal approach to the study of transition processes and modeling of transition mechanisms, topics that have become prominent, at least in the field of cognitive development, within the last few years.

The arguments are organized as follows. Because there are different uses of transition, transition principle, transition mechanism, and so forth, we will start with a clarification of concepts. To introduce a concrete, substantive point of reference for the discussion, we will then give a summary description of three transition models of cognitive development. A sketch of the field of developmental research strategies follows, with emphasis on the longitudinal approach. In the last section we discuss the interrelations between transition models and longitudinal data collection strategies. In large part these considerations are programmatic and prospective: What *would* be the strengths and the limits of the longitudinal approach if it *were* used? Although our analysis is restricted to the field of cognitive development, it may hold for other areas of developmental psychology as well.

Transitions, transition principles, and transition mechanisms

There is no consensus on a definition of psychological development. This is not surprising because research programs are based on different world views (Kuhn, 1962; Overton, 1984). But according to Nagel (1957) it is possible to delineate necessary (but not sufficient) constituents that are implicit in every definitional statement. When speaking about develop-

1

ment, we refer to "a system possessing a definite structure and a definite set of preexisting capacities; and . . . a sequential set of changes in the system, yielding relatively as well" (p. 17).[1] In agreement with these minimal criteria, we find developmentalists primarily engaged in describing the sequence of states $S1$, $S2$, . . . Sn through which the system passes. In the structuralist tradition the focus of analysis is on the sequence of structures, whereas in functionalist approaches it is on the system's ways of functioning (see Beilin, 1984, for more details of the structuralist vs. functionalist distinction of developmental theories). Or we find them analyzing "what happens in between" – that is, in the system's transition from $S1$ to $S2$, . . . to Sn.

Several authors have commented on this dichotomy of tasks (Case, 1985; Inhelder & Piaget, 1964; Siegel, Bisanz, & Bisanz, 1983; Sugarman, 1987). According to the Piagetian point of view, there is a strict order in resolving them: "In order to elucidate the causal mechanisms of a given process, we must first discover the structures which we are to begin with, and then show how and why these structures come to be transformed" (Inhelder & Piaget, 1964, p. 1). Others have equated it with the description versus explanation distinction (e.g., Lunzer, 1964); only the analysis of the transitions allows explanatory statements.

An inventory of the current uses of the notion of transition shows that at least two conceptions of the study of transitions and transition processes exist:

1. Studying the process of transition means to elaborate on a precise description of the steps (stages) of change from $S1$ to $S2$. This endeavor may result in the identification of (sub-) states $S1.1$, $S1.2$, . . ., $S1.n$ between $S1$ and $S2$ – that is, in a more precise process description.

2. Studying the process of transition means to locate the factors responsible for the change of the system from $S1$ to $S2$. We often refer to this second conception as the task of *explanation*. By one or the other kind of explanatory analysis we have to figure out the factors (determinants) that account for the structures or functions specific to the system in $S2$. The notion of *transition mechanisms* (or *mechanisms of change*) refers to this connotation. Thus, Sternberg (1984, p. vii) has this identification of explanatory factors in mind when he asks: "What are the mechanisms of development by which individuals pass from one state to another?"

In a loose way, the distinction between the descriptive and explanatory aspects of the study of transitions can be paraphrased as the how and the why questions of the transition process: *How* does the change in the developing system come about, and *why* does it come about? But recall that in everyday language answers to how questions sometimes are accepted as sufficient explanations, similar to answers to why questions –

for example, when we ask "How did the accident happen?" and the witness answers by giving a precise description of the event, we are gratified. As several observers have noted (e.g., Kessen, 1984), something analogous happens in science: the clear-cut distinction between descriptions on the one hand and explanations on the other does not work unless we restrict ourselves to a very limited concept of explanation, that is, to causal analysis.

Moreover, while studying transitions there is of course an interdependence between the specification of the steps of the transition process and the determination of the transition mechanisms. Take as an example the equilibration model, the transition mechanism proposed by Piaget (1977a/1975; 1977b), and accept for the time being (though several authors doubt it) that it is an explanatory construct. Besides explaining cognitive development the equilibration model includes statements for a more precise description of the emergence of new structures.

For clarity, we propose to use the terms transition (process), transition principle, and transition mechanism in the following way. A *transition* (*process*) is a change in a well-defined (developing) system; by *transition principles* we refer to the laws of change; and we define *transition mechanisms* as a subclass of principles that are primarily used to explain the transition.[2]

The terms transition, transition mechanism, and transition principle were brought to the field of cognitive development by proponents of an information processing and/or neo-Piagetian orientation. Take as an example Case's (1985) influential theory of intellectual development. A central part of this theory is an extended treatment of "the process of stage transition." Or take as another example Fischer's (1980) skill theory of development, part of which are "transition rules," which are "the heart of the mechanism for predicting specific sequences of development" (p. 497).

Maybe the focus on transition was a necessary next step in the elaboration of the information processing or the neo-Piagetian framework that promised to be "neo" exactly in going beyond structural descriptions to the study of the principles of the emergence of structures. But it may also be that the introduction of transitions is part of the larger conceptual endeavor observed by Sameroff: "The growth of developmental psychology has been accompanied by an increasing uneasiness. This discomfort is centered on the limitations of most current conceptual frameworks for dealing with change and transformations" (1982, p. 83).

But we should be careful to distinguish the use of the *term* transition from the *concept*. For sure, the popularity of the term reflects the current stress on the concept. But, on the other hand, even without talking explicitly about transitions, cognitive developmentalists have always speculated and theorized about the how and why aspects of ontogenetic changes. We are reminded of this for example by Kessen (1984), who in a historical survey distinguished directive, constrained, and open (transition) mechanisms. Note that as early as 1928 Kurt Koffka explicitly dealt with transitions. And Piaget's idea of the process of equilibration, as stated for example in *La naissance de l'intelligence* (1952/1936), was intended to describe and explain the transition from one structural level to the next.

Transitions and transition mechanisms in models of cognitive development

In this section we will sketch three of the transition models proposed in the field of cognitive development and thereby introduce a concrete point of reference for our arguments concerning the potential contributions of the longitudinal approach to the study of transition in the last section of this chapter.

For a long time research on cognitive development in childhood and adolescence was dominated by Piaget's genetic structuralism. But in the past 10 to 15 years this paradigm has been challenged by the information processing approach to development (Siegler, 1983; Sternberg, 1984). The information processing paradigm offers a variety of models that differ in their reliance on the computer as a metaphor of human cognition and vary in their openness to one or another structural–developmental premise. Thus, it would be misleading to refer to only one information processing model of cognitive development and to discuss it as representative of the approach in general. (On the other hand, there are elements common to all information processing models, established at a very general level.)

If you scan the whole spectrum of information processing approaches to cognitive development, at the one extreme there are the computer simulation models (e.g., Klahr, 1984; Klahr & Wallace, 1976). At the other extreme there are the so-called neo-Piagetian or neo-structural models. Although they rely heavily on information processing assumptions or concepts, these models are outlined as elaborations and/or modifications of the Piagetian view of development. Fischer's skill theory (1980; Fischer & Lamborn, this volume; Fischer & Pipp, 1984) and Case's neo-Piagetian stage theory (1984; 1985) are the most prominent representatives of these.

This is why we have sampled from the entire field of cognitive development three conceptualizations of the transition process: Piaget's new equilibration model, Klahr's concept of self-modification, and Fischer's two-component model of skill acquisition processes that are constrained by the optimal level parameter. My presentation does not intend to summarize these models, but is restricted to the concepts of transition. Thus, what follows cannot suffice as a basis for a general appraisal of these approaches.

K. W. Fischer: optimal level and transformation rules

According to Fischer's skill theory of cognitive development "two different types of processes are involved in developmental transitions" (Fischer & Pipp, 1984, p. 74): optimal level and skill acquisition processes.

1. *Optimal level* is the upper limit to the complexity of skills (concepts, structures)[3] that a person can construct. It denotes "the upper limit of a person's information processing capacity" (Fischer & Pipp, 1984, p. 47). That is, optimal level is a representational construct, and therefore Fischer's categorization of optimal level as a process seems to us to be misleading (for a detailed discussion of the uses and benefits of a strict structure–process distinction, see Siegler & Richards, 1983).

The capacity construct of optimal levels develops through a series of hierarchically organized levels – thirteen in the latest version of the theory (Fischer & Lamborn, this volume) – that seem to be closely tied to age. Sometimes Fischer refers to optimal level as the "true" developmental variable in his theory (Fischer & Lamborn, this volume), but note that he proposes the same two-component transition model for other than developmental changes, for example, for learning and problem solving (Fischer & Pipp, 1984, p. 46).[4]

2. The true developmental sequence of optimal levels has to be distinguished from intralevel sequences of steps of *skill acquisition*. Fischer's theory lists a limited set of transformation rules to explain the acquisition of new skills: substitution, focusing (or shift of focus), compounding, differentiation, and intercoordination. All of these five rules are formally specified as set-theoretic rewrite rules. Substitution, focusing, compounding, and differentiation describe (and explain?) the construction of skills of increasing complexity within a developmental level, whereas intercoordination in connection with optimal level explains how skills at one level are combined to produce a new skill at the next level. In addition to formalizing them as rewrite rules Fischer gives the following psychological interpretations of the five transformation processes. *Substitution,* the simplest within level transformation, is "a type of generalization, in which a skill is mastered through one task and then transferred to a second, similar task." This kind of transfer arises, "when all but one of

the components in the second skill structure are the same as those in the first structure" (Fischer & Pipp, 1984, p. 61). *Focusing* refers to the process of using two related skills in succession; they are simply strung together without being integrated. Not the person, who cannot apply both concepts at a time, but the situation is responsible for the shift of focus: it "tends to elicit both skills" (p. 64). By the process of *compounding*, two skills at a given level are combined to form a more complex skill that unifies the components at that level. Contrary to the shift of focus, here we have an integration of acts. *Differentiation* refers to the process of separating a skill into its distinct components. It seems always to accompany one of the aforementioned processes.

The fifth transformation rule, *intercoordination*, specifies in conjunction with optimal levels the change of skills to a higher level. Fischer and Pipp (1984, p. 65) describe the process as follows:

At the beginning of the process, the child has two well-formed skills at a given level. The two skills function separately from each other until some object or event in the world induces the child to relate the two skills. If at this point the child is capable of the next developmental level, he or she will unravel the relationship between the two skills, gradually intercoordinating them. This unraveling will include a series of microdevelopmental steps involving the other transformations, and it will culminate in the intercoordination.

Although the set of transformation rules is the same for all processes of developmental change, the sequences they produce may vary within a person from domain to domain, and from person to person, depending on the specific (idiosyncratic) kind of person–environment interaction; that is, they may cause different developmental pathways. Therefore, according to Fischer, development is intraindividually and interindividually domain specific, in that it includes different sequences of developmental steps for different domains. But at the same time a general course of development exists in that (a) the optimal level puts a general constraint on the skill acquisition processes, and (b) the same limited number of transformation rules is responsible for all the diversity of the domain-specific sequences.

To summarize, Fischer proposes two forms of transition, differing in "developmental dignity" (only one of them truly developmental): transitions from one step to the next within a developmental level, and transitions between developmental levels (optimal levels). Both are necessary components of the process of cognitive development. But whereas Fischer is explicit on the transition processes that account for the domain-specific skill-acquisition sequences, the problem of what brings about the transitions in the optimal-level construct itself is not discussed in any detail. Fischer is only explicit in rejecting working memory notions as explanatory for developmental changes in optimal level: "The growing efficiency [of a rise in optimal level] comes not from an increase in the number of items that can be held in working memory" (Fischer & Pipp, 1984, p. 71). From the few hints Fischer gives it is our impression that optimal level is not only age bound but also, in a stricter sense, a maturational construct, although he cautions "against thinking of ... biological changes as prerequisites in any simple sense for the psychological changes" (p. 58).

D. Klahr: self-modification in production systems

Klahr's (1982; 1984) model of transition processes and transition mechanisms is characterized by himself as a challenge to the classical Piagetian equilibration model, which he polemically rejects: "For 40 years now, we have had *assimilation* and *accommodation*, the mysterious and shadowy forces of *equilibration*, the 'Batman and Robin' of the developmental processes. What are they? How do they operate? ... What we need is a way to go beyond vague verbal statements of the nature of the developmental process" (1982, p. 80). But Klahr shares the fundamental assumption with Piagetian reasoning that the basic characteristic of the human cognitive system is its potential for self-modification.

Klahr's road to more explicitness and systematization in model formulation is computer simulation. The primary criterion of his models is that they can be run on a computer; thus they must be formulated in a suitable programming language. The language Klahr prefers for state descriptions of a developmental system as well as for the dynamic aspect of self-modification is the language of production systems (PS).

A production system consists of a set of rules, or *productions*, that are written in the form of condition–action pairs. The conditions stand as symbolic expressions for elements of knowledge. The whole system serves as a description of the knowledge state of a cognitive system. It works via a recognize–act cycle (for greater detail, see Klahr, 1984, and Klahr & Wallace, 1976). Each production within the production system has the ability to examine a data base and change it as a function of what it finds there.

According to Klahr production systems present in the first place those clear, explicit theories of knowledge states that are a prerequisite of acceptable transition theories, "because a transition theory can be no better than a theory of what it is that is undergoing transition" (1984, p. 104). It can be demonstrated that the formalism of production systems is equivalent to other formalisms (e.g., Klahr & Siegler, 1978), but Klahr points out that production systems have important practical and theoretical advances for modeling states and transitions. However, as early as 1973 Newell was critical about the value of production systems. He reminded us that programming languages such as PS are not only programming languages when applied in simulation but also serve as a theory of cognition (and cognitive development), and he stated that it is unclear what elements or parts of the programs are proposed to have psychological validity. (For a detailed discussion and critique of the use of computer programs as explanatory psychological theories, see Cummins, 1977; 1983.)

Self-modification processes in production systems operate on the time line, which is a temporally ordered record within which people preserve their goals, short-term memory (STM) contents, and outcomes (Klahr, 1984). In the course of elaborating their production system models as models of developmental change, Klahr and his co-workers have detected several self-modification mechanisms, that is, principles by which production systems modify themselves. The list includes designation, strengthening, generalization, discrimination, addition, merging of co-occurring conditions (Klahr, 1982), and, in a later formulation, discrimination, generalization, and composition (Klahr, 1984). *Discrimination*, for example, consists of taking an existing production and adding more tests on its condition side. *Composition* refers to the idea that whenever a set of productions repeatedly "fires" in the same sequence, it may be possible to combine the set into a single production.

Similar to Fischer, Klahr (1982) argued that these mechanisms are not specific to any sort of change but could be used for explaining learning as well as development: "There is little to be gained from believing that the mechanisms of learning are fundamentally different from the mechanisms of development" (p. 85). He has since modified this judgment, believing that "self-modifying systems appear to be more appropriately placed in the developmental than in the learning category" (1984, p. 130).

J. Piaget: assimilation, accommodation, and equilibration

Contrary to some critics' opinions, the structuralist model of the Genevan school from the beginning included a model of the process of ontogenetic change, that is, a transition model. The refined and revised formulation of this equilibration model also was the central aim of Piaget's work in his last years (Piaget, 1977a; 1977b). We will restrict our presentation to the revised version – what Furth (1981) calls Piaget's new equilibration model.

Piaget always emphasized (e.g., 1977a; 1977b; 1983; Inhelder & Piaget, 1964) that one origin of the equilibration model lies in the insufficiencies of the factors traditionally postulated in explanations of development. He lists three classical factors: influences of physical environment, hereditary program, and social transmission (including language), and convincingly argues that "no one of the three is sufficient in itself" (1977b, p. 3). The equilibration principle is the "critical" fourth factor, a factor that coordinates the others, and the only one that can account for the self-regulations that can be observed at all levels of development.

By *equilibration* Piaget (1977a; 1977b) refers to a process that may lead from one state of a cognitive equilibrium through a variety of disequilibrations and reequilibrations to the recurrence of the equilibrium at a higher, qualitatively different level – that is why Piaget introduces the term *equilibration majorante* (majoring, that is increasing or improved equilibration).[5]

The following summary description of the phases of the equilibration process has been adapted from Furth (1981, p. 257). Equilibration rests upon the existence of a cognitive system that is at the same time closed (i.e., an internally consistent whole) *and* open to an unlimited number of exchanges with its surroundings. Some of the exchanges lead to disturbances in existing balances. The disturbances are experienced as conflicts or gaps relative to the subject's cognitive system. The system responds to compensate for the disturbances, and this eventually leads to integrating them as parts into it. While the system proceeds, there is a reequilibration, which does not lead to the reestablishment of the old system but to the construction of an improved one.

Two components are included in each step of the equilibration process: assimilation and accommodation. *Assimilation* is a form of integration of external data into the structures of the subject. It is made possible by the existence of instruments for that very function – schemes of assimilation. Piaget underlines that "assimilation is clearly not a matter of passively registering what is going on" but an active process by the individual (1977b, p. 5). By *accommodation* Piaget refers to the fact that the subject in each act of assimilation has to take into consideration the specificities of the object that is to be assimilated and to adapt his schemes to that object.

The processes of assimilation and accommodation are simultaneously complementary and hierarchically ordered. They are complementary because at every moment of a cognitive system's activity, content is assimilated to the schemes and schemes accommodate to the content. And accommodation is subordinate to assimilation, because when it occurs it is always the accommodation of a scheme of assimilation.

Within the new equilibration model we have to distinguish between three kinds of equilibrium (Piaget, 1977a; 1977b). The first one is between the structures of the subject and the object. The object is assimilated to the structures and, as another part of the same adaptation process, the subject's structures accommodate to a new object. The second kind is an equilibrium between the subsystems of a subject's schemes. For example, there may exist a conflict between the subsystem dealing with logicomathematical operations and the subsystem dealing with spatial operations. The third kind of equilibrium, according to Piaget (1977a), is the most fundamental one. It is constructed step by step between the parts of the subject's knowledge and the totality of his knowledge system at any given moment. It can also be viewed as an equilibration between differentiation and integration of the subject's knowledge. The equilibration process that acts on this kind of equilibrium (or disequilibrium) in the total knowledge system leads to the construction of new operations upon previous operations – and this is "probably the secret of development and of the transition from one stage to the next" (Piaget, 1977b, p. 12).

The elaboration of the new equilibration model in Piaget's 1977 (originally 1975) book does not include empirical studies, not to speak of empirical tests of his theoretical propositions in the usual sense. But Piaget points to a number of former studies (e.g., Inhelder & Piaget, 1964; Inhelder, Sinclair, & Bovet, 1974) that demonstrate one or the other aspect of the theoretical system.

In the first section we distinguished two directions of the study of transition principles – one referring to the precise and elaborate description of the steps in the transition from one state to another, the other to the identification of the factors (mechanisms) responsible for the transition process. Obviously, the equilibration model is related to both tasks. In the first place, it serves as a precise process description (see the previous summary statement of the phases of the equilibration process): At the micro-level the ontogenetic process can be taken to be a series of ongoing equilibrations. Second, as Piaget explicitly noted, the equilibration process has explanatory force; it is proposed as a "causal mechanism" to "explain the development and even the formation of knowledge by a central equilibration process" (1977b, p. 11).

The explanatory function of the equilibration principle contrasts with the fact that there is no further need to explain the principle itself, because "the entire equilibration process is predicated on a biological (inborn) tendency for schemes of assimilation to do just that, to assimilate where and when it is possible, by extending and constructing new contacts in appropriate situations" (Furth, 1981, p. 255). But when going into detail, we actually have to distinguish two inborn tendencies of the scheme of assimilation: (a) the tendency to incorporate all external elements that are compatible with it, which "explains" why the subject is active; (b) the tendency to accommodate to the elements that it is assimilating. In other words, the schemes have the tendency to adapt to the specifics of the elements of experience without losing their continuity or potential for further assimilations, which "explains" why assimilation results in the construction of novelty.

The use of the equilibration principle as a transition model is not restricted to the Genevans (or the Piagetian school) but has been adopted by most structuralists in cognitive development. Social-cognitive structuralists in particular (e.g., Damon, 1983; Edelstein, Keller, & Wahlen, 1984; Furth, 1980; Langer, 1977; Turiel, 1983) have tried to elaborate the concept of equilibration by combining it with conceptions of the effect of social experience on development (see Damon, 1983, for a review). In this tradition the principle has not only been used as an adequate procedure to reconstruct step by step the successive construction of knowledge structures by an active subject at the micro level. It has also been used for modeling the long-term ontogenetic progress as a result of large-scale (macro) series of self-generated equilibriums and disequilibriums (Langer, 1977). But it seems to us that those authors are not always explicit about whether they use the model literally, that is, at the micro level, or more deliberately for the large picture of development.

From this survey of three models of transition processes in cognitive development we can learn that the current use of the transition concept is by no means restricted to qualitative models that view the course of development as an alternation of periods of fundamental restructurings and consolidations. The extensive definition in the first section that applies the notion of transition to all changes from one state to another in a well-defined developing system fits Fischer's and Klahr's as well as Piaget's use of the term. It also fits van den Daele's (1974) formal analysis of transition models within a set-theoretical interpretation of developmental structures and sequences. Mounoud (1982), who proposes a qualitative model of development, reserves a special term to refer to those periods of fundamental changes or disruptions in the system's organization – he speaks of *revolutions*.

The longitudinal approach to development

For conceptual clarification, Baltes and Nesselroade (1979) introduced the distinction between the general longitudinal-developmental design orientation and the variety of specific longitudinal methods. The criterion of repeated intraindividual observations (see the quotation from the Baltes & Nesselroade article in the introductory remarks) is the only common denominator to all specific methods – that is, it is the critical feature of the longitudinal design orientation. The spectrum of methods includes special designs as well as techniques for the statistical analysis of longitudinal data. Baltes and Nesselroade (1979), Kuhn and Phelps (1982), and others have convincingly argued that there can be no general preference for specific designs or statistical methods, because "the nature of longitudinal methodology is defined to a large extent by the nature of developmental theory" (p. 13). Several reviewers (e.g., Appelbaum & McCall, 1983; Baltes & Nesselroade, 1979; Schaie & Herzog, 1982) have documented that there have been notable advances in the technical know-how of planning (designing) and analyzing longitudinal studies. We will not deal with this aspect here.

Baltes and Nesselroade (1979, pp. 23ff.) identify five main rationales for longitudinal research in developmental psychology:

1. the direct identification of intraindividual change;
2. the direct identification of individual differences or similarities in intraindividual change;
3. the identification of interrelationships in behavioral change (identification of developmental patterns);
4. the analyses of causes or determinants of intraindividual change; and
5. the analysis of causes or determinants of interindividual differences in intraindividual change.

If we accept for the moment the description–explanation distinction and classify causal analysis as one type of explanation, the first three rationales correspond to the task of description and the fourth and fifth to the task of explanation. Thus, the characterization of the aims of the longitudinal approach by Baltes and Nesselroade clearly challenges a metatheoretical position that holds the aims and range of validity of the observational method to be restricted to description, and maintains that causal explanatory analyses can only be carried out within the strict experimental framework.

The concepts of cause and explanation are among the most ambiguous constructs in methodological analyses of the "logic" of the social sciences. The classical position identifies causal analysis with the experimental approach because only the experiment (by definition) allows for deliberate manipulation (Bunge, 1979; Cook & Campbell, 1979; von Wright, 1971). Through deliberate manipulation we can find out whether some factor f is a necessary and sufficient condition for the event e. By creating f it will be possible to produce all events (or states) e to which f is a sufficient condition, and by eliminating or preventing f, we can make sure that all events (states) e to which f is a necessary condition will not occur. According to the classical or essentialist view of causation, variables are causes when they are, taken together, both necessary *and* sufficient for the effect to occur (Cook & Campbell, 1979, p. 14).

Longitudinal designs are used to observe developmental functions (Wohlwill, 1973). The developmental function is a construct to relate change in some "interesting" dimension to age or some age-related variable. Because age is not an experimental variable (it cannot be manipulated deliberately), the typical application of the longitudinal approach is nonexperimental. This does not impede the combination of experimental and longitudinal design elements; for example, it may be useful to collect data longitudinally within an experimental follow-up design.

In search of a concept of cause that might be more adequate for the social sciences, Cook and Campbell (1979, pp. 14–15) have questioned the essentialist position: "We are convinced that observed causal relationships in the social sciences will be fallible rather than inevitable and that the connections between antecedents and consequences will be probabilistic" (p. 15). This weaker concept of causation is the tacit background for the popular approaches of "causal modeling" on the basis of correlational data by structural equation models (Mulaik, 1987).

It will be an interesting task for future analysts to find out the historical forces that maintained the experimental approach's strong position in developmental methodology and that are responsible for the recent shift to quasi-experimentation and a liberalized idea of causal explanation. According to Overton (1984) methodological preferences depend on the "world views" (in the sense of T. S. Kuhn) of the developmentalists. The experiment (in the strict sense) is connected with the mechanistic world view, which also determines the scientist's interest in external causes of development. Thus, we expect that the shift away from the strictly experimental study of causation will be accompanied by a focus on internal causes; both are related to the organismic world view.

Our definition of the longitudinal approach leaves open (a) the *timing* (spacing, frequency) of observations and (b) the kind of *sample(s)* to be included in a study. Of course, it has to leave the topics open, because reasons for decisions on these issues can only be stated in terms of the theory or the problem under study.[6] Take as an example the Berkeley Growth Study, initiated in 1928 by Nancy Bayley. The outstanding design includes the repetition of assessments at unequal intervals. The sample of $N = 74$ infants was assessed for the first time when the babies were 4 days old. Then the subjects were observed monthly from 1 to 15 months, every 3 months from 18 to 36 months, annually from 4 to 7 years, biannually from 8 to 18 years, and at 21, 26, and 36 (for more details, see Eichhorn, Clausen, Haan, Honzik, & Mussen, 1981). The unequal spacing of measurements points was "theory guided" – not by a developmental theory *sensu stricto*, but by the implicit theoretical consideration that there is a decrease in the density of significant developmental changes.

Of course, the general definition of the longitudinal approach does not specify in any way the range of sample sizes. In fact, it varies from $N = 1$ (see, e.g., the Lawler study mentioned later, or Fein & Moorin, 1985) to $N > 100$ (see, e.g., some of the studies reported by Bryant & Alegria, this volume; Magnusson & Stattin, this volume; or Hoppe-Graff & Keller, 1988). Probably the most important factor in deciding on the number of subjects is the access to financial, manpower, and organizational facilities. When the extent of support is fixed, the intensity of assessment (as can been seen from the number and elaborateness of observations) and the number of subjects relate reciprocally. What you invest in number you have to omit in intensity, and vice versa.

Theoretical considerations should, at least in the ideal case, lay the ground for sampling decisions. They concern, for example, the expected (or known) degree of interindividual variability of the developmental process under study, or expectations about cohort effects. As has been demonstrated by life-span developmental psychologists (see Baltes, Cornelius, & Nesselroade, 1979), there are some clusters of developmental variables that are influenced by the cohort factor, including psychometric intelligence and some personality traits. Within the life-span approach the relation of social change and individual development has become a topic of much interest (Nesselroade & von Eye, 1985). The focus on this interrelatedness generates new criteria for selecting samples (or subsamples), by comparing cohorts that are defined by varying experiences of social changes.

The longitudinal approach is often compared with the cross-sectional approach. A point that is made in introductory textbooks in favor of the longitudinal and against the cross-sectional approach states that the former asks for the observation of intraindividual change whereas the latter is restricted to the inference of intraindividual changes from the comparison of (interindividual) differences between groups of subjects (who differ in age or with regard to an age-related variable). Some developmental psychologists have doubted that it is possible to observe change; they have doubted it either in principle or that it is possible by realizable longitudinal studies (given the constraints in financial and institutional support). The question at issue appears to be, in some way, a pseudocontroversy. Everyone will agree that change is a fundamental concept (category), in analyses of epistemologists (e.g., Bunge, 1979; Whitehead, 1957/1929) as well as in the theoretical and empirical work of psychologists. Whether change is "directly" observable depends on one's concept (definition) of change. Take the example of Piaget's (1952) fascinating observations of the beginnings of the assimilation processes in newborns. Did he *observe* the growth (elaboration) of the sucking scheme out of the sucking reflex? We leave aside the problem that he only observed sucking behavior (and inferred the processes of assimilation and accommodation). Then it depends on your a priori conception of change whether you take the baby's sucking behavior at time n as a case of observing change, because it is different from the sucking behaviors at times $n - 1$ and $n + 1$, or (only) as a case of observing a specific mode of sucking behavior. If in the latter case the behavior is different from the sucking behaviors at times $n - 1$ and $n + 1$, then you *infer* the change of the sucking scheme because of these differences.

Some philosophers have made the point that there are different concepts of change more explicit (see Fetz, 1984, who connected Whitehead's process orientation with Piaget's inclination to the genetic method). In line with A. N. Prior, von Wright (1971) started exploring a logical calculus that includes the time dimension – and, thereby, change – in the formalism and thus seems to be more adequate for logical analyses of "modes of becoming" (Bunge, 1981). Leaving these metatheoretical considerations aside, there have been several attempts in the past years to study the process of change more directly by means of longitudinal studies. After objecting to the experimental strategy with some well-known arguments, Kuhn and Phelps (1982) suggest carrying out longitudinal research with a "dense" spacing of observations within a limited interval of observation. Lawler (1981) conducted a single case study with a similar aim and a similar logic. His "Intimate study" traces in detail the development of some mathematical skills ("addition-related matters") in school-age children.

Despite their similarity, when compared with the experimental design strategy, the longitudinal and the cross-sectional approaches differ in a number of aspects. This is brought out by a synopsis of their strengths and weaknesses. We do not present a detailed list here; it can be found in many introductory textbooks to developmental methods (e.g., Baltes, Reese, & Nesselroade, 1977; Hoppe, Schmid-Schönbein, & Seiler, 1977; Vasta, 1982). In our view, those properties of the longitudinal strategy that justify its expenses can be summed up in two points:

1. *There are some problems that can be addressed only by longitudinal observa-*

tions. Whether infancy determines or influences later development has been a problem of great concern to psychologists not only from the psychoanalytic camp (see, e.g., Kagan, 1978). Most of the time (but not necessarily so) the problem has been studied from a differential perspective: Do differences in subject and/or environmental variables in infancy relate to interindividual differences in late childhood, adolescence, and adulthood? This kind of differential prediction of developmental trajectories can only be addressed with intraindividual developmental data. Except for the collection of retrospective data – a method that may be classified as a substitution for repeated measurements – we have to observe individuals longitudinally. Or take as another example of the necessity of collecting longitudinal data the "genetic method" à la Piaget or à la Vygotsky (see Wertsch, 1985). We read it as a plea for the explanation of development by construction of the individual's ontogenesis. Despite their primary goal to explain development in general and their neglect of individual differences as the *explanans* of development, both theorists leave much place for idiosyncratic (i.e., individual specific) experiences. Thus, the reconstructive approach to explanation again calls for intraindividual observations (for more detail see the next section). Baltes and Nesselroade (1979, pp. 35ff.) seem to have some mode of explanation similar to the reconstructive approach in mind when they discuss historical (distal) explanations.

2. *The validity of the cross-sectional inference from group differences to intraindividual developmental changes depends on a number of assumptions that might not be fulfilled.* We will figure out some of the assumptions. (a) To arrive from cross-sectional difference data at a general change description we start with the computation of descriptive measures (mean, standard deviation, median, frequency distributions, etc.) for each of the groups included in the study. Next, these "point descriptions" are connected, which results in a description of the process of change. We assume that this gives us an account of development that is typical at least for most, if not all, individuals. More than 30 years ago, Sidman (1952) and Bakan (1954; 1967) pointed out that, in the case of quantitative variables, it cannot be deduced from mathematical theory that developmental curves constructed from group statistics will map the processes in most of the individual cases. (b) The Piagetian model of development and several of the recent approaches to cognitive development (e.g., Fischer & Lamborn, this volume) include predictions about the ordinality of developmental sequences. The developmental levels within a defined sequence should be acquired (and, in some cases, deleted) in the very same sequence by all individuals. To test the assumption of ordinality (invariant sequence), investigators have applied some sort of scalogram

analysis (Coombs & Smith, 1973; Green, 1956; Leik & Matthews, 1968; Lingoes, 1963) to the Individual × Developmental Level matrix based on cross-sectional data. If the coefficients of the scalogram methods (coefficient of reproducibility *Rep*, index of consistency *I*) are close to the maximum value, most authors infer that the ordinality assumption holds – that is, that all the subjects acquired the steps in the expected sequence.

Here we have exactly the case that an intraindividual process of change, as described by the developmental sequence, is inferred from the cross section (in the strict sense of the term). The decisiveness of the results of the scalogram analysis rests upon the validity of the inference; results in agreement with the invariant sequence hypothesis do not verify it. An example will help to clarify the rationale and the limits of testing sequence hypotheses by cross-sectional data.

Watson and Fischer (1977) studied the acquisition and deletion sequence of agent use (i.e., understanding other persons as agents) in early pretend play. In a cross-sectional study, they observed under several conditions the agent use skills of 36 subjects aged 12 to 25 months. Only 4 of them did not fit the predicted pattern of "passes" and "fails" of developmental levels. This result strongly supports the predicted sequence, but it does not unambiguously demonstrate the correctness of the reconstruction of the individual sequences from the cross sections. For purpose of illustration we will look at those children who show the data pattern $+++-$ for the tasks a, b, c, and d. This observation supports the predicted acquisition sequence $a \rightarrow b \rightarrow c \rightarrow d$ because we assume a priori that the pattern $+++-$ "means" that a was acquired before b, b before c, and d after c. But it might have happened that some of the children acquired level d before c and "grew out" of d first; the patterns are inconclusive about these possibilities.

A well-balanced evaluation of the approaches has to consider that the contrast between the observation of individual change by longitudinal studies and the reconstruction of individual change by cross-sectional studies is an idealized dichotomy. Whether the longitudinal approach makes possible the observation of intraindividual change depends not only on questions of conceptualization. It also depends on the density (spacing) of observations in relation to the rate of progress. If the spacing is inadequate it may happen that we observe the pattern $++++$ at $t1$ and $----$ at $t2$ (to take the extreme case). These longitudinal data tell us nothing about the acquisition sequence.

On the other hand, if a large cross-sectional sample includes subjects from very different developmental levels (as in the Watson & Fischer example), we are on firmer ground when going from data patterns to developmental sequences than with small homogenous samples because in the former case there is a greater chance to detect developmental irregularities.

To conclude, in spite of the fundamental differences in the data collection procedure, there is no general superiority of the longitudinal approach for each and any problem and for each and any specific design.

The longitudinal approach to transitions and transition mechanisms

In outlining the use of the term transition in the first section we made a distinction between two kinds of transition analysis:

1. The identification of internal or external factors that explain the system's transition from State 1 to State 2. This kind of analysis is the explanatory approach in the strict and traditional sense. It has been done for decades by developmentalists, but without referring explicitly to the concept of transition.

2. The step-by-step-description of the system's advance from State 1 to State 2. Above all, the transition models by Piaget, Klahr, and Fischer (see the second section) are of this kind. But at the same time they are more than this; they identify factors explaining the progress of the system. Thus, they show us that our distinction between two kinds of transitional analysis is not exclusive for one and the same theory.

In this section we will discuss the uses and potentialities of the longitudinal approach separately for each of the goals.

The contribution of the longitudinal approach to the identification of explanatory factors

In broad outline we find two classes of factors explaining development. They are either *organismic* (located inside the individual) or *environmental* (external to the individual). From an interactionist point of view, this separation is only artificial. In the real process of "causing development," internal and external sources interact; thus, they can only be brought out as isolated explanatory sources by means of our analytical methods of empirical study.

For purpose of illustrating the use of the longitudinal method and especially the combination of experimentation and the longitudinal strategy in explanatory transition analysis, we will refer to training studies of the class inclusion operation, that is, a concrete operational Piagetian task (see Hoppe-Graff, 1982, and Inhelder & Piaget, 1964, for analyses of the class inclusion problem, and Kuhn, 1974, for a fundamental critique of the training experiment in the study of cognitive development). In the simplest case we may assume that one single factor that may be manipulated by training is critical to the acquisition of the class inclusion competence. Suppose, again for illustration only, that the critical factor is explicit feedback about the correctness of the solution offered by the child. A simple pretest–posttest control-group design will suffice to test whether social feedback in fact is a sufficient causal factor. (This simple design does not suffice if our hypotheses do not specify the time of measurement. The experimental effect may remain undetected because we looked for it at the wrong time.)

The state of the art of research on the development of class inclusion and concrete operations in general, of course, does not ask for experimental work of the type just demonstrated (see Hoppe-Graff, 1982, and Winer, 1980, for reviews of the training study literature). A more realistic explanatory model of factors in class inclusion development may be of the following type. Let us assume:

1. A series of repeated encounters with explicit feedback to the individual's class inclusion behavior is needed as critical experience.
2. Each encounter may have only an incremental effect; whether it in fact has this effect depends on cofactors unknown yet.
3. The series of incremental effects "jumps" to the level of full class inclusion competence only with a time lag, that is, only after the training encounters have already stopped.
4. If there were no (or only some) incremental effects after each training session, there will be no large-step advance to full class inclusion after the time lag.

To study this table of hypotheses we necessarily have to observe subjects longitudinally. We suppose that, as our explanatory knowledge grows, we will have a growing number of manipulation studies embedded within the longitudinal data collection approach.

Cognitive development may be considered the product of the cooperation of necessary internal preconditions *and* (sufficient or necessary) external experiences. Therefore, every explanatory analysis that is restricted to external factors falls short from the goal of a comprehensive understanding of the laws and principles of ontogenesis. Within a philosophy of science framework, Bunge (1981) analyzed different modes of becoming. One is reciprocal causation, which takes the form of either cooperation or competition. Bunge states that "reciprocal causation, or interaction, is far more common than either pure randomness or one-sided causation. There are, of course, many kinds of interaction. While some have only quantitative effects, others *produce qualitative changes*" (Bunge, 1981, p. 39; emphasis added). We are convinced that Bunge's account is correct, especially for the inner and outer causal factors of cognitive development.

If we refer once more to the illustrating case of class inclusion, this means that the more realistic assumption is to propose that the influence of the external cause(s) e on the acquisition process cooperates with internal factors i, thereby creating new levels of cognitive competence (Bunge: qualitative changes). Probably, the four propositions given above should be supplemented by:

5. The process described by Propositions 1–4 takes place only in children who have already reached some initial level of transition.

Or we may suggest that the propositions hold only for children with information processing capacities at some specified level. The first suggestion takes evidence from the studies by Inhelder et al. (1974), the second has been expressed especially for the class inclusion acquisition by McLaughlin (1963), Pascual-Leone (1970; Pascual-Leone & Smith, 1969), and Halford and Wilson (1980).

Note that the assumption about internal explanatory factors takes the form of necessary conditions: Only when the internal factors i exist, will the developmental process take place. Jamison and Dansky (1979) proposed to use the term *prerequisite* to denote necessary internal conditions. Campbell and Richie (1983) in an analysis of the problems in the theory of developmental sequences made the distinction between *prerequisites* and *precursors*. Whereas each necessary (internal) condition for the development of a later ability is a prerequisite, "a precursor is a prerequisite ability that performs an analogous transformation on the world to the later ability" (Campbell & Richie, 1983, p. 156). Hence, according to Campbell and Richie we have to make a distinction between two classes of internal explanatory factors, depending on whether they are elements of the very same developmental sequence as the explanandum (precursor) or belong to a variable conceptually different but theoretically related (prerequisite).

In recent years, several techniques have been suggested as adequate data-analytical procedures in the study of precursor and prerequisite hypotheses (Froman & Hubert, 1980; Hildebrand, Laing, & Rosenthal, 1977; Hoppe-Graff, 1982; Rudinger, Chaselon, Zimmermann, & Henning, 1985). The general idea is always the same. The hypothesis that variable i is a necessary condition for event (state) c is mapped on a corresponding contingency table. This table includes all possible combinations of the values of the explanans and the explanandum, and by the hypothesis we specify all admissible cells and "error cells" within the table. Then some algorithm is defined on the basis of statistical theory to quantify the "degree" of evidence (number of cases) against the hypothesis.

Prerequisite hypotheses are different from covariation hypotheses, and they have to be tested by different procedures. As has been pointed out by several authors (Hildebrand et al., 1977; Hoppe-Graff, 1982; 1984; 1985), standard correlational procedures applied to assumptions of the prerequisite type may lead to wrong conclusions because they are designed for purposes other than figuring out the proportion of "errors" as an index for the compatibility of the data with the hypothesis.

The interpretation of factor i as a prerequisite or precursor always goes beyond the data in a covariation table. Even when assuming the weakest concept of causation, we implicitly suppose that i came into existence before the developmental product c.[7] Collecting the data cross-sectionally we can only infer from a one-point observation the time course of the individual's acquisition of prerequisite(s) and abilities to be explained, and, as we have already noted, the inference is valid only when several assumptions are fulfilled.

Being a bit more sophisticated about the cooperation of several internal conditions to the process of transition we may assume that not only some specified states are prerequisites to the generation of developmental products; specific developmental courses are necessary for progression. In this case it seems even more unjustified to infer ontogenetic relations from a snapshot at only one point of measurement. To conclude, in some cases of the search for internal factors responsible for transition processes, we may base our data analyses on cross-sectional observations, but we are no longer on firm ground.

The contribution of the longitudinal approach to the description of the transition process

As should be evident from the presentation in the second section, the transition models by Piaget, Fischer, and Klahr include rules (laws) that account for the step-by-step progression from one level of a developmental system to the next. That is, when applied correctly to the individual's history of experiences, they completely describe the developmental process. These far-reaching theoretical implications contrast sharply with the nature of the empirical work. As far as we know, the authors have not tried to validate their models by "direct" longitudinal observation of the transition processes. At least at first glance, this is surprising: What other method than the intensive observation of intraindividual change – that is, a longitudinal study – can be the adequate empirical test to step-by-step descriptions of processes of individual development? In what follows, we will try to find reasons for the absence of longitudinal work in testing transition models of the Piaget, Klahr, and Fischer type.

This process should help in understanding the empirical implications of transition models in general.

The reasons for the lack of longitudinal research on memory development according to Schneider and Weinert (this volume) can be generalized: Longitudinal studies suffer from (a) great financial and organizational expense and (b) some unresolved methodological problems (retest effects). But it seems that the application of the longitudinal orientation to transition models in addition suffers from (c) conceptual vaguenesses. What does it precisely mean to observe the transition process? This is the concept we must clarify.

Take as an example Fischer's transformation rules. Fischer proposes that a large (and interindividually different) number of microdevelopmental operations (processes), such as shift of focus and compounding, are carried out before a macrodevelopmental step (intercoordination) to the next developmental level can be made. In which way can we *observe* the processes of shift of focus or compounding? Let us look at Fischer's description of shift of focus: "In shift of focus, the person carries out one simple skill, and then he or she shifts to a second one. Thus, the co-occurrence leads to only a simple transformation, the systematic juxtaposition of two skills" (Fischer & Lamborn, this volume). Fischer and Lamborn continue: "For example, abstract honesty is first defined, and then separately abstract kindness is defined. This sort of juxtaposition of components that could be integrated is extremely common in development and seems often to be a transitional step to a genuine integration of components."

This passage from Fischer and Lamborn brings out several points. In particular the example shows that *in principle* it should be possible to observe each step of transition. But we do not know when these steps occur. When do children perform the juxtaposition of two skills? Each time they have the chance (environmental conditions) to do so – in the example case, each time they have the chance to define honesty first and kindness afterwards? Or does the operation of juxtaposition occur only in some of the cases where it could occur? We might even ask: When do children have the chance to perform the operation of juxtaposition? A far-reaching interpretation of the goal of process description calls for answers to these questions.

But perhaps we have gone too far in interpreting Fischer's model in this way. Another interpretation of the theory reads that it does not specify (or predict) in a deterministic way each and every microdevelopmental process within the individual but only the types of processes that are likely at some level of functioning and that are carried out sometimes. That is, Fischer's developmental rules do not predict each and every process in the individual's developmental activity (when it occurs exactly) but they rather allow for the reconstruction of the developmental sequence after it has taken place.

We think that the second interpretation of Fischer's model is the correct one. Although it exactly describes the kinds of the transition processes to occur at each developmental level, it does not include predictions about specific occurrences of the processes in some individual. But it allows for the reconstruction of the individual progressions in terms of his theoretical concepts after the developmental process took place.[8]

Whereas we are doubtful about the status of Klahr's mechanism of self-modification, we believe Piaget's equilibration model is similar to Fischer's position: It allows for the complete reconstruction of the developmental process, but it does not pretend to predict each molecular developmental step. We conclude from our considerations that the superiority of the longitudinal approach does not lie in the complete observation of the transition process. But we still suggest that it is a more direct test than the cross-sectional approach. For purposes of demonstration, we will again refer to Fischer's theory. Now we will consider the kind of empirical data he presents in favor of his transition model. Of the three authors discussed, Fischer is the only one who tried to carry out systematic (definite) empirical tests of his model, whereas Piaget's data are at best anecdotal (given the standards of empirical research in the field), and Klahr seems to be unaware of the need for empirical evaluation.

Fischer and Lamborn (this volume) report only on results from cross-sectional studies (Lamborn, 1987; Monsour, 1985) as empirical evidence for the transition mechanism proposed in skill theory, and if our review of the literature is complete, the same is true for Fischer's studies in general. He argues that the crucial step in relating cross-sectional data to the transition rules is the statistical data analysis by the "strong" scalogram method (Fischer & Lamborn, this volume; Fischer & Pipp, 1984; Fischer, Pipp, & Bullock, 1984; and the previous discussion in this section). Its use presupposes that for every step in a developmental sequence – that is, for every optimal level – a separate task has been designed a priori. The tasks are then given to a sample of children varying in age. Analyzing the pattern of passes and fails by the scalogram method and computing coefficients that describe the degree of ordinality – respectively invariability – of the sequence is all we have to do to test the assumptions of skill theory. A high degree of scalability is evidence enough not only for the correctness of the sequence hypothesis but for the transformation rules as well.

There are several shortcomings in this strategy. First, we think Fischer would agree that the data collected in this kind of study are directly mapping developmental products but not transition processes. For that reason they provide no direct evidence for testing the process assumptions empirically. We would have accepted the data as critical only if there were no other way of generating the sequences than by Fischer's transformation rules. But, of course, it is an easy task to think of other propositions that would result in the same sequences. One of the strengths of Fischer's model is that he formulated his model in propositions that can easily be transformed into observation procedures. In particular, this holds for the transformation rules. Thus, we suggest that the basic data should be observations of the processes of compounding, intercoordination, and so forth, and not of developmental products as in the scalogram studies. This suggestion does not contradict our skeptical notes on the possibility of observing the entire transition process.

Second, our arguments in the third section concerning the inference of developmental processes from cross-sectional data collections fits Fischer's strategy. If at the time of measurement the child passed the tasks from skill Levels 7, 8, and 9, we infer that the child developed from Level 7 through Level 8 to Level 9. We repeat that the confirmation of the ordinality assumption does not prove the correctness of the inference; on the contrary, testing sequence hypotheses on the basis of cross-sectional data presupposes it.

From our own research we know that fallacious inferences from group data to individual developmental processes are not only a vague possibility. In a longitudinal study on the development of the friendship concepts, the group data show a significant continuous increase in all aspects of friendship understanding throughout two age intervals, from 9 to 12, and from 12 to 15 years. But when going back to the individual patterns, we observe that more than 25% of the children stagnate (Hoppe-Graff & Keller, 1988).

But the longitudinal method might have even more merits when applied to the testing of skill theory. According to Fischer it is only under extraordinary environmental conditions that people perform close to or at the optimal level (see the second section). From our own experience with observations of social concepts, we agree that the task is an important factor to the child's performance. But do all children perform optimally under the same task conditions? Or should we expect a sort of trait–task interaction? If this speculation is correct, then we are in a much better position to obtain the best individual (idiosyncratic) environmental conditions when we get to know the child in more detail; and that is possible only in longitudinal studies.

In conclusion, there are several strong points in favor of the longitudinal approach to the study of transition models. Although I have tried to connect most of my arguments to the transition model of Fischer, some of the considerations are only programmatic, others are very general. This reflects the state of the art: Only future empirical studies and methodological reflections on transition processes can turn them from conjectures into propositions.

NOTES

1 These constituents do not suffice to separate, for example, processes of development from processes of learning. But they are useful here because they can serve as a starting point for the arguments to follow.
2 In the fourth section we will be more precise and show that the current usage of the term transition mechanism is restricted to a very specific class of explanations.
3 Although used in the theory's name, the concept of skill has never been rigorously defined by Fischer. It goes back to the theory's reliance on the learning theory tradition (see in detail Fischer, 1980), and in this sense Fischer uses the term skill to stress the person–environment interaction as the source of change: skill "connotes a transaction ... of organism and environment.... The skills in the theory are always defined jointly by organism and environment" (1980, p. 478). Formally skills are defined by means of a set-theory description.
4 In connection with the optimal level construct, Fischer argues in favor of investigations of the subject's competence under environmental conditions where she can perform near or at her best capabilities (Fischer, Pipp, & Bullock, 1984). This strategy seems to be very similar to the proposal by Baltes and his co-workers to use the testing-the-limits paradigm in the theory-guided analysis of mechanisms of development and aging (Kliegl & Baltes, in press).
5 There are different translations of the French *equilibration majorante* in the American literature. Furth (1981) prefers to speak of *increasing equilibration*, whereas Gelman and Baillargeon (1983) use the term *improved equilibration*.
6 This "rule" of course implies that there are no general guidelines for the timing and the composition of the sample in longitudinal studies of transition processes as well; again, it depends on the transition model in question how to design the empirical studies.
7 We exclude from our discussion the possibility of concurrent causation (but see Schneider, 1978; and von Wright, 1971).
8 If our interpretations are correct, the consideration of Fischer's model also helps to clarify and demonstrate the distinction between developmental prediction and reconstruction.

REFERENCES

Appelbaum, M. I., & McCall, R. B. (1983). Design and analysis in developmental psychology. In W. Kessen (Ed.), *Handbook of child psychology: Vol. 1.*

History, theory, and methods (P. Mussen, Gen. Ed.) (4th ed., pp. 415–476). New York: Wiley.

Bakan, D. (1954). Group and individual functions. *Psychological Bulletin, 51*, 63–64.

Bakan, D. (1967). *On method.* San Francisco: Jossey-Bass.

Baltes, P. B., Cornelius, S. W., & Nesselroade, J. R. (1979). Cohort effects in developmental psychology. In J. R. Nesselroade & P. B. Baltes (Eds.), *Longitudinal research in the study of behavior and development* (pp. 61–87). New York: Academic Press.

Baltes, P. B., & Nesselroade, J. R. (1979). History and rationale of longitudinal research. In J. R. Nesselroade & P. B. Baltes (Eds.), *Longitudinal research in the study of behavior and development* (pp. 1–39). New York: Academic Press.

Baltes, P. B., Reese, H. W., & Nesselroade, J. R. (1977). *Life-span developmental psychology: Introduction to research methods.* Monterey, CA: Brooks/Cole.

Beilin, H. (1984). Functionalist and structuralist research programs in developmental psychology: Incommensurability or synthesis? In H. W. Reese (Ed.), *Advances in child development and behavior* (Vol. 18, pp. 245–257). New York: Academic Press.

Bunge, M. (1979) *Causality: The place of the causal principle in modern science.* New York: Dover.

Bunge, M. (1981) *Scientific materialism.* Dordrecht: Reidel.

Campbell, R. L., & Richie, D. M. (1983). Problems in the theory of developmental sequences: Prerequisites and precursors. *Human Development, 26*, 156–172.

Case, R. (1984). The process of stage transition: A neo-Piagetian view. In R. J. Sternberg (Ed.), *Mechanisms of cognitive development* (pp. 20–44). New York: Freeman.

Case, R. (1985). *Intellectual development: Birth to adulthood.* New York: Academic Press.

Cook, T. D., & Campbell, D. T. (1979). *Quasi-experimentation: Design and analysis issues for field settings.* Boston: Houghton Mifflin.

Coombs, C. H., & Smith, J. E. K. (1973). On the detection of structure in attitudes and developmental processes. *Psychological Review, 80*, 337–351.

Cummins, R. (1977). Programs in the explanation of behavior. *Philosophy of Science, 44*, 269–287.

Cummins, R. (1983) *The nature of psychological explanation.* Cambridge: MIT Press.

Damon, W. (1983). The nature of social-cognitive change in the developing child. In W. F. Overton (Ed.), *The relationship between social and cognitive development* (pp. 103–141). Hillsdale, NJ: Erlbaum.

Edelstein, W., Keller, M., & Wahlen, K. (1984). Structure and content in social cognition: Conceptual and empirical analyses. *Child Development, 55*, 1514–1526.

Eichhorn, D. H., Clausen, J. H., Haan, N., Honzik, M. P., & Mussen, P. H. (1981). *Present and past in middle life.* New York: Academic Press.

Fein, G. G., & Moorin, E. R. (1985). Confusion substitution, and mastery: Pretend play during the second year of life. In K. E. Nelson (Ed.), *Children's language* (Vol. 5, pp. 61–76). Hillsdale: NJ: Erlbaum.

Fetz, R. (1984). Zur Genese ontologischer Begriffe: Für eine Verbindung Whiteheadscher und Piagetscher Ansätze. In H. Holz & E. Wolf-Gazo (Hg.), *Whitehead und der Prozessbegriff* (pp. 200–239). Freiburg: Alber.

Fischer, K. W. (1980). A theory of cognitive development: The control and construction of hierarchies of skills. *Psychological Review*, *87*, 477–531.

Fischer, K. W., & Pipp, S. L. (1984). Processes of cognitive development: Optimal level and skill acquisition. In R. J. Sternberg (Ed.), *Mechanisms of cognitive development* (pp. 45–79). San Francisco: Freeman.

Fischer, K. W., Pipp, S. L., & Bullock, D. (1984). Detecting developmental discontinuities. In R. Emde & R. J. Harmon (Eds.), *Continuities and discontinuities in development* (pp. 95–121). New York: Plenum Press.

Froman, T., & Hubert, L. J. (1980). Application of prediction analysis to developmental priority. *Psychological Bulletin*, *87*, 130–146.

Furth, H. G. (1980). *The world of grown-ups*. New York: Elsevier.

Furth, H. G. (1981) *Piaget and knowledge* (2nd ed.). Chicago: University of Chicago Press.

Gelman, R., & Baillargeon, R. (1983). A review of some Piagetian concepts. In J. H. Flavell & E. M. Markman (Eds.), *Handbook of child psychology: Vol. 3. Cognitive development* (P. Mussen, Gen. Ed.) (pp. 167–230). New York: Wiley.

Green, B. F. (1956). A method of scalogram analysis using summary statistics. *Psychometrika*, *21*, 79–88.

Halford, G. S., & Wilson, W. H. (1980). A category theory approach to cognitive development. *Cognitive Psychology*, *12*, 356–411.

Hildebrand, D. K., Laing, J. D., & Rosenthal, H. (1977). *Prediction analysis of cross classifications*. New York: Wiley.

Hoppe, S., Schmid-Schönbein, C., & Seiler, T. B. (1977). *Entwicklungssequenzen*. Bern: Huber.

Hoppe-Graff, S. (1982) *Bedingungsanalysen zur Genese der Klasseninklusion*. Unpublished doctoral dissertation, Technische Hochschule Darmstadt.

Hoppe-Graff, S. (1984) *Ist die Entwicklung der Informationsverarbeitungskapazität eine notwendige Bedingung für den Erwerb der Klasseninklusion?* (Report No. 31 from the Study Group "Language and Cognition"), Mannheim: Universität Mannheim, Lehrstuhl Psychologie III.

Hoppe-Graff, S. (1985). Probleme und Ansätze bei der Untersuchung von Entwicklungssequenzen. T. B. Seiler & W. Wannenmacher (Eds.), *Begriffs- und Wortbedeutungsentwicklung* (pp. 262–283). Berlin: Springer.

Hoppe-Graff, S., & Keller, M. (1988). Einheitlichkeit und Vielfalt in der Entwicklung des Freundschaftskonzeptes. *Zeitschrift für Entwicklungspsychologie und Pädagogische Psychologie*, *20*, 1–19.

Inhelder, B., & Piaget, J. (1964). *The early growth of logic in the child: Classification and seriation*. London: Routledge & Kegan Paul.

Inhelder, B., Sinclair, H., & Bovet, M. (1974). *Learning and the development of cognition*. Cambridge: Harvard University Press.

Jamison, W., & Dansky, J. L. (1979). Identifying developmental prerequisites of cognitive acquisitions. *Child Development*, *50*, 449–454.

Kagan, J. (1978). *The growth of the child*. New York: Norton.

Kessen, W. (1984). Introduction: The end of the age of development. In R. J. Sternberg (Ed.), *Mechanisms of cognitive development* (pp. 1–17). San Francisco: Freeman.

Klahr, D. (1982). Nonmonotone assessment of monotone development: An information processing analysis. In S. Strauss (Ed.), *U-shaped behavioral growth* (pp. 63–86). New York: Academic Press.

Klahr. D. (1984). Transition processes in quantitative development. In R. J.

Sternberg (Ed.), *Mechanisms of cognitive development* (pp. 102–139). San Francisco: Freeman.

Klahr, D., & Siegler, R. S. (1978). The representation of children's knowledge. In H. W. Reese & L. P. Lipsitt (Eds.), *Advances in child development and behavior* (Vol. 12, pp. 62–116). New York: Academic Press.

Klahr, D., & Wallace, J. G. (1976). *Cognitive development: An information processing view.* Hillsdale, NJ: Erlbaum.

Kliegl, R., & Baltes, P. B. (in press). Theory guided analysis of mechanisms of development and aging through testing-the-limits and research on expertise. In C. Schuler & K. W. Schaie (Eds.), *Cognitive functioning and social structure over the life course.* Norwood, NJ: Ablex.

Koffka, K. (1928). *The growth of the mind.* London: Routledge & Kegan Paul.

Kuhn, D. (1974). Inducing development experimentally: Comments on a research paradigm. *Developmental Psychology, 10,* 590–600.

Kuhn, D., & Phelps, E. (1982). The development of problem solving strategies. In H. W. Reese (Ed.), *Advances in child development and behavior* (Vol. 17, pp. 1–44). New York: Academic Press.

Kuhn, T. S. (1962). *The structure of scientific revolutions.* Chicago: University of Chicago Press.

Lamborn, S. (1987) Relations between social-cognitive knowledge and personal experience: Understanding honesty and kindness in relationships (Doctoral dissertation, University of Denver, 1986). *Dissertation Abstracts International, 47,* 2959A. (University Microfilms No. DA8626347)

Langer, J. (1977). Cognitive development during and after the preconceptual period. In M. H. Appel & L. S. Goldberg (Eds.), *Topics in cognitive development* (Vol. 1. p. 77–90). New York: Plenum Press.

Lawler, R. (1981). The progressive construction of mind. *Cognitive Science, 5,* 1–30.

Leik, R. K., & Matthews, M. (1968). A scale for developmental processes. *American Sociological Review, 33,* 62–75.

Lingoes, J. C. (1963) Multiple scalogram analysis: A set-theoretical model for analyzing dichotomous items. *Educational and Psychological Measurement, 23,* 501–524.

Lunzer, E. A. (1964) Translator's introduction. In B. Inhelder & J. Piaget, *The early growth of logic in the child: Classification and seriation.* London: Routledge & Kegan Paul.

McLaughlin, C. H. (1963). Psycho-logic: A possible alternative to Piaget's formulation. *British Journal of Educational Psychology, 33,* 61–67.

Monsour, A. (1985). The dynamics and structure of adolescent self-concept (Doctoral dissertation, University of Denver). *Dissertation Abstracts International, 46,* 2091B. (University Microfilms No. DA8517558).

Mounoud, P. (1982). Revolutionary periods in early development. In T. G. Bever (Ed.), *Regressions in mental development* (pp. 119–131). Hillsdale, NJ: Erlbaum.

Mulaik, S. A. (1987). Toward a conception of causality applicable to experimentation and causal modeling. *Child Development, 58,* 18–32.

Nagel, E. (1957) Determinism and development. In D. B. Harris (Ed.), *The concept of development* (pp. 15–34). Minneapolis: University of Minnesota Press.

Nesselroade, J. R., & von Eye, A. (Eds.). (1985). *Individual development and social change: Explanatory analysis*. Orlando: Academic Press.

Newell, A. (1973). Production systems: Models of control structures. In W. G. Chase (Ed.), *Visual information processing* (pp. 463–526). New York: Academic Press.

Overton, W. F. (1984). World views and their influence on psychological theory and research: Kuhn – Lakatos – Laudan. In H. W. Reese (Ed.), *Advances in child development and behavior* (Vol. 18, pp. 191–226). New York: Academic Press.

Pascual-Leone, J. (1970). A mathematical model for the transition rule in Piaget's developmental stages. *Acta Psychologica, 32*, 301–345.

Pascual-Leone, J., & Smith, J. (1969). The encoding and decoding of symbols by children: A new experimental paradigm and a neo-Piagetian model. *Journal of Experimental Child Psychology, 8*, 328–355.

Piaget, J. (1952). *The origins of intelligence in children*. New York: International University Press. (Original work published 1936)

Piaget, J. (1977a). *The development of thought: Equilibration of cognitive structures*. New York: Viking. (Original work published 1975)

Piaget, J. (1977b). Problems of equilibration. In M. H. Appel & L. S. Goldberg (Eds.), *Topics in cognitive development* (Vol. 1, pp. 3–13). New York: Plenum Press.

Piaget, J. (1983). Piaget's theory. In W. Kessen (Ed.), *Handbook of child psychology: Vol. 1. History, theory, and methods* (P. Mussen, Gen. Ed.) (4th ed., 103–128). New York: Wiley.

Rudinger, G., Chaselon, F., Zimmermann, E. J., & Henning, H. J. (1985). *Qualitative Daten*. Munich: Urban & Schwarzenberg.

Sameroff, A. J. (1982). Development and the dialectic. In A. W. Collins (Ed.), *The concept of development: Minnesota Symposia on Child Psychology* (Vol. 15, pp. 83–103). Hillsdale, NJ: Erlbaum.

Schaie, K. W., & Herzog, C. (1982). Longitudinal methods. In B. B. Wolman (Ed.), *Handbook of developmental psychology* (pp. 91–115). Englewood Cliffs, NJ: Prentice-Hall.

Schneider, H. J. (1978) Die Asymmetrie der Kausalrelation. In J. Mittelstrass & M. Riedel (Eds.), *Vernünftiges Denken* (pp. 217–234). Berlin: De Gruyter.

Sidman, R. S. (1952). A note on functional relations obtained from group data. *Psychological Bulletin, 49*, 263–269.

Siegel, A. W., Bisanz, J., & Bisanz, G. L. (1983). Developmental analysis: A strategy for the study of psychological change. In D. Kuhn & J. A. Meacham (Eds.), *On the development of developmental psychology* (Contributions to Human Development Series, Vol. 8, pp. 53–80). Basel: Karger.

Siegler, R. S. (1983). Information processing approaches to development. In W. Kessen (Ed.), *Handbook of child psychology: Vol. 1. History, theory, and methods* (4th ed., pp. 129–211). New York: Wiley.

Siegler, R. S., & Richards, D. D. (1983). The development of two concepts. In C. J. Brainerd (Ed.), *Recent advances in cognitive developmental theory* (pp. 51–121). New York: Springer.

Sternberg, R. J. (Ed.). (1984). *Mechanisms of cognitive development*. San Francisco: Freeman.

Sugarman, S. (1987). The priority of description in developmental psychology. *International Journal of Behavioral Development, 10*, 391–414.

Turiel, E. (1983). Domains and categories in social-cognitive development. In

W. F. Overton (Ed.), *The relationship between social and cognitive development* (pp. 53–89). Hillsdale, NJ: Erlbaum.

van den Daele, L. D. (1974). Infrastructure and transition in developmental analysis. *Human Development, 17,* 1–23.

von Wright, G. H. (1971). *Explanation and understanding.* Ithaca, NY: Cornell University Press.

Vasta, R. (1982). *Strategies and techniques of child study.* New York: Academic Press.

Watson, M. W., & Fischer, K. W. (1977). A developmental sequence of agent use in late infancy. *Child Development, 48,* 828–836.

Wertsch, J. (1985). *Vygotsky and the social formation of mind.* Cambridge: Harvard University Press.

Whitehead, A. N. (1957). *Process and reality: An essay in cosmology.* London: Macmillan. (Original work published 1929)

Winer, G. A. (1980). Class-inclusion reasoning in the child: A review of the empirical literature. *Child Development, 51,* 309–328.

Wohlwill, J. F. (1973). *The study of behavioral development.* New York: Academic Press.

I   Cognitive development

2 Mechanisms of variation in developmental levels: cognitive and emotional transitions during adolescence

KURT W. FISCHER AND SUSIE D. LAMBORN

The organization of behavior develops systematically, and simultaneously it varies across contexts and from moment to moment. These two sets of phenomena, systematic development and short-term variation, have conventionally been treated as opposed in the study of behavior, but their opposition is not necessary. Indeed, we believe that only a framework that integrates them can specify the mechanisms that produce cognitive development. The framework that we will outline for integrating development and short-term variation is based on skill theory (Fischer, 1980).

This framework applies both to what has traditionally been called cognition and to the organization of behavior more generally. What develops is not only behavior focused on the physical world, but any behavior that is subject to voluntary or operant control, including what has been conventionally categorized as social and emotional development. Different organizations produce both different cognitive capacities and different social–emotional capacities and vulnerabilities.

Over the months and years of childhood and adolescence, the organization of behavior develops through a series of levels, with each successive level involving more sophisticated and complex skills than the previous level. In moving from one level to the next, the person gradually constructs more complex skills, developing in small steps that eventually culminate in a major reorganization at the next level.

Concurrent with this systematic development, the individual's behavior varies in complexity across context and from moment to moment; he or she does not consistently show a single level. What shows true developmental levels is the upper limit on the complexity of skill that the person can construct and control. Only occasionally do people evidence this upper limit. At any one moment, a person is unlikely to demonstrate his or her upper limit but instead will use less advanced skills (Fischer & Pipp, 1984b).

The control system that produces the person's behavior at any one time is a skill, and several functional mechanisms affect the exact form and complexity of that skill. (a) The upper limit, called optimal level, increases systematically with age and experience. It is the process where development occurs in the most straightforward, stagelike way, much as Piaget's (1957) theory predicted. (b) The microdevelopmental transformation rules specify how skills are combined to form developmental steps within a level. These steps describe both progress within the optimal level and the ordering of performance below optimal level.

Variations below the upper limit occur routinely as a function of several other mechanisms as well. Especially important are (c) the degree of environmental support for high-level performance, (d) the task in which the person is engaged, and (e) the person's emotional state. Only when the environment supports high-level performance will people typically demonstrate their optimal level. Both at optimal level and in variations below it, the task organizes behavior, and changes in task produce powerful variations in both level and pattern of skill. Emotions affect variability too, motivating or interfering with behavior and organizing it in terms of a particular emotional constellation (Fischer, Shaver, & Carnochan, 1988; Scherer, 1984; Shaver, Schwartz, Kirson, & O'Connor, 1987).

Adolescent social-cognitive development provides an especially good example for introducing skill theory and illustrating the five functional mechanisms of variation in development. After presenting the skill-theory analysis, we conclude with a review of the evidence for emotional vulnerabilities in adolescence and an outline of a model of the development of those vulnerabilities.

Adolescent social-cognitive development: honesty and kindness

Adolescent social-cognitive development promises to be a fruitful arena for studying the mechanisms of variability in developmental level. Adolescents evidence major changes in their cognitive capacities (Fischer, Hand, & Russell, 1984; Inhelder & Piaget, 1958/1955) and also experience significant transformations in their close relationships (Youniss, 1980) and their senses of themselves (Harter, 1983). Close relationships and senses of self carry with them important emotional involvements. Consequently, we will focus on these topics to illustrate and analyze both how the organization of behavior develops over long periods and how it varies in the short term.

A topic of special relevance to close relationships and senses of self in adolescence is honesty and kindness in social interactions. When people characterize their close relationships or their own identities in relationships, honesty and kindness are two frequently occurring themes (Lamborn, 1987; Youniss, 1980). Honesty and kindness are also emotionally loaded constructs. Good relationships are supposed to involve both qualities, and violations of expectations of honesty and kindness can produce powerful negative emotions.

The concepts of honesty and kindness provide an especially promising domain for studying the interplay of cognition and emotion in adolescent development. Honesty and kindness are central both to the special social concerns of adolescents and to social interaction in general. They are highly valued in our culture and are the focal point of many emotional dilemmas in daily interactions.

Despite the value placed on these two qualities, intentions of being honest and kind can be undermined by the realities of day-to-day encounters. It is sometimes more convenient to be dishonest or unkind. Revealing one's mistakes or true feelings can be costly in many different ways: One can lose a job, a friend, or one's self-esteem. The concepts of a social lie, constructive criticism, and jealous truth capture some of the complexities of honesty and kindness. For example, a social lie involves a situation where honesty and kindness are in opposition. If one is honest, then one must be unkind. If one is kind, then one must be dishonest.

Consider a 15-year-old girl named Aurora, at the dawn of her adulthood. She is talking with her mother about a poem she has written. The mother reads the poem and tells her daughter that she likes it very much. In fact, the mother recognizes that the language in the poem is awkward and the ideas are adolescent. Aurora sees through her mother's social lie and becomes furious. "How could you lie to me? I am your daughter! I know that you don't like my poem! How could you be so dishonest?" Aurora has difficulty understanding her mother's analysis of the situation, which goes like this: If the mother is honest to her daughter and says what she thinks of the poem, she will hurt the girl's feelings – an unkind act. Because Aurora is just learning to write poetry, no one would expect her to write an elegant poem with a mature conception. To be kind, the mother lies and says that she likes the poem. But all that her daughter sees is that she lied, not that she was lying in order to be kind.

Later, Aurora is talking with her 20-year-old brother about the incident. He points out that her mother was trying to be kind, taking into account the fact that Aurora is just learning to write poetry. Although her mother did lie, she did it because of her love for Aurora, in order to be kind and encourage her daughter's efforts at poetry. Also, he points out that Aurora herself acted similarly with their 8-year-old brother the week before, when she praised him for kicking the soccer ball so well.

After a long discussion, Aurora moves beyond her initial anger and puts together the idea that her mother was telling a social lie, just as she did with her brother. It was dishonest, but it was also kind – not such a terrible act.

How collaboration of person and environment produces skill development

An adequate theory of development must be built upon the collaboration of person and environment in behavior. It is not enough to focus on person variables or environmental variables. People act in a world. The world and the person collaborate to produce behavior (Fischer & Bullock, 1984). Skill theory is built upon this principle of collaboration. All the constructs in the theory are specified in terms of both organismic and environmental contributions. The concept of skill itself implicates both person and environment, in contrast to concepts such as competence or capacity. In English usage, a skill involves an ability to carry out a set of actions in a particular context. A person has a skill for driving a car with a standard gearshift or a skill for sewing hems with a sewing machine. Even a switch to a different car or sewing machine changes the skill. Similarly, a person has skills for concepts such as honesty, kindness, and social lie, and a switch in task changes the skill.

Skills develop in particular task domains and must be generalized to other task domains (Fischer, 1980). That is, development does not automatically produce broadly applicable schemes but instead involves the construction of skills specific to task domains. Generalization to other domains is a gradual and laborious process (Fischer & Farrar, 1987). Predicting skill development therefore requires starting with a specific domain for analyzing skills.

Developmental levels

The concept of developmental level in skill theory fits this collaborative framework. A level is a characteristic not of a person but of a person-in-a-context. Within a restricted set of environments – those that support high-level performance – a person can function at his or her optimal level. From birth to 30 years of age, people develop through a hierarchical series of 13 optimal levels, moving through four vastly different tiers, from reflexes to sensorimotor actions to concrete representations and finally to abstractions (Fischer, 1980; Fischer & Pipp, 1984b). The levels specify one of the major mechanisms of development, an upper limit on the complexity of skill that a child can control. In this essay we will focus on the last 7 levels, which involve the development of representations

LEVEL

I

II

III

IV

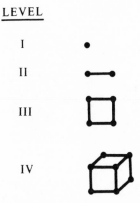

Figure 2.1. A metaphor for the cycle of four levels (from Fischer, 1980, © American Psychological Association)

and abstractions in childhood and adolescence. A clear description of the functional mechanisms producing development requires first a description of the nature of the skill structures for each level.

A cycle of levels. The 13 levels are generated by a repetitive cycle of 4 levels, which is reminiscent of what Piaget referred to as reflective abstraction (Beth & Piaget, 1966) and similar to Case's (1985) stages, Mounoud's (1976) revolutions, and Biggs and Collis's (1982) cycles. Each tier involves a repetition of the same basic 4-level cycle, with each successive tier building upon a more complex component. Figure 2.1 provides a metaphor for this cycle, and Table 2.1 shows how it is represented algebraically and how the cycle produces the last 7 developmental levels (the representational and abstract tiers).

The cycle begins at the first level with a single element, such as the dot in Figure 2.1, which serves as a building block for the more complex structures that follow. The single elements are combined to form the structures of the second level, simple relations of elements, which are similar to lines. Then these simple relations are combined to form the structures of the third level, more complex relations similar to planes. Finally, at the fourth level, the complex relations are combined to form still more complex structures similar to solids. With solids, a new building block is formed, and so the cycle can begin again, starting a new tier. In this way, the fourth level of one tier constitutes the first level of the next tier, as shown in Table 2.1 for representations and abstractions. The fourth level of the representational tier (systems of systems of representations) constitutes the first level of the abstract tier (single abstractions).

Table 2.1. *Seven levels of representations and abstractions*

Level in tier	Skill structure	Representational sets[a]	Abstract sets
RpI	Single representations	[R] or [T]	
RpII	Representational mappings	[R — T]	
RpIII	Representational systems	$[R_{j,k} \leftrightarrow T_{j,k}]$	
RpIV/AI	Systems of representational systems, which are single abstractions	$\begin{bmatrix} R \leftrightarrow T \\ \updownarrow \\ V \leftrightarrow X \end{bmatrix} \equiv$	$[\mathcal{E}]$
AII	Abstract mappings		$[\mathcal{E} — \mathcal{F}]$
AIII	Abstract systems		$[\mathcal{E}_{\mathcal{AB}} \leftrightarrow \mathcal{F}_{\mathcal{AB}}]$
AIV	Systems of abstract systems, which are single principles		$\begin{bmatrix} \mathcal{E} \leftrightarrow \mathcal{F} \\ \updownarrow \\ \mathcal{Q} \leftrightarrow \mathcal{H} \end{bmatrix}$

Note: Roman capital letters designate representational sets. Script capital letters designate abstract sets. Subscripts designate differentiated components of the respective set. Long straight lines and arrows designate a relation between sets or systems. Brackets designate a single skill.
[a] The structures of representational sets for Levels 8 to 10 have been omitted because the formulas become complex and bulky, but the representational sets can be filled in by substituting the representational structure of Level 7 for each of the abstract sets at Levels 8, 9, and 10.

The cycle is hypothesized to have not only cognitive characteristics but also emotional ones. In particular, the first 2 levels of the cycle carry with them intrinsic emotional instabilities that are eliminated in the later levels. The emotional labilities of both the young preschool child and the young adolescent stem in part from the nature of this cycle. The preschooler is developing through the first 2 levels of the representational tier, and the adolescent is developing through the first 2 levels of the abstract tier. There are thus very real cognitive-emotional parallels between preschooler and adolescent (Blos, 1962; Fischer & Pipp, 1984a). Here we will merely sketch the general nature of these levels. Later in the chapter, we will review the broader empirical and theoretical evidence for emotional instabilities in adolescence.

What produces the cognitive-emotional instabilities of the early levels in a tier is that the child cannot coordinate and differentiate many components. At the first level, understanding sometimes is similar to being in a fog, because the child cannot even compare one component to another, because he or she can deal with only one component at a time. As a result, confusion reigns in both the 2- to 3-year-old with single representations and the 10- to 14-year-old with single abstractions. For example, 2- to 3-year-olds show frequent wish-based distortions of thought (Fischer & Pipp, 1984a), and 10- to 14-year-olds are confused about who they are and how they fit into the world.

Substantial progress occurs with the construction at the second level of mappings coordinating two components, which allows simple comparisons of components (Case, 1985; Fischer, 1980). Still, however, there is cognitive-emotional instability because of the limitations of these simple structures. Strong stability requires the coordination of multiple elements in a single system, which occurs at Level 3. This progress relates closely to what Piaget (1975) called decentration and equilibration. For example, 4- and 5-year-olds begin to unravel the complexities of concrete social relationships, and in the process demonstrate major distortions of those relationships, as in the Oedipus conflict. To move beyond the distortions, they will need to consider multiple social categories simultaneously, including husband, father, wife, mother, child, and adult (Fischer & Watson, 1981). Similarly 14- to 16-year-olds show many confusions in their efforts to unravel the complexities of their own and other people's personalities, becoming distressed by, for instance, the contradictions they see in their own behaviors (Lamborn, 1987; Monsour, 1985).

Levels of development of honesty and kindness. Table 2.2 gives examples of each of the 7 levels of representations and abstractions, as well as the approximate ages of emergence of each new optimal level. Skills at each of these levels will be illustrated for the domain of honest and kind (or nice) social interactions, based on research in the Cognitive Development Laboratory at the University of Denver. Of course, these examples are specific to the contexts and methodologies used in our research, which involved concrete pretend stories about social interactions (Fischer, Hand, Watson, Van Parys, & Tucker, 1984).

The first 3 levels all involve concrete representations, in which the child can think about concrete characteristics of objects, events, or people. At the level of *single representations*, which first emerges at about 2 years of age, children can control single social categories, among other things. In pretend play, for example, children can demonstrate the social category of nice by making one character carry out several nice actions, such as giving someone candy and saying "I like you."

The level of *representational mappings*, which emerges at about 4 years of age, produces relations between social categories, such as simple reciprocity in pretend play: If one character is nice to a second one, then the second one will be nice in return, because of the first one's nice actions.

Representational systems, which first appear at about 6 years of age, are

Table 2.2. *Levels of development in childhood and adolescence*

Level	Age of emergence	Examples of skills
RpI: Single representations	18–24 months	Coordination of action systems to produce concrete representations of actions, objects, or agents: Pretending that a doll is walking. Saying, "Mommy eat toast."
RpII: Representational mappings	3.5–4.5 years	Relations of concrete representations: Pretending that two dolls are Mommy and Daddy interacting. Understanding that self knows a secret and Daddy does not know it.
RpIII: Representational systems (also called concrete operations)	6–7 years	Complex relations of subsets of concrete representations: Pretending that two dolls are both Mommy and Daddy as well as a doctor and a teacher simultaneously. Understanding that when water is poured from one glass to another, the amount of water stays the same.
RpIV/AI: Single abstractions (also called formal operations)	10–12 years	Coordination of concrete representational systems to produce general, intangible concepts: Concept of operation of addition. Evaluating how one's parents' behavior demonstrates conformity. Concept of honesty as a general quality of an interaction.
AII: Abstract mappings	14–16 years	Relations of intangible concepts: Understanding that operations of addition and subtraction are opposites. Integrating two social concepts, such as honesty and kindness, in the idea of a social lie.
AIII:[a] Abstract systems	18–20 years	Complex relations of subsets of intangible concepts: Understanding that operations of addition and division are related through how the numbers are grouped and how they are combined. Integrating several types of honesty and kindness in the idea of constructive criticism.

Table 2.2. (*cont.*)

Level	Age of emergence	Examples of skills
AIV:[a] Principles	25 years?	General principles for integrating systems of intangible concepts: Moral principle of justice. Knowledge principle of reflective judgment. Scientific principle of evolution by natural selection.

Note: Table is based on Fischer (1980), Kitchener (1982), and Lamborn (1987). Ages given are modal ages at which a level first appears based on research with middle-class American or European children. They may differ across cultures and other social groups.
[a] These levels are hypothesized, but to date there are too few data to test their existence unequivocally.

similar to what Piaget (1983) called concrete operations. Children can integrate several subsets of two representations. For example, they can demonstrate a concrete form of dual reciprocity, making two characters interact in such a way that both of them embody two social categories simultaneously: If one character acts toward another in ways that are simultaneously nice and mean, the second one will be reciprocally nice and mean. For instance, the first character hits the second one and says, "I'd like to be your friend. Let's play." The second one replies, "I'd like to be your friend too, but I won't be because you hit me."

The study of honesty and kindness began with this level of representational systems and assessed 3 levels beyond it, as shown in Table 2.3. For honesty (Step 1 in Table 2.3), children can coordinate their evaluations of two different individuals' social behaviors around a concrete concept of honesty, such as that honesty is telling the truth about one's grade on a mathematics test even when one did poorly. The child explains a story where two characters both do badly on their arithmetic test but one lies about it and the other tells the truth. In this story, as in the one about nice and mean behaviors, each character interacts with the other in terms of two types of behaviors – in this case, arithmetic test performance and lying or telling the truth. Lamborn (1987) provides formal descriptions of the skill structures for this step and all the others.

The fourth level of representations, which develops at about 10 years of age, constitutes both the end of the representational tier and the beginning of the abstract tier. The structure of this level is *systems of representational systems*, which are the same as *single abstractions*. With single abstractions, children can analyze social behaviors in terms of an in-

Table 2.3. *Development of the concepts of honesty and kindness in social interactions*

Level	Step	Description of skill	
		Honesty	Kindness
RpIII: Representa-tional systems	1	Concrete honesty, single instance: Honesty is telling the truth about your mathematics test grade.	Concrete kindness, single instance: Kindness is sharing your lunch with someone who forgot hers.
	2	Concrete honesty, shift between two instances: Honesty is telling the truth about getting in trouble at recess. Shift to: Honesty is telling the truth about breaking a watch.	Concrete kindness, shift between two instances: Kindness is sharing your paints with someone who does not have any. Shift to: Kindness is helping someone learn to play checkers.
	3	Concrete honesty, two instances integrated: Honesty is telling the truth about your English grade and about getting in trouble.	Concrete kindness, two instances integrated: Kindness is helping someone by fixing his watch and by sharing books when he forgot his.
RpIV/AI: Single abstractions	4	Abstract honesty: Honesty is being truthful to someone about your actions.	Abstract kindness: Kindness is caring by helping someone in need.
	5	Shift between abstract honesty and abstract kindness: Honesty is being truthful to someone about your actions. Shift to: Kindness is caring by helping someone in need.	
	6	Constructive criticism as mixture of honesty and kindness: In constructive criticism, a person is both honest by being truthful to others and kind by helping them to improve.	
AII: Abstract mappings	7	Social lie as opposition of honesty and kindness: In a social lie, honesty and kindness are related as opposites when being truthful is given up in order to be kind to others.	

Table 2.3. (*cont.*)

Level	Step	Description of skill	
		Honesty	Kindness
	8	Shift between social lie (as opposition of honesty and kindness) and constructive criticism (as integration of honesty and kindness):	
		In a social lie, honesty and kindness are related as opposites when being truthful is given up in order to be kind to others.	
		Shift to:	
		In constructive criticism, honesty and kindness are integrated when being truthful about someone's faults is used as a way of showing caring by helping them to improve.	
	9	Jealous truth as combination of honesty, kindness, and jealousy (opposition of honesty and kindness with integration of honesty and jealousy):	
		Sometimes honesty is the opposite of kindness and similar to jealousy when caring for others is given up in order to be truthful in a way that shows resentment toward another because of competition.	
AIII: Abstract systems	10	Constructive criticism as integration of two types of honesty (praising and criticizing) with two types of kindness (building confidence and helping to improve):	
		It is possible to be honest and kind at the same time by both praising and criticizing so as to help others with their needs for confidence and improvement, respectively.	

tangible (abstract) concept of honesty (Step 4 in Table 2.3): Honesty is being truthful to someone about your actions, even when it seems easier to be untruthful. This abstraction goes beyond a single concrete situation, such as telling the truth or lying about a mathematics grade. It integrates at least two such situations from the previous level, generalizing what they share in terms of a general, intangible concept.

For Piaget, this point marks the onset of formal operations, but according to skill theory the capacity that develops here is still far from the full formal-operational thought that Piaget hypothesized. Three more sophisticated levels develop after this one.

These higher levels must overcome major limitations of the first level of abstractions. With single abstractions, children cannot relate one abstraction to another. When they attempt to relate abstractions, they fall back into various confusions, such as mixing up the two concepts or reducing them to concrete instances (Fischer, Hand, & Russell, 1984). For example, they cannot understand how honesty and kindness are related in the social lie. The example of 15-year-old Aurora demonstrates one such confusion. She became upset with her mother's lie about her poetry because she did not understand the opposition of honesty and kindness for her mother. Instead, she focused on the (dis)honesty of her mother's statement and ignored the kindness underlying it. This kind of limitation contributes to the emotional confusion of pre- and early adolescence.

At about 15 years, adolescents develop the capacity to construct *abstract mappings*, in which two abstractions are related to each other. They can coordinate honesty and kindness in the concept of a social lie (Step 7), as Aurora did after her brother provided environmental support to help her sustain the mapping of honesty and kindness as opposites. In a different situation, mappings allow the understanding of a form of constructive criticism in which honesty and kindness are related as similar (Step 8, second part): One person is truthful about another's faults as a way of being kind by helping the other person to improve herself.

Mappings clearly involve a major advance in the understanding of abstractions, and yet they too are limited. With mappings, the adolescent cannot simultaneously relate multiple abstractions, and the result is continuing confusion. In the social lie, honesty and kindness are seen as opposites, but in constructive criticism they are seen as similar. Adolescents become confused by these apparent contradictions, and the confusion seems to contribute to the turmoil of adolescence.

The research of Monsour (1985) and Harter (1986) indicates that at the age when mappings are emerging, adolescents become intensely concerned with what they perceive as conflicts or contradictions in their own personalities. The ability to construct mappings makes it possible for them to recognize such conflicts. For example, a 15-year-old girl may be outgoing with her best friend but shy with boys, or she may see some of her beliefs as liberal and others as conservative.

The next level, *abstract systems*, seems to first develop at about 20 years, although more research is required to pin it down precisely. Young adults become able to coordinate several aspects of two abstractions into a single system. A sophisticated form of constructive criticism (Step 10) illustrates this type of skill. The person coordinates two types of honesty with two types of kindness, both praising and criticizing so as to help another person to both gain confidence and improve. With this sort of sophisticated understanding of the relations of honesty and kindness, mother and daughter would not fight over the mother's evaluation of the daughter's poetry. Such abstract systems can provide for greater emotional stability than single abstractions or abstract mappings.

The final level, which is hypothesized to emerge at about 25 years of age, involves *systems of abstract systems*, which are the same as *general principles*. Two or more abstract systems are coordinated in terms of some general principle that integrates them. Of all the levels in Table 2.2, this one has the least data available to test it. Also, we did not test for it in the study of honesty and kindness. Nevertheless, the research evidence that does exist indicates that several such general principles emerge in the mid to late 20s (Fischer, Hand, & Russell, 1984). For example, it is in this age period that adults first demonstrate an understanding of the principle of reflective judgment (Kitchener & King, 1981). This principle specifies how despite the relativity of knowledge one can judge the probable truth of conclusions based on the quality of the arguments and the evidence, thus comparing several different abstract systems of knowledge.

Skill theory predicts that there are no additional levels beyond general principles. It also predicts that while most adults are capable of constructing abstract systems and general principles, they often do not use these highest cognitive levels.

Transformation rules

Besides the large changes specified by the levels, people also show microdevelopmental changes within a level, which are called steps, as shown in Table 2.3. The developmental mechanism that produces these steps is skill combination, which occurs in several forms specified by transformation rules. (In addition, the movement from level to level can be described by a macrodevelopmental rule, which involves coordinating two skills from one level to form a new skill at the next level.)

For skill combination of any type to occur, the person must first experience the co-occurrence of two skills. That is, in carrying out some task, he or she attempts to perform both skills close together in time. This co-occurrence induces attempts to coordinate the two skills. Usually the first coordinations involve microdevelopmental combinations, and some labor is required before the person can achieve a coordination advancing the skill to the next level (Fischer & Farrar, 1987).

Of course, the likelihood of co-occurrence is affected by many factors, including task, optimal level, environmental support, and emotion. These same factors also facilitate or interfere with the performance of a particular step. Only by analyzing the factors inducing variation in developmental level can researchers unravel the functional mechanisms of development (Fischer & Canfield, 1986; Fogel & Thelen, 1987).

For the sequence of honesty and kindness in Table 2.3, there are three microdevelopmental steps for each of the first 3 levels assessed. The exact number of steps per level is not fixed but can range from one to as many as can be empirically discriminated. That is, the transformation rules can be used to predict an unlimited number of steps. This fact represents an important difference between skill theory and many other stage theories. According to skill theory, the number of steps varies with context, domain, and person.

The transformation rules specify types of skill combination that produce changes in skill complexity within a level. One of their uses is that the researcher can rewrite simpler skills at a given level to specify how more complex skills can be formed at the same level. In the reverse process, they can be used to specify how skills can be simplified by rewriting complex skills into simpler ones. We will illustrate just the two rules used in the study of honesty and kindness – shift of focus and compounding.

In shift of focus, the person carries out one simple skill, and then he or she shifts to a second one. Thus, the co-occurrence leads to only a simple transformation, the systematic juxtaposition of two skills. At step 5 in Table 2.3, for example, abstract honesty is first defined, and then separately abstract kindness is defined. This sort of juxtaposition of components that could be integrated is extremely common in development and seems often to be a transitional step to a genuine integration of components.

In its reverse form, shift of focus also describes one of the most common ways that people simplify tasks that are too difficult for them (Fischer, Hand, & Russell, 1984). When they are called upon to relate two components, such as abstract honesty and kindness (Step 7), they spontaneously simplify the task by dividing it into two separate parts, one involving honesty and one involving kindness (Step 5). In this way, they control the pieces but not the integration.

The transformation of compounding is more sophisticated than shift of focus because it involves a genuine integration of components (but one that still keeps the skill at the same developmental level as the components). In Step 6, honesty and kindness are put together in a simple version of constructive criticism: A person is simultaneously honest by telling another person the truth and kind by helping him to improve himself. Honesty and kindness are thus combined in the same story, but the combination does not involve a clear differentiation of them and specification of an articulated relation. In the more advanced versions of constructive criticism in Steps 8 and 10, the relation is specified more precisely.

In research in the Cognitive Development Laboratory, the transformation rules have been tested repeatedly in studies of predicted developmental sequences. More than 20 such sequences have been tested, and all of them have been strongly supported. Tests of how subjects spontaneously simplify tasks that they perform incorrectly have also supported the transformation rules (Fischer, Hand, & Russell, 1984; Fischer, Hand, Watson, Van Parys, & Tucker, 1984). The studies have mostly involved cross-sectional designs, but they have used methods that share some of the most important characteristics of longitudinal research.

Methods for testing developmental sequences in cross-sectional and longitudinal research

One of the main strengths of longitudinal research is that it provides independent assessments of individual performance at different points in development. In much cross-sectional research on cognitive development, the investigators hypothesize a developmental sequence, but they do not assess that sequence directly in individuals. For example, in a common method that we will call the single-task scaling procedure, they use one task to assess people of different ages and assume that differences in performance on that task across age groups reflect a developmental sequence. The lack of independent assessments of different steps in the sequence in the same individuals is a major weakness. Longitudinal studies deal with this weakness by assessing the same people at several different points in time, thus potentially providing independent assessments of different steps in the sequence.

Longitudinal research is not, however, the only method that provides independent assessments of developmental steps. The method of scalogram analysis provides independent assessment even within cross-sectional studies, as illustrated in Table 2.4 (Fischer & Bullock, 1981). Separate tasks are used to assess every step in the sequence. With at least one independent task assessing each step, the sequence can be tested by analysis of the profiles of performance across tasks. In the simple case shown in Table 2.4, where people either pass or fail each task, the profiles predicted for a sequence are simple: Every person should pass the tasks for every step up to some point in the sequence and fail the tasks for every step beyond that point. If more than one task is used to assess a step, then the predicted profiles involve passing at least one of those tasks, as shown for Steps 4 and 9.

Table 2.4. *The strong scalogram method: predicted profiles for hypothetical developmental sequence*

Developmental step	Tasks designed a priori											
	A	B	C	D	E	F	G	H	I	J	K	L
0	−	−	−	−	−	−	−	−	−	−	−	−
1	+	−	−	−	−	−	−	−	−	−	−	−
2	+	+	−	−	−	−	−	−	−	−	−	−
3	+	+	+	−	−	−	−	−	−	−	−	−
4	+	+	+	−	+	−	−	−	−	−	−	−
	+	+	+	+	−	−	−	−	−	−	−	−
	+	+	+	+	+	−	−	−	−	−	−	−
5	+	+	+	+	+	+	−	−	−	−	−	−
6	+	+	+	+	+	+	+	−	−	−	−	−
7	+	+	+	+	+	+	+	+	−	−	−	−
8	+	+	+	+	+	+	+	+	+	−	−	−
9	+	+	+	+	+	+	+	+	+	−	+	−
	+	+	+	+	+	+	+	+	+	+	−	−
	+	+	+	+	+	+	+	+	+	+	+	−
10	+	+	+	+	+	+	+	+	+	+	+	+

Note: Each step is assessed by a single task except for Steps 4 and 9, which are each assessed with two parallel tasks. Passing a task is indicated by +, and failing it by −.

Traditionally researchers have not used the scalogram technique to test developmental sequences but instead have used it in its weakest form, to describe tasks that happen empirically to show such scalogram patterns in a particular study. To take full advantage of the scalogram to provide independent assessments of developmental steps, researchers can use the strong scalogram method, designing a separate task a priori to test every developmental step as shown in Table 2.4. Then, each subject is given every task in the region of the sequence appropriate for his or her age, and every subject should show one of the predicted profiles.

We used the strong scalogram method to test the developmental sequence for honesty and kindness (Table 2.3) (Lamborn, 1987; Lamborn, Fischer, & Pipp, 1988). A total of 113 subjects were tested; half were male and half female, and they were distributed evenly over the age range from 9 to 20 years. They were tested initially in a high-structure condition, in which they were shown a videotape of the story for a step in the sequence and were immediately asked to retell and explain the story. This procedure was repeated with a different story for each step. Steps 1 to 4 were each assessed with two stories, designed to test separately the concepts of honesty and kindness. The stories embodied the kinds of scripts sketched in the descriptions of the developmental sequence in Table 2.4. On the videotape, a narrator first described each story in general terms, and then the story was acted out through a set of realistic cardboard figures. For example, here is the narrator's description of the story for abstract honesty (Step 4 in Table 2.3):

> This story shows that honesty is being truthful to someone about your actions, even when it seems easier to be untruthful. Sara and Tom both can't go to a party, but Tom lies about why he can't go, while Sara tells the truth. At the same time, Sara and Mark realize that they have lost Mary's notebook. Mark wants to tell her that someone stole it, but Sara thinks they should tell her what really happened. Honesty is being truthful to someone about your actions, even when it seems easier to be untruthful. And that means telling someone the truth about why you can't come to a party and about losing a notebook.

After the high-structure condition, subjects were also tested in a low-structure, spontaneous condition, in which they made up a story of their own about honesty and kindness. Two weeks later, they were again tested in both conditions. In addition, they were also given several questionnaires assessing their social skills and their close social relationships.

The scalogram results from the high-structure condition are shown in Table 2.5. Of 113 subjects, 98 matched the predicted profiles perfectly for the first session, and 107 did so for the second session. By Green's (1956) index of consistency, the results showed high scalability, $I = .81$ and .93, respectively.

Although this study was cross-sectional, the strong scalogram method makes possible the rigorous testing of a hypothesized developmental sequence with either a cross-sectional or a longitudinal design (Fischer & Bullock, 1981). In a cross-sectional design, the sequence is tested via the synchronic pattern of passes and failures as shown in Table 2.3. In a longitudinal design, it is tested via both this synchronic pattern and the diachronic pattern of passes and failures over time.

Traditionally, longitudinal studies have used the single-task scaling procedure rather than the scalogram method. In that traditional design, the repeated sessions provide potentially independent assessments of each step in a developmental sequence, but whether the independent assessments are realized is in part a matter of luck: Individuals may develop through one step to another between assessment times, so that they show no evidence of a step that is in fact part of the sequence. The scalogram method eliminates this problem, providing a more powerful assessment of sequence in longitudinal studies.

The method allows the precise testing of many hypotheses about

Table 2.5. *Predicted profiles for understanding honesty and kindness*

Developmental sequence of profiles	Tasks for understanding honesty and kindness										Session I		Session II	
	1	2	3	4	5	6	7	8	9	10	N	Mean age	N	Mean age
0	−	−	−	−	−	−	−	−	−	−	0	—	1	9.05
1	+	−	−	−	−	−	−	−	−	−	4	9.31	0	—
2	+	+	−	−	−	−	−	−	−	−	1	12.07	1	9.03
3	+	+	+	−	−	−	−	−	−	−	1	11.00	3	10.05
4	+	+	+	+	−	−	−	−	−	−	7	10.90	1	12.07
5	+	+	+	+	+	−	−	−	−	−	11	11.41	10	10.85
6	+	+	+	+	+	+	−	−	−	−	20	13.40	14	12.91
7	+	+	+	+	+	+	+	−	−	−	9	15.05	10	12.46
8	+	+	+	+	+	+	+	+	−	−	16	17.62	17	15.29
9	+	+	+	+	+	+	+	+	+	−	26	17.59	40	17.01
10	+	+	+	+	+	+	+	+	+	+	3	20.71	10	18.74
Nonscalable profiles											15		6	
Total											113		113	
Index of consistency											.81[a]		.93[a]	

[a] Values range from 0 to 1, with 1 indicating perfect scalability. Any value above .50 is considered statistically significant (Green, 1956).

development (Fischer, Pipp, & Bullock, 1984). For example, with the even distribution of ages in our sample, we can assess what might be called *developmental distance* between steps in the predicted sequence – the interval separating development of successive steps. Many key developmental concepts, such as that of stage, make predictions about the developmental distances between steps. Skill theory predicts that before the emergence of a new optimal level, optimal performance will proceed slowly through new steps. Then when the new level emerges, optimal performance will show rapid movement through a series of steps characteristic of the new level. That is, when the assessment conditions provide high environmental support, the developmental distances between these steps will be large before emergence of the optimal level and small after it.

Longitudinal designs can be more powerful than cross-sectional ones because they provide both synchronic and diachronic tests of sequence. Yet that is only part of the story: Treatments of longitudinal methods tend to emphasize their advantages and deemphasize their limitations (Schneider, in press; Wohlwill, 1973). They definitely have limitations as well as virtues. The limitation most often emphasized is the bias in subject selection: Many types of people simply do not participate in longitudinal studies or drop out before completion (Horn & Donaldson, 1976). (Hoppe-Graff [this volume] provides a particularly thoughtful analysis of the role of longitudinal methods in the study of developmental transitions.)

An equally significant problem in cognitive research is the effects of repeated testing. Longitudinal designs typically provide practice in the skills being assessed and thus push performance toward optimum. Cross-sectional designs typically provide better assessments of ordinary, nonoptimal performance. Researchers cannot simply assume, therefore, that performance is comparable across cross-sectional and longitudinal studies. The two designs will produce dramatically different portraits of cognitive development.

The ideal study would seem to combine cross-sectional and longitudinal designs, in order to deal with the limitations of each. For most developmental questions, both types of designs provide important information. With the scalogram method, both designs can provide strong assessments of developmental sequences, but for some questions one design is clearly superior over the other. Cross-sectional designs are best for assessing spontaneous performance in unfamiliar domains, and longitudinal ones are best for following individuals over time.

Mechanisms that produce change

As illustrated in the honesty-and-kindness study, the levels and transformation rules of skill theory can be used to predict developmental sequences in detail. Armed with such sequences and with methods such as strong scalogram analysis, we have been able to study the important problem of the functional mechanisms of variation and development.

One of the most persistent findings in the developmental literature is what Piaget (1941) called horizontal decalage. With changes in task or domain, children show unevenness in developmental level. Instead of consistently showing Piagetian concrete operations across 10 tasks, for example, they show wide variations in stage of performance. There have been so many documentations of this unevenness that several theorists have suggested that decalage is the rule in cognitive development (Biggs & Collis, 1982; Fischer, 1980; Flavell, 1982).

Decalage occurs not only when there are changes in task or domain, but also from moment to moment. From 1 minute to the next, performance varies substantially in the same person for the same sequence in the same domain assessed in the same context. At 1 minute the person may show a high step of performance, a minute later he may show a much lower step of performance, and then still later he may show an intermediate step. Performance thus varies across a number of developmental steps in a developmental sequence for a single domain (Fischer & Elmendorf, 1986).

There is order to the diverse types of decalages or variations, order determined by the functional mechanisms of development. Skill theory is designed to explain and predict such variations. First, they follow the developmental sequences predicted by the transformation rules. Second, the variations occur systematically as a function of at least four other mechanisms or sources besides the transformations: task, optimal level, environmental support, and emotion.

Task

The particular task being performed by the person is not just a passive aliment for his or her skills. It actively contributes to them, helping to organize the person's behavior. That is one of the implications of the collaboration of person and environment, and it is consistent with the growing ecological literature demonstrating the important organizing effects of the environment on behavior (Gibson, 1979; Fogel & Thelen, 1987). When the task is changed, the skill is changed.

Consequently, one of the basic tenets of skill theory is that developmental sequences cannot be predicted in detail *across* task domains, except under limited circumstances. Detailed predictions of microdevelopmental sequences such as that for honesty and kindness are not possible if the task domain is changed from one step to the next. Prediction of developmental sequences requires that tasks remain within the same task domain because only then are the skills similar enough to show consistent microdevelopmental ordering.

On the other hand, global sequences can be predicted, with large distances between steps. For example, the development of a single abstraction in one familiar domain, such as honesty, will generally precede the development of a skill at the next level in another familiar domain, such as a mathematics skill requiring abstract mappings.

Also generalizations can occur from one task domain to another, but the person must work to bring about this change in a skill (Fischer & Farrar, 1987). When Aurora praised her younger brother for his soccer playing even though she knew he was still not playing well, she understood the concept of social lie in this domain. But when her mother praised her poem, she could not yet apply the concept of social lie to that domain. Her older brother helped her to generalize the concept from the first domain to the second.

Tasks are thus one of the major contributors to variations in developmental step, actively contributing to the organization of behavior.

Optimal level

Although tasks and other factors produce wide variations in developmental level, there is a limit to how high in any developmental sequence people's performance can go. The use of independent tasks to assess every step in a sequence allows precise testing of whether performance goes beyond a specific step. Even under ideal testing conditions, the person's performance does not move beyond his or her optimal level, the upper limit on the complexity of skills that he or she can construct and control. When children or adolescents are given instructions in how to perform a task, they do not learn the task when it is beyond their optimal level (e.g., Jackowitz, 1988; Moshman & Franks, 1986; O'Brien & Overton, 1982). One of the primary sources constraining variation in developmental step, then, is optimal level.

Optimal level is evidenced in not only an upper limit but also in a rapid spurt in performance upon emergence of a new optimal level. That is, there are stagelike spurts at certain age periods, but only in optimal, not in ordinary performance. Across task domains, the spurts in optimal performance occur during limited age bands, reflecting a general reorganization in behavior. Of course, other factors besides optimal-level changes also produce spurts in performance in specific domains (Fischer & Bullock, 1981).

For example, two studies at the University of Denver have demonstrated such spurts for abstract mappings. In a study assessing the understanding of abstract relations of two similar arithmetic operations, such as division and subtraction, optimal performance abruptly jumped from nearly 0% correct at 14 and 15 years of age to over 80% correct at 16 years – a dramatic spurt (Fischer, Pipp, & Bullock, 1984). At the same time, performance under nonoptimal conditions did not show any spurt at all but slow, gradual improvement, as shown in Figure 2.2.

The second study showed a similar spurt that involved self-concepts. In Harter's (1986) and Monsour's (1985) study, a high-structure technique was used to elicit self-characterizations by 13- to 17-year-olds. At 15 years of age, adolescents showed a sharp spurt in both the perception of contradiction in their own personalities and the feelings of conflict about the contradictions. This increased sense of conflict had been predicted because of the emergence of the level of abstract mappings, which allows comparison of abstract characterizations of one's own personality and thus the recognition of contradictions.

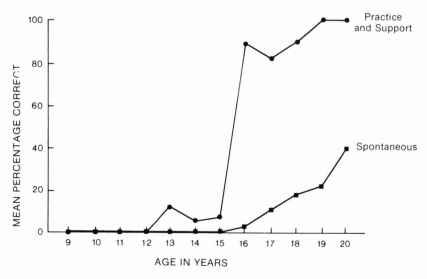

Figure 2.2. Developmental changes in the percentage of problems passed involving abstract mappings (from Fischer, Pipp, & Bullock, 1984, © Plenum)

The results on honesty and kindness also suggested a spurt in abstract mappings during the same age period, although the study was not designed to provide a definitive test for such a spurt (Lamborn, 1987). The developmental distance was greater for steps between levels than for those within a level. In addition to the spurt in understanding, there was an associated increase in perception of problems with parents as well.

Functional level and degree of environmental support

Optimal level is reliably evident only under environmental conditions that provide strong support for high-level performance. Such environmental support is one of the most important factors affecting level of performance within a task domain. High-support conditions include the presence of aids or cues that minimize memory demands, the use of familiar materials, the clear definition of task demands, and the opportunity for practice (Brown & Reeve, in press; Lamborn & Fischer, 1988).

High support, however, does not include direct intervention in the person's performance by a knowledgeable adult. Vygotsky (1978) pointed out that children's performance improves substantially when adults provide scaffolding of high-level performance. In cases of scaffolding, the adult typically intervenes directly to do part of the task for the child. That improvement is beyond the variations in performance that we are investigating, which all involve the production of a response by a person without any direct intervention by another. That is, high support involves indirect aid rather than direct performance of part of the task for the child.

When people are not in high-support conditions, their behavior is typically below their optimal level. Most spontaneous situations and most developmental and educational assessment procedures do not provide high environmental support. In a number of studies we have found a persistent gap in performance between high- and low-support conditions (Fischer & Canfield, 1986; Lamborn & Fischer, 1988). For example, in the honesty-and-kindness sequence, the average 10-year-old performed at Step 5 or 6 (single abstractions) with high support, but showed only Step 3 (representational systems) with low support. Other studies have found even larger gaps (Fischer, Hand, & Russell, 1984). These gaps do not merely reflect a preponderance of low-step responses mixed in with a few high-step responses. Instead, they reflect a general lowering of performance, a move to an earlier part of the developmental sequence.

The persistence of the gap between high- and low-support conditions reflects what is called the child's *functional level*, the highest step that he or she shows consistently under specific low-support conditions for a task domain. Fifteen-year-old Aurora's oversimplification of her mother's social lie about her poem illustrates the persistence of the gap. Her functional level was a simplification of an abstract mapping for a social lie into a single abstraction for dishonesty. Her optimal level was abstract mappings, but she could not easily move her understanding up to that level, even when her 20-year-old brother attempted to explain the nature of her mother's social lie. When he provided high support for understanding the social lie, she finally did put together the necessary mapping.

The persistence of the gap as well as the consistency of functional level for a specific task domain has been demonstrated repeatedly in over a dozen studies in the Cognitive Development Laboratory. We have assessed children's behavior on various developmental sequences under two different low-support (spontaneous) conditions. Consistently, the highest steps that the children showed under these several low-support conditions were similar for each child in a given domain. However, as soon as environmental support was increased, children showed an immediate jump in developmental step (Fischer, Hand, Watson, Van Parys, & Tucker, 1984; Lamborn & Fischer, 1988). Changes in domain also affected functional level.

These findings, we propose, support the collaborational view of the development of the organization of behavior. Both person and environment contribute to children's "competencies." People do not have fixed competencies that they carry with them everywhere they go. To the contrary, their competence varies with the context (Fischer & Bullock, 1984). Changes in the task and changes in environmental support, as well as other factors such as emotions, affect their competence.

Emotions

Emotions are obviously an important part of behavior, and they deserve to be included in any theory of mechanisms of development. Recent breakthroughs in emotion theory and research promise to facilitate developmental analysis (Fischer, Shaver, & Carnochan, 1988). People possess a set of basic, prototypical emotions, including anger, fear, sadness, joy, love, and a few others (Ekman & Oster, 1979; Izard, 1977). These emotions can be grouped into positive and negative sets or differentiated into more situation-specific emotion categories, such as jealousy, resentment, and nostalgia (Shaver, Schwartz, Kirson, & O'Connor, 1987).

Emotions have a potent direct effect on the organization of behavior, an effect analogous in some ways to that of tasks (Fischer & Elmendorf, 1986). Emotions can alter what might be called the *organismic context*, thus drastically affecting the organization of behavior.

The organizations that emotions produce are best understood in terms of the basic emotions, which seem to be species-specific behavioral organizations that arise when a particular goal of the organism is advanced (producing a positive emotion) or impeded (producing a negative emotion). These organismic states bias the person toward one kind of organization, such as anger, and away from others, such as joy (Scherer, 1984; Shaver et al., 1987). (See Carey, 1985, for a discussion of other sorts of biases, or constraints, on the organization of behavior.)

When a person is strongly experiencing one of these emotions, it sharply alters the organismic context: It directly affects the organization of his or her behavior in terms of a specific prototypical pattern or script for anger, as shown in Table 2.6. The person's developmental step is produced by the interaction of this script with other factors such as task, optimal level, and environmental support.

When 15-year-old Aurora became angry with her mother, the script for anger became predominant in organizing her behavior. Once she was behaving in the anger context, she was predisposed to notice potential wrongs or insults, to respond aggressively, to be upset, and to refuse to consider her mother's viewpoint. Consequently, it became extremely

Table 2.6. *Prototypic script for anger*

Antecedents:
Something interferes with the person's plans or goals or threatens to harm him or her.
This interference or harm is illegitimate or unfair.

Responses:
The person becomes energized to fight or verbally attack or imagine attacking the agent
    causing the anger so that he or she can rectify the injustice or physical harm.
The person looks angry and moves in a heavy, tight, or exaggerated way.
The person focuses on the anger-inducing situation, convinced that he or she is right.

Self-control procedures:
The person may try not to show his or her emotion or to redefine the situation so that it no
    longer makes him or her angry.

Source: Based on Shaver, Schwartz, Kirson, & O'Connor (1987).

difficult for her to perform at her optimal level for honesty and kindness
and understand her mother's social-lie motivation. Her functional level
in that domain was perforce well below her optimal level.

For her to move up to her optimal-level understanding, she needed
environmental support for integrating the concepts of honesty and kindness (support which her brother supplied). In addition, she needed to
shift away from her anger mode to an emotional state that would
facilitate the components necessary to understand her mother's social lie.
When her brother helped her evoke the love she and her mother shared,
then the emotion of love facilitated her taking her mother's perspective
and understanding the social lie behind her mother's behavior.

In this way, specific emotions such as anger, love, fear, and joy have
potent effects on developmental step within a domain. If the emotion is
consonant with the demands of the domain, it can facilitate understanding and promote high-level behavior. But if it is dissonant with the
demands, it can interfere with understanding and produce low-level
behavior.

In addition to these effects of emotional prototypes on the organization
of behavior, there are also developmental changes in emotions. Each
developmental level brings changes in the understanding of emotions
and the conditions that elicit them. As we noted in the description of the
cycle of levels, certain levels bring special emotional vulnerabilities. In
the preschool years, the onset of representational mappings at about 4
years helps produce the emotional turmoil of the Oedipus conflict (Fis-

cher & Watson, 1981). In early adolescence, the onset of single abstractions helps produce a generally confused, emotional state. At each level, there are significant complexes of emotional change, just as there are significant cognitive and social changes. These changing complexes have been one focus of our research on adolescent development.

Emotional vulnerability in adolescence

Our analysis so far has focused on the general pattern of cognitive development. Still needed is a portrait of emotional-cognitive development during adolescence. Several forces converge to produce a special emotional vulnerability during adolescence. Besides developing new cognitive capacities, adolescents are becoming mature sexually, building new kinds of close, personal friendships (Youniss, 1980), and beginning to leave the world of childhood, redefining their roles in the family and in the world outside the home. Research provides strong evidence for vulnerability to emotional turmoil in adolescence, despite some assertions that the "storm and stress" of adolescence do not really exist.

Social changes that produce vulnerabilities in adolescence

One of the most important forces that produces special emotional vulnerabilities during adolescence is change in close social relationships. According to Blos (1962), Erikson (1968), and Sullivan (1953), the emotional transitions of adolescence are connected with changes in emotional investments in the adolescent's relationships, with a focus on the issue of autonomy. A central goal of adolescence is to give up parents as the primary relationship and develop important emotional connections outside the family, eventually establishing romantic relationships with peers as well as a strong sense of identity and self-esteem.

Prior to adolescence, children are emotionally invested in their familial ties, especially with their parents. During pre- and early adolescence the separation from the family begins. The child's idealistic conceptions of the parents are gradually replaced by more realistic views (Blos, 1962). The initial awareness of failings on the parents' part can result in disappointment and anger. Also, the move away from parents can be facilitated by the adolescent becoming overly critical of the parents.

This transition is mediated by a shift to idealized friendships and intimate relationships that replace the idealized relationships with parents. The shifts in emotional investments to different relationships are often accompanied by loneliness, isolation, and depression. As the young person gives up both the idealized parents and idealized friends, a void is often left before achieving the transition to extrafamilial relationships. She may feel insecure about her parents' feelings for her, both because of the instability and confusion in her own self and because of the distance from parents that she is encouraging in order to achieve autonomy. Without an emotional connection either inside or outside the family, the adolescent is self-oriented, and self-esteem becomes unsteady, tending to be either overly high or overly low. The adolescent is likely to feel unsure of herself and critical of any actions that can be viewed as inconsistent.

Late adolescence is characterized by consolidation of a sense of individuality that encompasses work, love, and a value system. As the life tasks that will be implemented during adulthood are defined, stability of emotions and self-esteem and commitment to extrafamilial sexual relationships become apparent.

It is our contention that these emotional patterns in adolescence generally fit the findings on adolescent emotional-cognitive development and that they make sense in terms of not only the social and biological changes in the adolescent's life but also the cognitive developments.

Evidence for emotional vulnerabilities during adolescence

In recent years, some scholars have claimed that adolescence does not really involve any special emotional turmoil or vulnerability (Conger, 1981; Weiner, 1976). This claim is based, among other things, on the fact that most people do not report serious upset while they are adolescents. Yet when adults look back to adolescence, they report that it was a difficult, emotional time (Pipp, Shaver, Jennings, Lamborn, & Fischer, 1985; Woodruff & Birren, 1972). Many other data, ranging from the frequency of conflict to the incidence of suicide, indicate that for many adolescents at least, it is an unstable time (Coleman, 1974; Hakim-Larson et al., 1985).

Some of the vulnerabilities seem to relate to the cognitive "advances" of early abstractions, as indicated by two of the studies we have mentioned from the University of Denver. Adolescents demonstrate a vulnerability in both their understandings of themselves and their perceptions of their relationships with parents.

To assess adolescents' understandings and feelings about the self, Monsour (1985) asked 64 adolescents, 13 to 17 years old, to describe themselves in different roles, such as at home, at school, with friends, or with a boyfriend or girlfriend. Then each description was written on a small piece of paper, and the adolescent placed it in a figure representing the self. The figure was composed of three concentric circles, with the innermost one representing the qualities most central to the self, the outermost one representing the qualities most peripheral, and the one in the middle representing the qualities intermediate in importance.

Working with this figure of their own personality, the adolescents were asked to identify inconsistencies in their self-descriptions and to report their emotional reactions to the inconsistencies. Recall that abstract mappings emerge at about 15 years of age, and with this ability to compare two abstractions, adolescents are predicted to experience more conflicts in their own personalities.

The prediction was strongly supported. There was a dramatic spurt in both inconsistencies and feelings of conflict over the inconsistencies. The 15-year-olds reported feeling mad, confused, worried, and pressured over the inconsistencies they noticed in themselves. The spurt was present for both sexes, but it was stronger for girls than for boys. One adolescent reported, "I am an understanding person, but I can get so inconsiderate with my friends. I feel really bad about it afterwards, and don't know why I did it. It really bothers me that I can be so different. It's not like me" (Monsour, 1985, p. 59). By age 17, the perception of inconsistencies had decreased somewhat, and the feelings of conflict about them had decreased substantially. Harter (1986) reports several further studies replicating these findings.

The study of honesty and kindness produced evidence for the development of conflict and turmoil even earlier in adolescence (Lamborn, 1987). In the beginning teenage years, adolescents reported a drop in the quality of their parental relationships, and the drop was especially strong for girls. They rated their relationships with each parent as lower in regard and higher in punishment, and they rated their relationships with their father as also lower in disclosure and control.

A model of adolescent emotional vulnerabilities

These changes in emotional reactions, together with the evidence for cognitive and social changes, provide foundations for building a general model of the development of emotional vulnerabilities in the period from preadolescence to late adolescence (9 to 20 years). During this time, there seems to be a general spurt and subsequent decrease in emotional vulnerabilities, which relates closely to the developing understanding of self and of social relationships, including the concepts of honesty and kindness.

During the years just before adolescence (approximately 9 to 12), there is a *blossoming of social comparison*, in which children consolidate their ability to compare themselves with other people as well as to compare other people with each other (Ruble, 1983). Concrete social comparisons occur commonly with skills at the level of representational systems, but the emergence of single abstractions at about 10 years adds new power and generality to the comparisons. Indeed, the tasks assessing single abstractions about honesty and kindness (Steps 4, 5, and 6 in Table 2.3) all involved comparing two people's differing reactions to some social situation and judging one to be better. Social comparison is permeating the personality system.

In the study, children in this age range who showed higher steps of understanding honesty and kindness demonstrated the (short-term) negative effects of these developments. Better understanding correlated with greater dissatisfaction with both one's relationships with others and one's own skills.

With the emergence of adolescence (approximately 13 to 16 years), the dissatisfaction and conflict emerge full-blown, and adolescents show a period of *storm and stress*. This is the period when Lamborn (1987) found a decrease in perceived quality of relationships with parents and Monsour (1985) found an increase in feelings of conflict about oneself. A study by Buhrmester (1981) showed a general increase in reports of anxiety about a number of domains, including personal appearance, popularity, and the future.

At the same time adolescents are showing a *shift toward peers*. In Lamborn's study, they reported more disclosure with peers, and the level of disclosure was especially high for same-sex peers. Better understanding of honesty and kindness related to satisfaction with same-sex peers; it no longer predicted greater dissatisfaction, as it had earlier. Apparently same-sex peer relationships are the arena where new emotional commitments are being worked through, as Erikson (1968), Blos (1962), and Sullivan (1953) have suggested.

During late adolescence (17 to 20 years), these young adults went through a period of quieting down and moving out into the world. They showed a return to better relationships with their parents. At the same time, better understanding of honesty and kindness related to satisfaction with parental relationships, especially with mothers. Of course, they also became more interested in opposite-sex relationships. In Monsour's study, they showed a decrease in feelings of conflict about their own inconsistencies.

The emergence and development of abstractions provides part of the explanation for these changes in emotional vulnerabilities. Recall that the early levels of abstractions bring with them special instabilities and confusions. Single abstractions are advances when compared to sensorimotor and representational skills, but they are the most primitive forms of abstract thought. They do not even allow the comparison of two abstractions, and so when a person tries to think of several abstractions simultaneously, a fog of confusion reigns.

By middle adolescence, abstract mappings become common. These new skills constitute an enormous leap forward, in that they allow the adolescent to think about and relate two abstractions at the same time. The fog of single abstractions begins to lift as the adolescent compares and sorts out many relations among abstractions.

Nevertheless, the abstract comparisons made are often crude and simple, because the limitations of mappings preclude the consideration of multiple relevant abstract concepts. For example, when the adolescent compares her own characteristics in different situations or compares herself with her parents, differences are likely to be viewed as conflicting, opposing, or clashing. The primitiveness of mappings can thus still lead to emotional confusion.

Of course, much of an adolescent's actual behavior will be below his or her optimal level. After the emergence of the capacity for abstract mappings, it still takes years for adolescents to work out all they need to know about simple relations among abstractions. For example, a 15-year-old will often be functioning with single abstractions even though she is capable of using abstract mappings under ideal conditions. In Aurora's argument over her mother's social lie, she demonstrated this common phenomenon.

The ability to understand nuances or multiple components of abstract relations is characteristic of later skill levels. These abstract systems and general principles bring with them the potential for greater stability. Thus, older adolescents and adults can build more sophisticated understandings of themselves and their relationships that promote emotional stability. Of course, even adults frequently function below their optimal level, and presumably their low-level functioning also contributes to their emotional vulnerabilities. The stabilization in late adolescence and early adulthood is hypothesized to relate to the elaboration of advanced abstract mappings and the emergence of abstract systems.

In conclusion, the age-related cognitive changes of adolescence seem to contribute to the vulnerabilities in self-concept and relationships with parents that are characteristic of this period. The period of greatest vulnerability and turmoil seems usually to be the early teenage years, when single abstractions dominate the cognitive profile and abstract mappings are beginning to emerge. By the late teenage years, stability seems to become more common. Of course, the social and biological changes of adolescence also contribute to these developmental patterns.

Summary

What changes with development is the organization of behavior. The changes in organization involve both microdevelopmental transformations of skills and large-scale shifts to new optimal levels. All changes require the coordination of a number of skill components to form a more complex skill. At least five major functional mechanisms affect whether the components are available and thus whether the complex skill will occur: optimal level, emotion, task, environmental support, and skill transformations. These factors are the sources of both long-term development and short-term variations in developmental step.

The optimal level sets an upper limit on the complexity of skill that the person can produce. The person's emotions act as an organismic context, producing predispositions for certain prototypical organizations of behavior. The task evokes a set of component behaviors based on the context it provides. The degree of environmental support for high-level behavior affects the functional level of the behavior. For all these mechanisms of variation, the skill transformation rules indicate the ordering of steps along developmental scales.

In adolescence, the emergence of the early, primitive levels of abstractions predispose the youth toward emotional vulnerabilities, in which cognitive confusions lead to emotional lability. The several functional mechanisms of variation affect exactly when these cognitive confusions will occur and when they will be resolved. Of course, the social and biological changes of adolescence join with these cognitive changes to produce the storm and stress of adolescence.

NOTE

Preparation of this essay was supported by a grant from the Spencer Foundation and a fellowship from the Cattell Fund to the first author as well as NIMH predoctoral and postdoctoral fellowships to the second author. The authors would like to thank Dorothy Haltiwanger, Susan Harter, Ann Monsour, and Phillip Shaver for their contributions to the work here.

REFERENCES

Beth, E. W., & Piaget, J. (1966). *Mathematical epistemology and psychology* (W. Mays, Trans.). Dordrecht: D. Reidel. (Original work published 1961)

Biggs, J., & Collis, K. (1982) *Evaluating the quality of learning: The SOLO taxonomy (structure of the observed learning outcome)*. New York: Academic Press.

Blos, P. (1962). *On adolescence: A psychoanalytic interpretation.* New York: Free Press.

Brown, A. L., & Reeve, R. (in press). Bandwidths of competence: The role of supportive contexts in learning and development. In L. S. Liben (Ed.), *Development and learning: Conflict or congruence?* Hillsdale, NJ: Erlbaum.

Buhrmester, D. (1981). *Developmental changes in third- through ninth-graders' worries.* Paper presented at the Rocky Mountain Psychological Convention, Denver, Co.

Carey, S. (1985). *Conceptual change in childhood.* Cambridge: MIT Press.

Case, R. (1985). *Intellectual development: Birth to adulthood.* New York: Academic Press.

Coleman, J. C. (1974). *Relationships in adolescence.* London: Routledge and Kegan Paul.

Conger, J. J. (1981). Freedom and commitment: Families, youth, and social change. *American Psychologist, 36,* 1475–1484.

Ekman, P., & Oster, H. (1979). Facial expressions of emotion. *Annual Review of Psychology, 30,* 527–554.

Erikson, E. H. (1968). *Identity, youth, and crisis.* New York: Norton.

Fischer, K. W. (1980). A theory of cognitive development: The control and construction of hierarchies of skills. *Psychological Review, 87,* 477–531.

Fischer, K. W., & Bullock, D. (1981). Patterns of data: Sequence, synchrony, and constraint in cognitive development. In K. W. Fischer (Ed.), *Cognitive development* (New Directions for Child Development No. 12, pp. 69–78). San Francisco: Jossey-Bass.

Fischer, K. W., & Bullock, D. (1984). Cognitive development in school-age children: Conclusions and new directions. In W. A. Collins (Ed.), *The years from six to twelve: Cognitive development during middle childhood* (pp. 70–146). Washington, DC: National Academy Press.

Fischer, K. W., & Canfield, R. L. (1986). The ambiguity of stage and structure in behavior: Person and environment in the development of psychological structures. In I. Levin (Ed.), *Stage and structure: Reopening the debate* (pp. 246–267). New York: Plenum.

Fischer, K. W., & Elmendorf, D. (1986). Becoming a different person: Transformations in personality and social behavior. In M. Perlmutter (Ed.), *Minnesota Symposium on Child Psychology* (Vol. 18, pp. 137–178). Hillsdale, NJ: Erlbaum.

Fischer, K. W., & Farrar, M. J. (1987). Generalizations about generalization: How skills transfer across tasks in development. *International Journal of Psychology, 22,* 643–677.

Fischer, K. W., Hand, H. H., & Russell, S. L. (1984). The development of abstractions in adolescence and adulthood. In M. Commons, F. A. Richards, & C. Armon (Eds.), *Beyond formal operations* (pp. 43–73). New York: Praeger.

Fischer, K. W., Hand, H. H., Watson, M. W., Van Parys, M., & Tucker, J. (1984). Putting the child into socialization: The development of social categories in preschool children. In L. Katz (Ed.), *Current topics in early childhood education* (Vol. 5, pp. 27–72). Norwood, NJ: Ablex.

Fischer, K. W., & Pipp, S. L. (1984a). Development of the structures of unconscious thought. In K. Bowers & D. Meichenbaum (Eds.), *The unconscious reconsidered* (pp. 88–148). New York: Wiley.

Fischer, K. W., & Pipp, S. L. (1984b). Processes of cognitive development:

Optimal level and skill acquisition. In R. J. Sternberg (Ed.), *Mechanisms of cognitive development* (pp. 45–80). San Francisco: Freeman.

Fischer, K. W., Pipp, S. L., & Bullock, D. (1984). Detecting discontinuities in development: method and measurement. In R. Emde & R. Harmon (Eds.), *Continuities and discontinuities in development* (pp. 95–121). New York: Plenum.

Fischer, K. W., Shaver, P., & Carnochan, P. (1988). From basic- to subordinate-level emotions: A skill approach to emotional development. In W. Damon (Ed.), *Child development today and tomorrow* (New Directions for Child Development No. 40). San Francisco: Jossey-Bass.

Fischer, K. W., & Watson, M. W. (1981). Explaining the Oedipus conflict. In K. W. Fischer (Ed.), *Cognitive development* (New Directions for Child Development No. 12, pp. 79–92). San Francisco: Jossey-Bass.

Flavell, J. (1982). On cognitive development. *Child Development, 53,* 1–10.

Fogel, A. & Thelen, E. (1987). The development of communicative and expressive action in the first year: Reinterpreting the evidence from a dynamic systems perspective. *Developmental Psychology, 23,* 747–761.

Gibson, J. J. (1979). *The ecological approach to visual perception.* Boston: Houghton-Mifflin.

Green, B. G. (1956). A method of scalogram analysis using summary statistics. *Psychometrika, 21,* 79–88.

Hakim-Larson, J., Livingston, J., & Tron, R. (1985). *Mothers and adolescent daughters: Personal issues of conflict and congruency.* Paper presented at the meetings of the Society for Research in Child Development, Toronto, Canada.

Harter, S. (1983). Developmental perspectives on the self-system. In E. M. Hetherington (Ed.), *Handbook of child psychology: Vol. 4. Socialization, personality, and social development* (P. Mussen, Gen. Ed.) (pp. 275–385). New York: Wiley.

Harter, S. (1986). Cognitive-developmental processes in the integration of concepts about emotions and the self. *Social Cognition, 4,* 119–151.

Horn, J. L., & Donaldson, G. (1976). On the myth of intellectual decline in adulthood. *American Psychologist, 31,* 701–719.

Inhelder, B., & Piaget, J. (1958). *The growth of logical thinking from childhood to adolescence* (A. Parsons & S. Seagrim, Trans.). New York: Basic Books. (Original work published 1955).

Izard, C. E. (1977). *Human emotions.* New York: Plenum.

Jackowitz, E. R. (1988). *The effects of self-instruction and environmental support on understanding mean and nice social interactions in children.* Unpublished doctoral dissertation, University of Denver.

Kitchener, K. S. (1982). Human development and the college campus: Sequences and tasks. In G. R. Hanson (Ed.), *Measuring Student Development. New Directions for Student Services* (No. 20, pp. 17–45). San Francisco: Jossey-Bass.

Kitchener, K. S., & King, P. M. (1981). Reflective judgement: Concepts of justification and their relation to age and education. *Journal of Applied Developmental Psychology, 2,* 89–116.

Lamborn, S. D. (1987). Relations between social-cognitive knowledge and personal experience: Understanding honesty and kindness in relationships (Doctoral dissertation, University of Denver, 1986). *Dissertation Abstracts International, 47,* 2959A. (University Microfilms No. DA8626347)

Lamborn, S. D., & Fischer, K. W. (1988). Optimal and functional levels in cognitive development: The individual's developmental range. *Newsletter of the International Society for the Study of Behavioral Development, 2* (Serial No. 14), 1–4.

Lamborn, S. D., Fischer, K. W., & Pipp, S. L. (1988). Constructive criticism and social lies: A developmental sequence for understanding honesty and kindness. Unpublished manuscript.

Monsour, A. (1985). The dynamics and structure of adolescent self-concept (Doctoral dissertation, University of Denver). *Dissertation Abstracts International, 46,* 2091B. (University Microfilms No. DA8517558)

Moshman, D., & Franks, B. A. (1986). Development of the concept of inferential validity. *Child Development, 57,* 153–165.

Mounoud, P. (1976). Les revolutions psychologiques de l'enfant. *Archives de Psychologie, 44,* 103–114.

O'Brien, D. P., & Overton, W. F. (1982). Conditional reasoning and the competence-performance issue: A developmental analysis of a training task. *Journal of Experimental Child Psychology, 34,* 274–290.

Piaget, J. (1941). Le mécanisme du developpement mental et les lois du groupement des opérations. *Archives de Psychologie, Genève, 28,* 215–285.

Piaget, J. (1957). Logique et équilibre dans les comportements du sujet. *Études d'Épistemologie Génétique, 2,* 27–118.

Piaget, J. (1975). L'equilibration des structures cognitives: Problème central du developpement. *Études d'Épistemologie Génétique, 33.*

Piaget, J. (1983). Piaget's theory. In W. Kessen (Ed.), *Handbook of child psychology: Vol. 1. History, theory, and methods* (P. Mussen, Gen. Ed.) (4th ed., pp. 103–126). New York: Wiley.

Pipp, S. L., Shaver, P., Jennings, S., Lamborn, S., & Fischer, K. W. (1985). Adolescents' theories about the development of their relationships with parents. *Journal of Personality and Social Psychology, 48,* 991–1001.

Ruble, D. N. (1983). The development of social comparison processes and their role in achievement-related self-socialization. In E. T. Higgins, D. N. Ruble, & W. W. Hartup (Eds.), *Social cognition and social development: A sociocultural perspective.* Cambridge: Cambridge University Press.

Scherer, K. R. (1984). Emotion as a multicomponent process: A model and some cross-cultural data. In P. Shaver (Ed.), *Review of personality and social psychology* (Vol. 5, pp. 37–63). Beverly Hills, CA: Sage.

Schneider, W. (in press). Problems of longitudinal sudies with children: Practical, conceptual, and methodological issues. In M. Brambring, F. Losel, & H. Skowronek (Eds.), *Children at risk: Assessment and longitudinal research.* New York: De Gruijter.

Shaver, P., Schwartz, J., Kirson, D., & O'Connor, C. (1987). Emotion knowledge: Further exploration of a prototype approach. *Journal of Personality and Social Psychology, 52,* 1061–1086.

Sullivan, H. S. (1953). *Interpersonal theory of psychiatry.* New York: Norton.

Vygotsky, L. (1978). *Mind in society: The development of higher psychological processes* (M. Cole, V. John-Steiner, S. Scribner, & Ellen Souberman, Trans.). Cambridge: Harvard University Press.

Weiner, I. B. (1976). The adolescent and his society. In J. R. Gallagher, F. P. Heald, & D. C. Garell (Eds.), *Medical care of the adolescent* (3rd ed.). New York: Appleton-Century-Crofts.

Wohlwill, J. F. (1973). *The study of behavioral development.* New York: Academic Press.

Woodruff, D. S., & Birren, J. E. (1972). Age changes and cohort differences in personality. *Developmental Psychology, 6,* 252–259.

Youniss, J. (1980). *Parents and peers in social development.* Chicago: University of Chicago Press.

3 Universal trends and individual differences in memory development

WOLFGANG SCHNEIDER AND FRANZ E. WEINERT

The study of cognitive development has been one of the most active disciplines within developmental psychology for some time. Within this discipline, the study of memory development has received much attention over the past 20 years. In the present essay, we will focus on the major achievements as well as some limitations of research into memory development conducted during that period.

Although we will concentrate on recent trends in memory development, there are earlier studies of memory development that were conducted before the information processing approach was introduced into developmental psychology about two decades ago. It is unfortunate that these studies, conducted almost a century ago, have been completely forgotten by contemporary European and American memory researchers. Although we do not intend to provide an overview of these studies, a summary of the main findings from that early period seems in order (see Schneider & Pressley, 1988, for a more detailed account). In our view, a juxtaposition of what was known then and what we know now may provide a more precise reading of the advances actually made.

Most early studies of memory development were stimulated by Hermann Ebbinghaus's pioneer work. One of its major goals was to obtain information about *general* or *universal* trends in memory development across the life-span. Thus, the main interest was in what Wohlwill (1973) called the "developmental function" of memory performance, or its value plotted over age. In many studies, memory performance was equated with achievement in memory-span tasks using meaningless syllables, words, or numbers as stimuli (cf. Braunshausen, 1914, for an overview). In other studies, the inclusion of meaningful materials (words, sentences) led to the insight that factors like word meaning and familiarity of material play a significant role in determining the amount of material recalled. For example, it was demonstrated that schoolchildren's memory for long sentences was considerably better than that for short lists of meaningless words, and that as a rule the "skeleton," that

68

is, the core unit of the sentence, was retained best (Binet & Henri, 1894; Netschajeff, 1902). Comparisons of results from different assessment procedures (e.g., recognition vs. recall) clearly showed that the developmental function varied with the type of materials and the output demands used. Further major findings of that time can be summarized as follows:

1. In general, memory performance (immediate recall) improves over the school years and continues to increase until about the age of 25 years;
2. A particularly steep, linear increase in level of performance can be observed between the ages of 7 and 11, whereas a stagnation first sets in at the ages of 13 to 16 years;
3. A sharp distinction must be made between the developmental processes of immediate and long-term retention. Contrary to the findings for immediate recall, children's long-term retention skills are better than those of adults (cf. Radossawljewitsch, 1907).

Although this early period was characterized by a strong interest in general laws and universal developmental memory functions, this does not mean that the second realm of developmental inquiry, the study of individual differences, was totally ignored. On the contrary, the present-day reader is struck with the numerous studies on sex differences or on children of different "memory types" (e.g., acoustic, visual, tactile–motor). Interestingly enough, most of these studies were stimulated by the dominating issues of educational theory and practice. For example, many influential opponents of coeducation claimed that it would be "a sin against nature" to educate jointly boys and girls because of the girls' inferior intellectual aptitudes (see Braunshausen, 1914). Consequently, many studies compared boys' and girls' memory performances to test the assumption that girls cannot keep up with boys. The findings were unequivocal: regardless of the age group and memory function studied, girls' memory performance levels on the average tended to be higher than those of boys. Needless to say, these findings helped introduce the coeducation principle, at least in German schools.

Similarly, the study of "memory types" was mainly stimulated by the idea that children of different "memory types" should receive different instructional treatments, or optimal combinations of visual and auditory instructional methods (cf. Kirckpatrick, 1894). The major problems with this approach, however, were that it was difficult to find "clear-cut" or pure memory types (most subjects were classified as "mixed" types), and the individual differences detected were not stable over time (cf. Offner, 1924). Although the idea of "memory types" remained attractive during this early period, no changes in educational practices were made mainly as a consequence of these unsatisfactory results.

Thus, experimental research in memory development was active long before the term *memory* was rediscovered and developmental research was reestablished within the past two decades. What are the major differences between the early and the contemporary approaches? Although there are many, we think that the most crucial difference concerns the way the dependent variables were determined: Whereas the early studies focused on various aspects of memory performance and their developmental trends, the contemporary approach can be characterized as redirecting attention from overt memory products to the cognitive activities that generate them (cf. Flavell, 1985). Current research efforts concentrate on the identification of factors that "cause" variations in memory performance in different contexts or domains. Of course, one should not overlook the fact that the concept of "mechanisms" of developmental change was also used by theorists of the early period, particularly by those strongly interested in learning theory. Their assumption was that the organism provides the framework of mechanism within which learning and remembering occur (McGeoch & Irion, 1952). According to this view, changes in memory with age are primarily dependent on organic growth and decline, and less on previous learning. The problem of how factors like maturation and degeneration can change the framework of mechanisms remains unsolved within this approach (see Weinert, Schneider, & Knopf, 1988, for a more thorough treatment of this topic).

Theories of memory development derived from the information processing approach provide a much more detailed account of sources of memory development. In particular, four sources of memory development have received considerable attention within this approach: basic capacities, strategies, content knowledge (i.e., domain-specific knowledge), and metamemory. Most studies of memory development conducted within the past twenty years dealt with the role of one or more of these four sources in describing and explaining age differences in memory development.

In the following discussion, we will first give an overview of the major outcomes of this line of research. Given the multitude of empirical studies published in the past few years, we will not present a comprehensive picture of the state of the art, but rather focus on selected recent empirical findings and opinions concerning progress in this area. Although all these sources undoubtedly contribute to memory development, we think that there are still some issues that deserve special treatment that are typically neglected in the literature. Some of these central issues will be explicated in detail in this essay. In our view, one of the major shortcomings of most experimental studies is that it is almost impossible to determine the *relative* impact of the four sources and their interactions in predicting and explaining memory development. To achieve this goal, the experimental approach must be substituted or complemented by nonexperimental assessment procedures and more sophisticated data analysis techniques. A few examples will be given to illustrate how this can be done.

A further problem with the present view of memory development is that these four sources represent "within-the-child" parameters. A particular weakness of this approach is that it ignores possible explanatory factors in children's environments. As a consequence, the generality or universality of developmental trends is usually overestimated. This problem can best be illustrated by examining the impact of cultural factors like schooling or instructional differences on memory development.

Another neglected issue concerns the study of individual differences. Compared with research in memory development during the early period, only a few studies focus on interindividual as well as intraindividual differences. In our view, the few available studies seem suited to qualify the findings obtained from typical experimental studies on the "developmental function" sensu Wohlwill.

Our final point refers to the problem that more than 99% of the studies on children's memory have been cross-sectional in nature. Thus, all these studies must face the criticism that they are not truly developmental (Wohlwill, 1973). Development means change – more specifically, change over time within organisms. Developmental *changes* can only be assessed via longitudinal designs, whereas cross-sectional studies are restricted to the assessment of developmental *differences*. According to Appelbaum and McCall (1983), the phrase *individual differences* refers to the variability of performance between individuals about their group mean. Within a developmental perspective, the stability or instability of individual differences is of major interest. Individuals are stable if they maintain about the same relative ordering within their group at one age as they do at another age. This means that not only general developmental change but also the development of individual differences can be only observed within the framework of a longitudinal study. As a consequence, in the remainder of this essay we will present a series of arguments for a revival of longitudinal studies in the area of memory development, and also provide some empirical examples that seem suited to demonstrate the special relevance of such studies for our better understanding of memory growth.

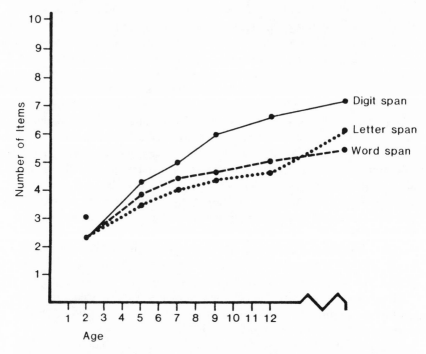

Figure 3.1. Developmental differences in digit span, letter span, and word span (data from Dempster, 1981, Figs. 1 to 3).

Sources of memory development: an overview

Basic capacities

One of the earliest views of memory development relied heavily on the concept of capacity. In its simplified version, memory development was exclusively seen as a function of memory capacity: According to this "container" model (Brown & DeLoache, 1978), young people have small boxes in their heads, whereas older people have bigger boxes. Translated into terms of a computer analogy, this model suggests that what develops is the *hardware* of the memory system conceptualized as absolute capacity, rather than its *software*, that is, the specific procedures to memorize material. At first glance, the data obtained from various studies concerning development of the memory span seem to support such a "container" model. For example, the data aggregated by Dempster (1985) indicate a continuous increase in different indicators of memory span from early childhood to adulthood (cf. Fig. 3.1). However, the major problem with this view is that memory span cannot be equated with "capacity" in the sense of memory "hardware"; there is evidence that performance in memory span tests is also influenced by "software" operations like rehearsal and grouping strategies (cf. Dempster, 1985) and by the familiarity and meaningfulness of the learning material. Thus, it does not make much sense to use the memory span as a measure of memory capacity.

Before analyzing the role of basic capacity in memory development, we should be more explicit about how basic capacity is conceptualized within the information processing approach. In general, this approach is based on the assumption that there are stable memory and processing limitations that individuals have to overcome by using either internal or external memory aids. According to this view, basic capacities are the building blocks of cognitive activity, in the sense that more complex cognitive activities are built up by combining them in different ways (Siegler, 1986). Given their frequent use, developmental differences in basic capacities could account for a number of developmental differences in memory performance. The memory model by Atkinson and Shiffrin (1968) with its division of memory into sensory, short-term, and long-term stores provided the first useful framework for describing basic capacities and their development. In short, experimental work conducted within this approach indicates that the absolute capacities of the three storage systems seem to be rather constant across childhood and adolescence. On the other hand, however, ample evidence indicates that parameters of information processing speed increase with age. This is true for the speed with which sensory representations are formed, and also holds for the speed with which objects can be represented in short-term memory or retrieved from long-term memory (cf. Keating & Bobbitt, 1978; Siegler, 1986). This finding seems in accord with Dempster's (1981; 1985) assumption that age differences in memory span are mainly due to nonstrategic factors like item identification speed or automatic item sequencing.

It follows, then, that we have to distinguish between an invariant total capacity of the memory system and basic operating functions that develop with age. There is an increasing tendency in the literature to accept the tentative model developed by Case (1985; Case, Kurland, & Goldberg, 1982) that tries to delineate these two constructs. In this model, a distinction is made between a storage space and an operating space. The term *storage space* refers to the hypothetical amount of space available for storing information; *operating space* refers to the hypothetical amount of space available for executing intellectual operations. Finally, *total processing space* is defined as the sum of an individual's storage space and operating space. The core assumption is that the total processing space available does not change over time, but just the proportions allocated to storage and operative processing. That is, as children grow older less and less memory space is necessary for the operative space, leaving more space for the storage of information. Case (1985) proposed that a child's ability to hold more information in short-term memory is mainly due to increasing automatization and perhaps biological maturation.

To illustrate the model's implications, Siegler (1986) used the analogy of a car trunk:

> The capacity of a car's trunk does not change as the owner acquires experience in packing luggage into it. Nonetheless, the amount of material that can be packed into the trunk does change. Whereas the trunk at first might hold two or three suitcases, it might eventually come to hold four or five. As each packing operation is executed more efficiently, trunk space is freed for additional operations. (p. 82)

According to this view, age-correlated improvements on short-term memory tests are due to shifts in the two space allotments rather than changes in total processing capacity. Does this mean, then, that basic memory capacities do not have any impact on memory performance? Of course, this is not the case. It is important here to note that the hypothesized invariance of total memory capacity is concerned with *intraindividual* characteristics. However, *interindividual* capacity differences are certainly not negligible when it comes to explaining differences in actual memory performance. Suppose, for example, that you want to predict young children's free recall for unrelated words by using a measure of basic memory capacity. Undoubtedly, a considerable amount of variation found in the memory performance measure could be explained by the variation in the memory capacity measure. In other words, individual differences in memory capacity are accurate predictors of individual differences in memory performance within and between age groups (cf. Schneider, 1986, for an empirical demonstration). It appears, however, that the predictive power of basic memory capacity depends on both the nature of the memory task and the age of the subjects. Its influence will be restricted whenever the task allows for compensatory operations (e.g., mnemonic strategies), or whenever the subjects are old enough to use mnemonic aids efficiently. It is thus reasonable to assume that the role of memory capacity in explaining age differences in memory performance generally decreases with the increasing age of the subjects.

Memory strategies

Since the early 1970s, numerous studies have investigated the role of strategies in memory development. According to these studies, strategy use was not only an important source of developmental differences but probably the major source (cf. Lange, 1978; Moely, 1977, for reviews). As will be noted, these researchers somewhat overstated the case. One fundamental problem typically neglected in the 1970s concerns a clear definition of memory strategies. In the 1980s, this question became a controversial issue. Whereas some authors defined strategies exclusively as *conscious* memory activities (cf. Naus & Ornstein, 1983; Paris, Lipson, & Wixson, 1983), others preferred a less strict definition that also subsumed *automatic* processes, particularly in the case of reading strategies (cf. Brown, Bransford, Ferrara, & Campione, 1983; Flavell, 1985). The detailed conceptualization provided by Pressley, Forrest-Pressley, Elliott-Faust, and Miller (1985) can be regarded as an acceptable compromise:

A strategy is composed of cognitive operations over and above the processes that are natural consequences of carrying out the task, ranging from one such operation to a sequence of interdependent operations. Strategies achieve cognitive purposes (e.g., comprehending, memorizing) and are potentially conscious and controllable activities. (p. 4)

Although children's acquisition of memory strategies varies with the particular strategy, certain characteristics seem to be common to all strategies (cf. Brown et al., 1983; Waters & Andreassen, 1983). For example, memory strategies first appear under task conditions that are optimal for processing the to-be-remembered material (e.g., conditions that provide sufficient time to study the items). Further, strategies first appear with materials that encourage their use (e.g., semantically related materials that are particularly easy to interrelate in the case of organization strategies). The dependence of strategic behavior on task and procedural conditions changes with development. Older children are more active in initiating strategy use in different memory situations, including those that do not strongly encourage optimal processing, making the strategy difficult to execute. In short, they become more flexible in tailoring their strategy use to the demands of the particular situation.

The majority of studies of strategy use investigated children's use of rehearsal, organization, and elaboration strategies in laboratory tasks. Typically, these strategies were not observed in children younger than 6 or 7. This absence of strategic behavior was attributed to a "production deficiency" (Flavell, 1970); according to this hypothesis, young children do not engage in memory strategies because they simply do not know how and when to do so. Although evidence abounds for young children's production deficiencies concerning many memory strategies, more recent research has shown that the ages of strategy acquisition are relative, and variable between and within strategies. For example, it has been demonstrated that even preschool and kindergarten children are able to use intentional memory strategies, both in ecologically valid settings like hide-and-seek tasks (cf. DeLoache, Cassidy, & Brown, 1985; Sophian, 1984) and in the traditional context of a laboratory task (cf. Baker-Ward, Ornstein, & Holden, 1984; Sodian, Schneider, & Perlmutter, 1986). It appears, then, that very young children use rudimentary strategies whenever the task is either simply structured or extremely motivating for them.

It should be emphasized, however, that most developmental changes in children's strategy use can be observed during the elementary school years. In the remainder of this section, we will focus on the acquisition of the more prototypical memory strategies, namely, rehearsal and organizational strategies (see Pressley, 1982, for a detailed account on elaboration strategies). With regard to rehearsal, the typical difference between younger and older schoolchildren is that the younger subjects use a passive and inefficient single-item repetition strategy, whereas the older children put more items together in a "rehearsal set" and prefer cumulative rehearsal strategies (see Naus & Ornstein, 1983; Ornstein & Naus, 1985, for detailed reviews). Although young schoolchildren were able to use a cumulative rehearsal strategy when instructed to do so, they nonetheless did not employ this more complex strategy spontaneously. Recent work by Guttentag (1984; 1985) suggests that the main reason for this production deficiency is the "mental effort" requirement of the cumulative rehearsal strategy. Guttentag used a dual-task procedure: In addition to the usual "overt rehearsal" of to-be-recalled items, a motor task (key tapping) was performed simultaneously. The amount of interference was measured as the difference between the normal tapping during a baseline phase (without rehearsal) and tapping during rehearsal. Guttentag reported that the degree of interference experienced in motor performance was impaired more by simultaneous rehearsal among younger as compared with older children. However, age differences in interference did not occur when children used a passive, one-item repetition strategy. Thus, age differences in the spontaneous use of cumulative rehearsal strategies may in part be due to the enormous effort required of young children to employ complex strategies.

A subsequent study by Ornstein, Medlin, Stone, and Naus (1985) not only confirmed this assumption, but also provided a more exact indication of which components of cumulative rehearsal cause special difficulties for younger children. In this study the efficiency of second graders' cumulative rehearsal improved considerably when the previously presented items continued to be visible as they rehearsed. Apparently, a particular difficulty of cumulative rehearsal strategies for younger children is that the stimuli must be maintained internally during the repetition of learning material. Such maintenance requires great exertion, often exceeding the capacity of young grade-school children. In our view, this finding squares well with the proposal of several Russian investigators (e.g., Smirnov & Zinchenko, 1969) that a skill must be well developed in its own right before it can be effectively deployed as a strategic means to a memory goal.

Our second example concerns semantic grouping or categorization, one of the most frequently studied strategies. Developmental changes in children's organization of material parallel developmental changes in rehearsal, although it appears that the organizational strategy is acquired somewhat later in development. In its traditional form, the sort–recall task requires that a number of semantically related but randomly ordered stimuli should be remembered within a certain time interval. The subjects are usually instructed to do anything they want with the items in order to recall them better. The optimal strategy is to sort the items completely into categories and to use the category names as retrieval cues during recall. Thus, the amount of clustering during study as well as during recall is usually taken as an indicator of an organizational strategy.

Although this assessment procedure appears very elegant, there are nonetheless several problems with it. For example, the mere presence of clustering in subjects' recall does not prove that they indeed had intentionally used an organizational strategy when retrieving the items. We now have ample evidence suggesting that clustering during recall can represent automatic processes mainly stimulated by high interitem associativity (cf. Bjorklund, 1985; 1987; Frankel & Rollins, 1985; Lange, 1978). Similarly, sorting items into semantic categories is not always reflective of a conscious, deliberate organizational strategy. Instead, it may be that subjects are able to detect the categorical structure of an item list and sort items into categories, but do not know that this procedure enhances recall. These problems notwithstanding, the sort–recall task has generally proved valuable in demonstrating age differences in the intentional use of organizational strategies.

How can these age differences best be described? Recent studies (Schneider, 1986; Schneider, Körkel, & Vogel, 1987) have demonstrated considerable developmental differences during encoding of information. While second graders rarely sorted the items by categorical relations, fourth graders did so spontaneously. More important, whereas the majority of the younger children only looked at the items or labeled them when asked to learn the stimulus list, the older subjects used more sophisticated learning strategies like rehearsal or self-testing. Taken together, these developmental differences in encoding stimuli explain a considerable amount of age differences in recall. In addition, substantial developmental differences also appear in retrieval strategies, and encoding and retrieval strategies not only contribute independently to increased memory performance but also in interaction with one another (cf. Ackerman, 1985, for a detailed account on this problem).

Although the *interaction* of encoding and retrieval strategies and their joint effect on memory performance can be assessed through systematic manipulation in experimental designs, it is practically impossible to determine the *relative* roles of encoding and retrieval process, because comparable measures for the two do not exist. It should be noted that mathematical models for the separation of encoding and retrieval processes in memory tasks have been recently developed independently by several research groups (cf. Brainerd, 1985, for a review). Unfortunately, the results obtained for the various mathematical models are not consistent, and thus do not permit clear-cut conclusions. All in all, the results indicate that retrieval processes, unlike storage processes, seem to develop more from the early elementary school phase to adulthood; however, further research is clearly needed to validate this impression.

The impact of knowledge on memory

Recent theoretical statements have suggested that influences of the knowledge base or content knowledge are highly important for the development of strategic behavior and memory performance in children (cf. Bjorklund, 1985; Ornstein, Baker-Ward, & Naus, 1988; Ornstein & Naus, 1985). According to this view, the fact that children acquire specific information about particular content areas every day should influence their memorizing. It is an everyday observation that people who know more about an area than others find it easier to remember new information linked to that area. Although this fact is certainly recognized by most researchers in memory development, the measure usually taken to control for influences of prior knowledge – that is, selecting learning materials well known even to the youngest subjects – seems insufficient. The faulty logic of such an approach lies in the assumption that *knowledge* of stimuli names can be equated with *familiarity* with the learning material. As was impressively demonstrated by Chechile and Richman (1982), variations in meaningfulness of identical learning material in various age groups can explain age differences in memory performance: When meaningfulness values were equated, age differences in recall were minimized.

In addition, what a child knows about the materials to be remembered can have a strong impact on strategic manipulation of those items. This contention is supported by several experiments that systematically varied the meaningfulness of items across experimental conditions. For example, Tarkin, Myers, and Ornstein (cited in Ornstein et al., 1988), compared third graders' rehearsal in two experimental conditions. Although the stimuli of the word lists were all known to the children, subjects in one condition studied highly meaningful items – that is, words that elicited many associations – whereas subjects in the other condition rehearsed words that were low in meaningfulness. The data indicated marked differences in rehearsal as a function of condition. Rehearsal sets of the low-meaningfulness group were relatively small (fewer than two different items), whereas the high-meaningfulness group rehearsed more than three items together, a value characteristic of sixth graders. These outcomes suggest that the observed strategies are to some extent "stimulus driven": highly meaningful materials may facilitate rehearsal (and subsequently recall) because of an associative activation of the knowledge base.

Similar effects due to age-related increases in associative connections and the developing knowledge of hierarchical conceptual relations were demonstrated for the utilization of organizational (clustering) strategies in sort–recall tasks (Frankel & Rollins, 1985; Schneider, 1986). In both experiments, word lists were generated that varied in terms of strength of associations between category exemplars and the strength of category relationships. The combination of these two variables yielded four different list conditions: high category relatedness/high interitem associativity; high category relatedness/low interitem associativity; low category relatedness/high interitem associativity; and low category relatedness/ low interitem associativity. Typical exemplars of the "high/high" lists were dog, cat, horse, and cow, and those of the "low/low" lists were beaver, walrus, squirrel, and giraffe. Frankel and Rollins (1985) reported that 10- and 16-year-old subjects evidenced high levels of clustering during recall under conditions of either high category relatedness or high interitem associativity; lower levels of clustering were only obtained when both variables were low in strength. On the other hand, 6-year-old children showed elevated clustering during recall only under conditions of high interitem associativity. These findings were basically replicated by Schneider (1986), working with 8- and 10-year-olds, and are consistent with the hypothesis that young children's clustering during recall is more a function of interitem associativity than of intentional strategy use. However, it is important to note that in Schneider's study, second graders demonstrated sorting strategies under conditions of either high category relatedness or high interitem associativity, with cluster scores approaching values usually obtained with fourth graders. In our view, this can be regarded as another example of "stimulus-driven" strategy use, that is, the impact of the knowledge base on the activation of memory strategies.

Probably the most dramatic demonstrations of the impact of the knowledge base on memory stems from experiments that focused on the relationship between domain-specific knowledge and memory performance. The most suitable way to demonstrate effects of the knowledge base is to contrast the performance of experts and novices in a specific domain. A now classical, clever experiment by Chi (1978) provided evidence for how greatly the knowledge base can influence children's memory performance. Chi compared the memory ability of chess experts and novices. Her twist was that knowledge was negatively correlated with age. That is, the 10-year-old children were the experts, whereas the adults were chess novices. Both groups were tested on two tasks. One was a standard digit-span task; the other was a chess reproduction task, which involved replacing chess pieces correctly in their positions. Chi (1978) found that her young experts outperformed the novices in the chess reproduction task, both in terms of actual memory performance and in predicting in advance how well they would perform. On the digit-span task, the adults, as expected, were better. Chi's conclusion was that differences in the knowledge base can outweigh all other memory differences between children and adults.

In a series of related experiments conducted in our laboratory (Körkel, 1987; Schneider, Körkel, & Weinert, 1987a; Weinert, Knopf, Körkel, Schneider, Vogel, & Wetzel, 1984), performances of soccer experts and of novices recruited from samples of third, fifth, and seventh graders were compared. Subjects read a story about a soccer game and were tested for their recall and comprehension of the text. Not surprisingly, soccer experts showed better recall of text details than novices, regardless of age. Moreover, experts were better at identifying contradictions in the text and in drawing text-specific inferences – that is, in reconstructing information that had not been explicitly included in the text. Younger experts outperformed older novices on all outcome measures, demonstrating the specific importance of a highly articulated knowledge base on text comprehension and recall.

In view of these findings, it seems that the knowledge base explains a great deal about why older children remember more efficiently than younger ones. The knowledge base not only influences the way children prepare for recall, but also what and how much they can recall. However, the question of *how* the knowledge base influences memory remains a controversial issue. For example, Ornstein and Naus (1985) emphasized the fact that an association between expert–novice status in a specific domain and differential patterns of recall of this material does not provide an explanation of how such differences arise. That is, findings of this sort do not tell us anything about the underlying mechanisms that could explain how experts are able to use their better-structured knowledge during remembering. According to Siegler (1986), two mechanisms – networks of association that link different items to each other, and the encoding of distinctive features – seem of major importance. Although empirical evidence from case studies (e.g., Chi & Koeske, 1983) supports such a view, in-depth analyses of the mechanisms by which the knowledge base mediates memory are still badly needed. In such analyses, the possible involvement of motivational and interest factors should also be considered. In our view, the work by Rabinowitz and colleagues (Rabinowitz & Chi, 1987; Rabinowitz & Glaser, 1985) represents a good starting point for more comprehensive theoretical and empirical analyses.

The impact of metamemory on memory development

As already noted, children's knowledge about particular domains increases as a function of daily experience. It also seems reasonable to assert that children's knowledge and understanding of memory processes develop simultaneously and that this kind of knowledge may be similarly related to improvements in strategy use and memory performance. Knowledge of this sort was labeled "metamemory" by Flavell (1971) and broadly defined as knowledge about different aspects of memory processing. Subsequent attempts to define this "fuzzy" concept more precisely (Wellman, 1983) led to the construction of taxonomies of metamemory that roughly distinguished between two basic types, namely conscious, verbalizable knowledge concerning memory, and implicit, probably unconscious knowledge about how to monitor and regulate memory (for more detailed accounts, see Brown et al., 1983; Flavell & Wellman, 1977; Wellman, 1983; 1985).

Factual knowledge about memory was further subdivided into knowledge about *persons*, *tasks*, and *strategy variables* that influence performance on a memory task, and the interaction of these variables. The person category refers to what children know about themselves and others as mnemonic beings, whereas the task category includes children's knowledge about what makes some memory tasks more difficult than others. The strategy variables category refers to children's verbalizable knowledge about various encoding and retrieval strategies, as distinguished from actual "on-line" strategy use in memory situations.

The second type of knowledge – regulation and monitoring of cognitive activities – refers to judgment of feelings about the ease or difficulty of remembering something. Here, the assumption is that children become more and more attuned to internal "mnemonic sensations" with development. They develop a sensitivity to the objective need for effort at present retrieval or additional storage activities for purposes of future retrieval. Examples of situations suitable to assess children's metacognitive experiences concerning memory include the prediction of one's own memory span or the decision about when one is ready to attempt recall of an item list.

Space constraints do not allow us to give a representative account of the development of declarative and procedural metamemory (for reviews, see Brown et al., 1983; Flavell, 1985; Schneider & Pressley, 1988). In brief, evidence from metamemory interviews and experimental tasks supports the general view that both components of metamemory seem to develop between preschool age and adolescence, with particularly rapid increases observable during the elementary school period.

Since the beginning of research into metamemory, a hypothesis that stimulated many studies was that children's metamemory is closely linked to their behavior and performance in various memory situations. For example, it was assumed that the "production deficiencies" frequently observed in younger children could be explained by their lack of specific strategy knowledge and a lack of knowledge concerning the appropriate conditions for controlled strategy use. Children's increasing knowledge about the memory system was thought to lead them to think and remember more and more effectively.

Early investigations into the metamemory–memory behavior relationship revealed only modest support for such a position, particularly where the relationship between declarative (factual) knowledge about memory and behavior in memory tasks was concerned (cf. Cavanaugh & Perlmutter, 1982; Schneider, 1985). Theoretically, several factors could contribute to the weak relations observed (cf. Flavell, 1978; Flavell & Wellman, 1977). For example, children who know that a strategy is useful might think that an alternative strategy is even better in a particular situation, or that the task is much too simple to use a memory strategy. Further, they may have abstract knowledge about strategies but not be very good at executing them. Finally, we can think of situations where strategy use is clearly needed for optimal performance, but where we decide that it is somehow not worth the effort. Flavell and Wellman (1977) termed this the "original sin" hypothesis.

Although it is intuitively reasonable to believe that these factors can attenuate the correlations among metamemory, memory behavior, and memory performance, they do not completely account for the negative findings. A major problem is that children's metamemory was only insufficiently and unreliably assessed in most of the early studies.

In the "second generation" of metamemory studies, precautions were taken to assess adequately the kind of metamemory relevant for the memory situation under investigation. As a consequence, closer relationships were found among knowledge, behavior, and performance (cf. Borkowski, 1985; Pressley, Borkowski, & O'Sullivan, 1985; Weinert, 1986). The findings further indicated that the intercorrelations among metamemory, memory behavior, and performance increased with age, probably due to the metamemory of older children. The aforementioned study by Schneider (1986) seems suited to illustrate this point. As noted, the second graders in this study sorted the items into semantic categories only when either category relatedness or interitem associativity was high, whereas the fourth graders were more flexible in using the organizational strategy. Additional metamemory assessments clearly showed that young children's knowledge about organizational strategies was generally poor and inconsistent across different assessment procedures. Thus, it was not surprising that rather low correlations between metamemory and memory behavior were found in this age group. On the contrary, most fourth graders knew about the efficiency of organizational strategies, and the metamemory scores obtained were highly consistent across measures. Even more important, significant intercorrelations among metamemory, memory behavior, and memory performance were found for this age group. Results of multiple regression analyses further indicated that fourth graders' recall could be best predicted by both their task-related metamemory and sorting strategies, whereas second graders' recall was not influenced by either metamemory or strategy variables. It suggests, then, that age differences in children's metamemory can be regarded as an important source of age differences in memory performance.

It should be noted, however, that we know too little about the developmental mechanisms involved. The question of how we should conceive of the functional and developmental connections between metamemory and strategies is a controversial issue. Although empirical evidence is still scarce, the so-called bidirectionality hypothesis (Flavell, 1978) has intuitive appeal. Accordingly, initial strategy use leads to some dim knowledge of the strategy's usefulness, which in turn stimulates more strategy use, which then leads to greater knowledge of the strategy's utility, and so on. This principle of reciprocal mediation is also central in the model of knowledge about strategies developed by Pressley, Borkowski, and O'Sullivan (1985) and depicted in Figure 3.2.

The fundamental elements of the model are the learner's strategies,

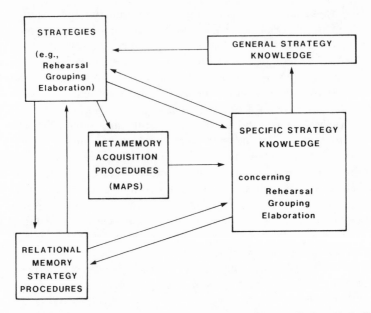

Figure 3.2. A model of metamemory about strategies (Pressley, Borkowski, & O'Sullivan, 1985; slightly modified).

which may share subprocesses. These commonalities among strategies are "detected" by a set of relational strategy procedures that are conceptualized as meta rules (Chi, 1987) in that they take other rules as input. Another important aspect of knowledge about strategies (MAS) is the general strategy knowledge component, consisting of general principles relevant to all or most strategies. The model implies that the reciprocal mediation process between strategy employment and specific strategy knowledge also adds to general strategy knowledge. We think that the inclusion of so-called metamemory acquisition procedures (MAPS) makes the MAS model particularly interesting. Like relational memory strategy procedures, they are conceptualized as meta rules in that they take as input other rules; their output is conceived of as an appropriate evaluation resulting in new knowledge. The various components of the model are not seen in isolation but in close interaction. Thus the MAS model is characterized as *dynamic* and *interactional*.

Although the validity of the MAS model has not yet been tested in detail, there is already promising evidence supporting the view that MAPS (e.g., self-testing procedures) play a central role in metacognitive approaches to strategy instruction (cf. Pressley et al., 1985; Pressley,

Forrest-Pressley, & Elliott-Faust, 1988). In particular, the training of MAPS has been proved successful in young learners, teaching them to compare the efficacy of different strategies and to use that information to make strategy decisions. From this kind of intervention research, it can be concluded that MAPS not only feed in specific strategy knowledge, but also provide learners with more general monitoring skills, thus demonstrating that they are not tied to any particular strategy. Given the positive empirical evidence for at least some components of the model, one can be optimistic that future research will lead to theoretical refinements in the concept of metamemory and demonstrate its educational utility.

The four sources of memory development in a life-span perspective

It has been shown that memory development can be explained in four different ways: changes in basic capacities, in strategies, in the knowledge base, and in various components of metamemory. In the overview presented so far, we occasionally referred to the fact that some of these sources seem to have larger effects than others, and that some seem to contribute significantly in certain age periods but not in others. A systematic summarization of the types of contributions that these four sources make to memory growth during different periods of development was given by Siegler (1986) and is depicted in Table 3.1. According to Table 3.1, performance differences in the early developmental period (age 0–5) may be best explained by differences in memory capacity and content knowledge (the knowledge base). From age 5 to age 10, all four sources can account for developmental differences, with memory capacity declining in importance. Finally, from late childhood to adulthood, it seems that knowledge factors generally contribute more than both strategy and capacity components; Siegler (1986) assumes that factual (declarative) memory knowledge may exert most of its effect on memory performance within this later phase of memory development, whereas the impact of memory monitoring and regulation skills as well as of the knowledge base already contribute to memory development from early in life.

Although such a view is generally supported by the empirical evidence presented so far, it is nevertheless speculative in many aspects. For example, few empirical studies have directly investigated the relative impact of the four sources of memory on memory performance during different developmental periods, that is, for different age groups. Moreover, the summary given in Table 3.1 suggests a "natural," univer-

Table 3.1. *Contributions of four sources of memory development during different periods of development*

Source of development	Age		
	0–5	5–10	10–adulthood
Basic capacities	Many capacities present: association, generalization, recognition, etc. Absolute capacity already at adultlike levels by age 5	Speed of processing increases	Speed of processing increases
Strategies	Little evidence of strategy use	Acquisition of many strategies: rehearsal, organization, etc.	Increasing use of elaboration. Continuing improvement in quality of all strategies
Metamemory	Little factual knowledge about memory. Some monitoring of ongoing performance	Increasing factual knowledge about memory. Improved monitoring of ongoing performance	Continued improvement in factual knowledge, monitoring and regulation skills. Factual knowledge may exert increasing effects on memory behavior and performance
Content knowledge	Steadily increasing content knowledge helps memory where the knowledge exists	Steadily increasing content knowledge helps in acquiring new strategies, and helps memory where the knowledge exists	Continuing improvements as in the 5–10-year period

Source: Modified after Siegler, 1986.

sal course of development primarily caused by internal, "in-the-child" mechanisms. Indeed, most research discussed so far has completely ignored the problem of how external, environmental factors like cultural differences or instructional experiences can influence the impact of the four major sources of memory development. Finally, the literature summarized in Table 3.1 usually neglected the issue of individual differences. The importance of these neglected issues will be discussed in the following section.

Sources of memory development: neglected issues

Relative contribution of the four sources to memory development

It is not surprising that the problem of how to assess the relative or simultaneous impact of memory capacity, strategies, the knowledge bases, and metamemory has not been dealt with adequately in previous research. Appelbaum and McCall's (1983) criticism that developmental psychology has spent the past two decades in methodological narcissism is particularly true for the area of memory research. As most studies were devoted (or should we say restricted) to the experimental approach, the emphasis was on study memory development in a methodologically precise manner, and not on asking "bigger" questions requiring either many observed variables, or large samples, or both. In our view, exploring the relative contributions of those four sources to memory development as well as their complex interactional pattern means asking such a "bigger" question. Thus, to treat this problem appropriately, we need to replace the experimental approach by a methodological strategy that allows us to deal simultaneously with many variables and with large samples. We want to illustrate how the problem can be handled by using the causal modeling or structural equation approach based on correlational data.

One particular advantage of causal modeling procedures is that they can use latent variables instead of observed indicators. In causal models using latent variables, the measurement model defines the relationships between observed variables and the unmeasured hypothetical constructs via factor analytical procedures, whereas the structural equation model ("causal" model) is used to specify the causal links among the latent variables. Thus, a regression type of analysis is conducted on the basis of latent variables instead of manifest indicators, which means a more powerful explanatory approach.

The causal model developed by Hasselhorn (1986) may serve as an illustration of how this methodological approach can be used to integrate all variables considered relevant for the prediction of memory performance and to assess their relative impact on memory behavior and performance (cf. Fig. 3.3). The task chosen to illustrate the role of the four sources was the sort–recall paradigm. Various indicators of information processing speed were used to represent memory capacity, and several measures of semantic knowledge represented children's knowledge base. Sorting strategies in the sort–recall task indicated the strategy component (memory behavior) in the model. The two different components of metamemory – declarative and procedural metamemory – were con-

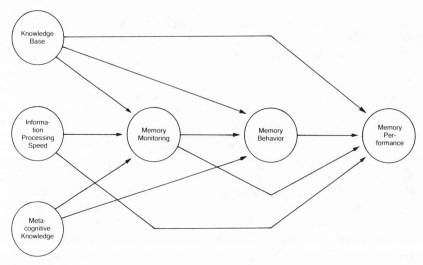

Figure 3.3. The structural equation model developed by Hasselhorn (1986) to illustrate the interplay of different sources in predicting memory performance.

ceptualized as two different constructs in Hasselhorn's model. Meta-cognitive knowledge included general declarative metamemory as well as knowledge concerning the sort–recall task. Memory monitoring, on the other hand, comprised measures tapping children's procedural knowl-edge (e.g., prediction of memory performance). As can be seen from Figure 3.3, the knowledge base, information processing speed, and meta-cognitive knowledge were used as exogeneous variables in the model, that is, they were not further explained or interrelated. They were assumed to influence memory monitoring in the sort–recall task, and also to influence memory behavior – that is, strategy use as well as memory performance. It was further assumed that memory monitoring should affect both memory behavior and performance, whereas memory behavior should directly influence the amount of recall. Hasselhorn (1986) estimated this model by using the data from 176 fourth graders. As a main result, metacognitive knowledge, information processing speed, the knowledge base, and memory behavior were shown to contri-bute independently to the prediction of memory performance. Moreover, in comparison with metacognitive knowledge and information processing speed, the knowledge base had by far the strongest impact on children's memory behavior.

Similar analyses based on structural equation modeling procedures and using data from third, fifth, and seventh graders and elderly adults (Schneider, Körkel, & Weinert, 1987b; Weinert et al., 1984) by and large confirmed these findings. In addition, it could be demonstrated in these studies that the structural patterns obtained in the analyses were similar across age groups in that metamemory always affected strategy use, which in turn significantly influenced memory performance. Although these models were not completely specified as they did not include the knowledge base, the striking similarity of interrelationships among metamemory, memory behavior, and performance obtained for the different age groups suggests that the basic structural or interactional relationship remains stable over time. As the empirical evidence is still confined to cross-sectional studies into the sort–recall paradigm, additional longitudinal analyses are needed to test the generalizability of these findings.

Of course, generalizability can only be expected if the problem of the specific "memory type" under investigation can be neglected – that is, if individual differences across various memory tasks do not matter at all. As already noted, the question of whether the memory concept represents a general, unitary human faculty or rather a variety of independent abilities certainly was a controversial issue a century ago, but it has not attracted much attention since then. The more recent empirical evidence will be summarized next (see Knopf, Körkel, Schneider, & Weinert, 1988, for a more detailed account).

The problem of individual differences

It should be noted that only a few studies conducted within the information processing approach have addressed the issue of intraindividual consistency in performance across several memory tasks. The hypothesis was that individual differences in memory reflect a general, strategic factor (Kail, 1979). According to this assumption, some people may use memory strategies consistently and perform well, whereas others may use strategies poorly, and thus show low levels of recall. Kail (1979) used a factor analytic procedure to test the hypothesis that third and sixth graders' memory performance in different tasks could be explained by a general strategic factor. Although he claimed to have found empirical support for such an assumption, a closer inspection of the intercorrelations among tasks and strategy measures revealed that they were generally small.

There is evidence, however, that the degree of intraindividual consistency across memory tasks strongly depends on the similarity–

Table 3.2. *Intercorrelations among various memory performance measures obtained for 4-year-old children (N = 185)*

Variables	(2)	(3)	(4)
(1) Memory span	.21	.20	.25
(2) Recall in a sort–recall task		.23	.36
(3) Text recall 1 (birthday party)			.64
(4) Text recall 2 (playing with friends)			—

Source: Data from Weinert, Schneider, & Knopf, 1988.

dissimilarity of task requirements. That is, high intraindividual consistency can be found for memory tasks tapping similar strategic skills. For example, substantial intertask correlations were found for free recall tasks that either used different stimulus lists or different procedures (Cavanaugh & Borkowski, 1980; Knopf et al., 1988). On the other hand, only weak intercorrelations were obtained when children's memory for text and memory for word lists were compared (Knopf et al., 1988; Weinert & Schneider, 1986; 1987). It seems important to note that this pattern of results holds for different age groups. In the study by Cavanaugh and Borkowski (1980), comparably high intertask correlations were found for kindergartners and first, third, and fifth graders. This was also true for the similar recall tasks in the study by Knopf et al. (1988), where high stability scores were observed for third, fifth, and seventh graders. Conversely, the correlations among dissimilar memory tasks (e.g., digit span and memory for prose tasks) were comparably low for all age groups in the study by Knopf et al. This finding can also be generalized to the four-year-old subjects of the Munich Longitudinal Study (Weinert & Schneider, 1986; 1987), as illustrated in Table 3.2. In this study, several memory tasks were presented to the children. While a word span task similar to that used by Case et al. (1982) tapped memory capacity, a simple sort–recall task was given to assess rudimentary sorting strategies and their impact on recall. Finally, two similar stories were presented to assess children's memory for prose. Given the large number of subjects, it is not surprising that all correlations shown in Table 3.2 are statistically significant. However, the data indicate that, with the exception of the interrelationship between recall for the two similar stories, intertask consistency of children's memory performance was reasonably low.

It appears, then, that subjects' memory behavior and performance differ as a function of the memory paradigm under investigation. Only for memory tasks belonging to the same class or type (e.g., free recall tasks, memory for prose tasks) can high intertask consistency be expected across a broad range of age groups. Obviously, there is no evidence for generally strategic or mnemonically sophisticated subjects. As a consequence, we doubt that a single structural model concerning the interplay of capacity, strategy, and knowledge variables can be constructed that is equally suited to explain performance in different memory paradigms.

The impact of cultural and instructional differences

One problem with our knowledge about memory development is that it is based on findings obtained in Western societies. In this connection, it is interesting to note that, according to these findings, the most active period in memory development coincides exactly with the period of formal education in Western societies. Thus, it has been pointed out many times that formal education may be significantly implicated in advanced memory development, and that the case is one of educational rather than maturational development (cf. Brown, 1977; Paris, Newman, & Jacobs, 1985). Schools represent cultural institutions in modern societies where remembering as a distinct skill is routinely undertaken in isolation from possible applications (Cole & Scribner, 1977). Although deliberate remembering as an end in itself rather than as a means to achieve a meaningful goal is an activity typical of Western schools, it may not play a major role in unschooled populations. The only way to test this assumption is to investigate cultures in which the degree of formal schooling and chronological age are not hopelessly confounded as in Western societies. Although the results from cross-cultural studies dealing with this problem are not always consistent (cf. Rogoff & Mistry, 1985; Wagner, 1981, for reviews), they give important information on the question of whether universal trends in memory development can be assumed.

First of all, they unequivocally support the position that the development of verbal memory strategies is closely connected to schooling. It has been repeatedly shown that verbal rehearsal and organizational strategies are not spontaneously available to subjects with no formal education. As a consequence, they usually show poor performance in verbal recall tasks. In fact, the impact of schooling on verbal memory tasks is so strong that it can easily outweigh factors like age or social class.

On the other hand, probably the clearest evidence for culturally invariant developmental trends was obtained for tasks where familiar, meaningful materials are used, and where the instructions focused on activities that are close to daily experiences in each of the widely differ-ing cultures. In particular, the recall of stories or fairy tales whose structure seems comparable across varying cultures belongs to this category. Similarly, memory for location seems comparable in subjects with differing cultural backgrounds. In addition, the mediating effect of the knowledge base on children's memory performance seems to be comparably high in schooled and unschooled populations. As demon-strated by Kearins (1983), it is even possible that unschooled children can outperform schooled children in verbal recall tasks when the stimu-lus lists are highly familiar. In this example, Australian aboriginal chil-dren and white Anglo-Australian children recalled a word list consisting of the names of wild animals (known to both groups). Interestingly, recall of the aboriginal children was superior independently of whether only the names of the animals were read aloud ("name-only task") or pictures of the objects were given simultaneously ("picture–name task"). Subsequent interviews revealed that both groups in the "picture–name task" had mainly used imagery strategies, but that their learning styles differed in the "name-only task": whereas rehearsal strategies dominated in the Anglo-Australian children, the aboriginal children were apparent-ly capable of spontaneously employing imagery. This seems to be a nice example of the compensatory effects that the knowledge base and in-terest factors can have on children's memory performance. Although an efficient verbal memory strategy was not available to the aboriginal children, their detailed knowledge and particular interest in wildlife led to superior performance in the verbal recall task.

Taken together, however, the findings from cross-cultural studies clearly demonstrate that the emergence of verbal memory strategies is a function of schooling. As a consequence, the development of memory strategies and their impact on memory performance is not a universal phenomenon but is confined to Western societies.

However, even within Western societies, differences in instructional practices can mainly determine the degree to which verbal memory strategies are spontaneously used. For example, mainly as a consequence of instructional differences, it may be observed that some children spon-taneously employ strategies, whereas other children of their age do not. In a study by Schneider, Borkowski, Kurtz, and Kerwin (1986), sub-stantial differences in the use of organizational strategies were found between American and German third graders. Whereas the German children clustered the picture stimuli almost perfectly according to their semantic categories, American subjects showed only low levels of spon-taneous sorting. Interestingly, only a short training procedure was neces-sary to overcome the American subjects' production deficiencies. In a subsequent study (Kurtz, Schneider, Turner, & Carr, 1986), similar trends were found for American and German second graders. Here, the most important finding was that differences in children's strategy use covaried with the different emphasis put on memory strategies by teachers and parents. That is, the analysis of teacher and parent interviews clearly indicated that German teachers and parents spend more time teaching and explaining memory strategies to their children.

Additional evidence comes from recent studies by Moely and her research group (Moely, Hart, Leal, Johnson-Baron, Santulli, & Rao, 1986; Moely, Leal, Pechman, Johnson, Santulli, Rao, Hart, & Burney, 1986). In these studies, it could be demonstrated that individual differences in the use of memory strategies by elementary school children are substantially related to teachers' use of strategy suggestions in the classroom. Children whose teachers often suggested strategies were better able to maintain strategies and also improved recall performance more than children from classrooms with teachers low in strategy suggestions.

All in all, these findings indicate that the development of memory strategies does not follow a "natural" pattern predominantly caused by maturational factors. Instead, the speed and amount of developmental change clearly depends on the degree of formal education and other environmental factors (e.g., parental influences). Of course, formal education does not operate like a constant, invariant factor: Individual differences in educational practices have an enormous impact on when and how children acquire memory strategies. As a consequence, even in schooled environments, individual differences in strategy use are still observed.

Developmental differences versus developmental changes: the need for longitudinal studies

Usefulness and shortcomings of cross-sectional studies in research on memory development

Given the empirical findings reported so far, there is little doubt that research in memory development has made enormous progress during the past two decades. As a consequence, our knowledge concerning developmental differences in memory performance as well as the sources of those differences has increased considerably. However, such a positive evaluation of the state of the art must be qualified in several respects.

Research in memory development has been limited in that (a) only a few experimental paradigms (in most cases, short-term recognition or free recall of word lists and text materials) have been considered; (b) the focus has been on the assessment of (age-correlated) developmental differences in basic memory capacities, memory behavior, and performances, whereas developmental changes have been typically ignored; (c) most studies have examined linear relationships between developmental differences in memory performance on the one hand and developmental differences in memory processes on the other hand, which have typically been inferred from findings based on different age groups; (d) research has focused on universal aspects of memory development, thus neglecting intraindividual and interindividual differences in developmental changes, and possible causes for these differences; and (e) research has concentrated on the description of developmental differences in the relationship between memory processes and memory performance, and typically ignored the problem of how to conceptualize developmental (explanatory) mechanisms.

Because of these limitations, most contemporary theories and models of memory development appear *idealistic*. That is, the traditional research strategy of comparing average, isolated memory performances with average performance-related memory processes in two or more age groups supports a tendency to overestimate the universality, intraindividual homogeneity, and interindividual consistency of developmental sequences. Thus, according to this approach, memory development is viewed as a regular, rule-bound sequence of changes in cognitive competencies and related memory skills. Typically, deviations from this ideal sequence have been ignored. If not ignored, they have been either treated as error variance or interpreted as individual acceleration or retardation, compared to a prototypical developmental sequence.

Despite these problems, the research approach we have described has certain theoretical advantages that should not be overlooked. In particular, many recent studies conducted within the experimental paradigm were well suited to illustrate interrelationships among differences in memory performance and differences in specific mental capacities. Undoubtedly, this experimental approach can provide a solid basis for generating important hypotheses concerning memory development. However, the validity and generalizability of these hypotheses are restricted by the cross-sectional designs used. In our view, it is mainly because of the restricted range of experimental designs (used by most cognitive developmental psychologists) that the predominant models of memory development are idealistic in nature.

A different developmental pattern has emerged whenever the classical experimental approach is replaced by field-experimental studies using several memory tasks in identical samples. Here, a typical finding is that memory performance varies considerably within individuals and between subjects of the same age group. As mentioned previously, the intertask correlations are generally low. They are particularly low for different classes of memory tasks (e.g., word span, memory for prose), and somewhat higher when similar memory tasks (e.g., word lists using different stimulus materials) are used. It is safe to state that all efforts to establish a taxonomy of memory performances and their underlying dispositions based on factor analytical approaches have failed. Thus we have reason to adopt the conclusion provided by Campione, Brown, and Bryant:

> The picture is not as simple as had originally been thought, however, since no single, unitary learning or memory faculty of great generality has been revealed. Rather, both learning and memory are complex processes, incorporating a wide array of subprocesses, together with procedures for overseeing those subprocesses. (1985, p. 121)

Note that this conclusion is also in accord with the theoretical approach presented by Ericsson (1985), who inferred from his analysis of exceptional memory performance that "all systematic differences in memory performance are due to acquired memory skill" (p. 214).

According to Ericsson (1985), the skill hypothesis is not restricted to memory experts but also might describe the memory development of normal subjects. This hypothesis was confirmed through a series of training studies conducted by Baltes and his co-workers (Kliegl, Smith, & Baltes, 1986). In these studies, it was demonstrated that intensive training of elderly people in the utilization of complex but specific memory skills had impressive effects on their performance in a digit-span task. Do these results imply that memory development is best viewed as a function of several independent processes concerning the acquisition, improvement, and automatization of memory skills? Recent empirical evidence based on performances on various memory tasks does not confirm such a position. This evidence includes studies concerning the transfer of procedural knowledge (Brown & Campione, 1984), the (de-contextualized) use of memory strategies (Naus & Ornstein, 1983), and the impact of general metacognitive skills on memory performance in different memory tasks (Campione et al., 1985).

Given the empirical evidence, realistic or "true" models of memory development should be located somewhere between the two poles of "the big picture of development" (Fischer, 1980) on the one hand, and a model representing memory development as the acquisition of many independent, specific skills on the other hand. Undoubtedly, memory development is much more variable and fragmentary than many idealistic models of development and intuitive developmental theories suggest. We believe that, in order to come to more realistic conceptualization of memory development, we must complement our cross-sectional data with empirical evidence from longitudinal studies.

Why longitudinal studies into memory development?

We would not go so far as to say that all those problems described in the previous section can be solved by focusing on the longitudinal approach. Nonetheless, it is indeed surprising that there are almost no longitudinal studies in the area of memory development. Of course, several disadvantages of longitudinal studies may have contributed to this situation (cf. Schneider, in press). They are extremely expensive and difficult to organize. Further, it is not an easy task to develop tasks that can be repeatedly used over a long period of time without producing floor and ceiling effects. Other methodological problems include the issue of how to substitute tasks with equivalent procedures at a later point in development, and how to control for retest effects. These problems seem particularly important in the context of learning and memory tasks, which are often repeatedly presented over a longer time period.

The lack of longitudinal studies may also be caused by the predominance of metatheoretical principles in the information processing approach: Most studies within this approach have been conducted in the area of memory development, an area that suggests the study of between-group differences (Kail & Bisanz, 1982). Despite these methodological and practical differences, however, an increasing number of social scientists consider longitudinal studies in the area of memory development to be a *necessary* complement to cross-sectional studies. In support of this judgment, the following reasons are frequently given:

1. In comparison with cross-sectional analyses, within-subject assessment of skill acquisition and performance changes are advantageous in that they allow for the description of developmental sequences. However, this advantage of longitudinal studies is of benefit only if individual data curves are considered instead of group means. Of course, the identification of typical or prototypical patterns of change is a major goal of developmental sequential analyses based on individual curves.

2. Longitudinal assessment of developmental change is particularly useful when there is evidence that cognitive competencies or performances do not continuously increase during childhood but may stagnate or even regress for a short period. Such U-shaped curves have been repeatedly observed (cf. Hoppe-Graff, 1985; Strauss & Stavy, 1982). According to Karmiloff-Smith's (1984; 1986) three-phase model of cognitive development, these U-shaped curves can be regarded as one of several "behavioral indices of representational change" (1986, p. 108).

For example, Lesgold (1984) observed such U-shaped performance changes when adult learners acquired domain-specific expertise, thus demonstrating the broad range of empirical examples for this phenomenon.

3. Longitudinal studies that not only include several memory measures but also additional cognitive indicators provide opportunities to go beyond the typical analysis of synchronous and asynchronous patterns of change. That is, they give information about interactional patterns in the development of different domains. According to Wohlwill (1973), this is the only way to assess homogeneity versus heterogeneity of individual memory development.

4. In our view, it is particularly informative to include specific training programs in the course of a longitudinal study because this allows the investigation of preconditions of successful intervention. Analyses of this kind are valuable as part of a comprehensive analysis concerning the preconditions and precursors of developmental changes in memory performance and the changes in related memory competencies (cf. Campbell & Richie, 1983). Although the longitudinal design is a necessary precondition, it may not be always sufficient for conditional analyses or prognostic studies of this type, mainly because of its nonexperimental character (cf. Hoppe-Graff, 1985). Given the very complicated cumulative or compensatory effects observed in the interactions among different sources of memory performance (e.g., domain-specific knowledge, general memory strategies, intelligent processing of information), it is probably difficult to identify necessary and/or sufficient conditions for memory development (see Hasselhorn, 1986; Kintsch, 1986; Körkel, 1987).

5. The assessment of stable interindividual differences in intraindividual change has been considered one of the most important tasks of longitudinal studies. As a matter of fact, these invariants are always masked by the effects of variable individual experiences; thus, it seems difficult to measure stable differences in operative abilities (e.g., differences in intelligence) and basic capacities in isolation, as emphasized by Estes (1982). Obviously, the only way to analyze the consistency of individual differences across tasks and their persistence over time is to use longitudinal designs.

To meet these theoretical expectations, longitudinal studies should be designed in a way that allows for the consideration of two different goals: On the one hand, the inclusion of a broad range of variables allows the empirical identification of complex interrelationships, isolated developmental trends, and age-dependent as well as age-independent developmental sequences (inductive approach). On the other hand, the hypotheses to be tested through longitudinal studies are best derived from theoretical knowledge about memory development obtained from cross-sectional studies (deductive approach). If it is also possible to vary conditions of development by using training programs or similar intervention procedures, then longitudinal studies could not only help in generating a broad descriptive knowledge, but could also provide conditional knowledge in the sense of theoretically postulated and empirically testable mechanisms of development. Given the present state of the art, however, this possibility seems restricted. The question of *why* changes occur cannot be adequately addressed by simply answering questions concerning which processes change how and under what conditions: Here, additional speculations are still needed.

Empirical evidence for developmental change: first results of longitudinal studies on memory development

We do not want to conclude without giving at least a short demonstration of how results from the few available longitudinal studies can enrich our knowledge about memory development.

In a short-term longitudinal study by Kunzinger (1985), the overt rehearsal and free-recall performance of 18 children was analyzed in two experimental testing sessions, initially when the children were 7 years of age and again 2 years later when they were 9. The impact of rehearsal frequency and rehearsal set size on subsequent recall was assessed in both sessions. The longitudinal results confirmed previous cross-sectional findings in that both rehearsal frequency and rehearsal set size increased with age, and that recall was more closely related to rehearsal set size than to rehearsal frequency. In addition, however, two interesting observations were made: First, it could be shown that rehearsal set size assessed at measurement Point 1 was not related to recall at measurement Point 1, but significantly predicted recall assessed 2 years later. This finding suggests that early differences in strategy use are better suited to predict future performance than to predict concurrent memory performance. According to Kunzinger, this finding may be due to the fact that production deficiencies dominant in the early assessment period were no longer a problem at age 9.

The second interesting finding concerns the relatively high stability over time observed for most memory variables. This stability was found for individuals' relative standing within their group between age levels (*group* stability) as measured with the correlation coefficient (r between .60 and .80) as well as for the level of *individual* stability. Here a "lability score" was computed to measure the amount of across-age variability shown in an individual's relative standing within the referent group. A high lability score indicated a high level of instability. The particularly high level of stability for rehearsal set size indicates that those children with initially larger set sizes were also those showing the largest set sizes 2 years later. Although these findings should be interpreted cautiously because of the small sample size, they give evidence of impressive interindividual stability over time, at least during the elementary school years.

However, as first evidence from our Munich Longitudinal Study (Weinert & Schneider, 1986; 1987) demonstrates, the picture of memory development may be different in preschool years. Our findings from the first two measurement points, when the subjects were 4 and 5 years of age, revealed considerable intraindividual inconsistency in performance across similar memory-for-prose tasks as well as individual instability with regard to the two measurement points. Lability scores were computed to assess the across-age stability in text recall, verbal intelligence, and motor skills. As a main result, we found that lability scores were almost three times as high as those obtained by Kunzinger (1985), and that they were absolutely comparable across the three tasks considered. It seems, then, that at that particular age high levels of instability are not only typical of memory performance but can be generalized across different domains. Although the reasons for the high levels of instability observed for most preschool measures of the Munich Longitudinal Study are not entirely clear, there are several possibilities (cf. Schneider, in press). For example, assessing true competence in preschool children is very difficult because situational factors seem to play an important role. That is, performance in a cognitive task may vary as a function of children's interest in the task, their familiarity with the experimenter, or their actual mood. On the other hand, it is also possible that the phenomenon under study is less stable over time than is typically the case for such variables in older children. This may even be true for traitlike variables (e.g., intelligence).

As a consequence, it is extremely important to make sure that variables are reliably assessed in order to evaluate the findings of considerable change over time. Whenever possible, coefficients of internal consistency should be obtained. If this turns out to be difficult, multiple measurements concerning the variable of interest should be available that allow for an evaluation of short-term stability.

Because sufficient internal consistency and/or short-term stability could be demonstrated for the measures in our longitudinal study, it appears that various memory phenomena indeed change considerably over time. Taken together, however, longitudinal evidence from memory studies is still too scarce to allow far-reaching conclusions. We believe that future longitudinal studies will be helpful in increasing our understanding of the emergence of how skilled remembering appears and develops.

NOTE

We would like to thank Beth Kurtz and Mitch Rabinowitz for helpful comments on the chapter.

REFERENCES

Ackerman, B. P. (1985). Children's retrieval deficits. In C. J. Brainerd & M. Pressley (Eds.), *Basic processes in memory development* (pp. 1–46). New York: Springer-Verlag.

Appelbaum, M. I., & McCall, R. B. (1983). Design and analysis in developmental psychology. In W. Kessen (Ed.), *Handbook of child psychology: Vol. 1. History, theory, and methods* (P. Mussen, Gen. Ed.) (4th ed., pp. 415–476). New York: Wiley.

Atkinson, R. C., & Shiffrin, R. M. (1968). Human memory: A proposed system and its control processes. In K. W. Spence & J. T. Spence (Eds.), *The psychology of learning and motivation* (Vol. 2, pp. 90–197). New York: Academic Press.

Baker-Ward, L., Ornstein, P. A., & Holden, D. J. (1984). The expression of memorization in early childhood. *Journal of Experimental Child Psychology, 37,* 555–575.

Binet, H., & Henri, V. (1894). La memoire des phrases. *L'Année Psychologique, 1,* 24–59.

Bjorklund, D. F. (1985). The role of conceptual knowledge in the development of organization in children's memory. In C. J. Brainerd & M. Pressley (Eds.), *Basic processes in memory development* (pp. 103–142). New York: Springer-Verlag.

Bjorklund, D. F. (1987). How age changes in knowledge base contribute to the development of children's memory: An interpretive review. *Developmental Review, 7,* 93–130.

Borkowski, J. G. (1985). Signs of intelligence: Strategy generalization and metacognition. In S. Yussen (Ed.), *The growth of reflection in children* (pp. 105–144). New York: Academic Press.

Brainerd, C. J. (1985). Model-based approaches to storage and retrieval development. In C. J. Brainerd & M. Pressley (Eds.), *Basic processes in memory development* (pp. 143–208). New York: Springer-Verlag.

Braunshausen, N. (1914). *Die experimentelle Gedächtnisforschung – Ein Kapitel der experimentellen Pädagogik.* Langensalza: Beyer & Mann.

Brown, A. L. (1977). Development, schooling, and the acquisition of knowledge about knowledge: Comments on chapter 7 by Nelson. In R. C. Anderson, R.

F. Spiro, & W. E. Montague (Eds.), *Schooling and the acquisition of knowledge* (pp. 241–258). Hillsdale, NJ: Erlbaum.

Brown, A. L., Bransford, J. D., Ferrara, R. A., & Campione, J. C. (1983). Learning, remembering, and understanding. In J. H. Flavell & E. M. Markman (Eds.), *Handbook of child psychology: Vol. 3. Cognitive development* (P. Mussen, Gen. Ed.) (pp. 177–276). New York: Wiley.

Brown, A. L., & Campione, J. C. (1984). Three faces of transfer implications for early competence, individual differences, and instruction. In M. E. Lamb, A. L. Brown, & B. Rogoff (Eds.), *Advances in developmental psychology* (Vol. 3, pp. 143–192). Hillsdale, NJ: Erlbaum.

Brown, A. L., & DeLoache, J. S. (1978). Skills, plans and self-regulation. In R. S. Siegler (Ed.), *Children's thinking: What develops?* (pp. 3–36). Hillsdale, NJ: Erlbaum.

Campbell, R. L., & Richie, D. M. (1983). Problems in the theory of developmental sequences. *Human Development, 26*, 156–172.

Campione, J. C., Brown, A. L., & Bryant, N. R. (1985). Individual differences in learning and memory. In R. J. Sternberg (Ed.), *Human abilities: An information processing approach* (pp. 103–126). New York: Freeman.

Case, R. (1985). *Intellectual development: Birth to adulthood.* New York: Academic Press.

Case, R., Kurland, D. M., & Goldberg, J. (1982). Operational efficiency and the growth of short-term memory span. *Journal of Experimental Child Psychology, 33*, 386–404.

Cavanaugh, J. C., & Borkowski, J. G. (1980). Searching for metamemory-memory connections: A developmental study. *Developmental Psychology, 16*, 441–453.

Cavanaugh, J. C., & Perlmutter, M. (1982). Metamemory: A critical examination. *Child Development, 53*, 11–28

Chechile, R. A., & Richman, C. L. (1982). The interaction of semantic memory with storage and retrieval processes. *Developmental Review, 2*, 237–250.

Chi, M. T. H. (1978). Knowledge structures and memory development. In R. S. Siegler (Ed.), *Children's thinking: What develops?* (pp. 73–96). Hillsdale, NJ: Erlbaum.

Chi, M. T. H. (1987) Representing knowledge and metaknowledge: Implications for interpreting metamemory research. In F. E. Weinert & R. H. Kluwe (Eds.), *Metacognition, motivation, and understanding* (pp. 239–266). Hillsdale, NJ: Erlbaum.

Chi, M. T. H., & Koeske, R. D. (1983). Network representation of a child's dinosaur knowledge. *Developmental Psychology, 19*, 29–39.

Cole, M., & Scribner, S. (1977). Cross-cultural studies of memory and cognition. In R. V. Kail & J. W. Hagen (Eds.), *Perspectives on the development of memory and cognition* (pp. 239–271). Hillsdale, NJ: Erlbaum.

DeLoache, J. S., Cassidy, D. J., & Brown, A. L. (1985). Precursors of mnemonic strategies in very young children's memory. *Child Development, 56*, 125–137.

Dempster, F. N. (1981). Memory span: Sources of individual and developmental differences. *Psychological Bulletin, 89*, 63–100.

Dempster, F. N. (1985). Short-term memory development in childhood and adolescence. In C. J. Brainerd & M. Pressley (Eds.), *Basic processes in memory development* (pp. 209–248). New York: Springer-Verlag.

Ericsson, K. A. (1985). Memory skill. *Canadian Journal of Psychology, 39*, 188–231.

Estes, W. K. (1982). Learning, memory, and intelligence. In R. J. Sternberg (Ed.), *Handbook of human intelligence* (pp. 170–224). Cambridge: Cambridge University Press.

Fischer, K. W. (1980). A theory of cognitive development: The control and construction of hierarchies of skills. *Psychological Review, 87,* 477–531.

Flavell, J. H. (1970). Developmental studies of mediated memory. In H. W. Reese & L. P. Lipsitt (Eds.), *Advances in child development and behavior* (Vol. 5, pp. 181–211). New York: Academic Press.

Flavell, J. H. (1971). First discussant's comments: What is memory development the development of? *Human Development, 14,* 272–278.

Flavell, J. H. (1978). Metacognitive development. In J. M. Scandura & C. J. Brainerd (Eds.), *Structural/process models of complex human behavior* (pp. 213–245). Alphen a.d.Rijn: Sijthoff & Noordhoff.

Flavell, J. H. (1985). *Cognitive development* (2nd ed.). Englewood Cliffs, NJ: Prentice-Hall.

Flavell, J. H., & Wellman, H. M. (1977). Metamemory. In R. V. Kail & J. W. Hagen (Eds.), *Perspectives on the development of memory and cognition* (pp. 3–33). Hillsdale, NJ: Erlbaum.

Frankel, M. T., & Rollins, H. A. (1985). Associative and categorical hypotheses of organization in the free recall of adults and children. *Journal of Experimental Child Psychology, 40,* 304–318.

Guttentag, R. E. (1984). The mental effort requirement of cumulative rehearsal: A developmental study. *Journal of Experimental Child Psychology, 37,* 92–106.

Guttentag, R. E. (1985). Memory and aging: Implications for theories of memory development during childhood. *Developmental Review, 5,* 56–82.

Hasselhorn, M. (1986). *Differentielle Bedingungsanalyse verbaler Gedächtnisleistungen bei Schulkindern.* Frankfurt: Lang.

Hoppe-Graff, S. (1985). Probleme und Ansätze der Untersuchung von Entwicklungssequenzen. In B. Seiler & W. Wannenmacher (Eds.), *Begriffs- und Wortbedeutungsentwicklung* (pp. 262–284). Heidelberg: Springer-Verlag.

Kail, R. (1979). Use of strategies and individual differences in children's memory. *Developmental Psychology, 15,* 251–255.

Kail, R., & Bisanz, J. (1982). Cognitive development: An information-processing perspective. In R. Varta (Ed.), *Strategies and techniques of child study* (pp. 209–243). New York: Academic Press.

Karmiloff-Smith, A. (1984). Children's problem solving. In M. E. Lamb, A. L. Brown, & B. Rogoff (Eds.), *Advances in developmental psychology* (Vol. 3, pp. 39–90). Hillsdale, NJ: Erlbaum.

Karmiloff-Smith, A. (1986). From meta-processes to conscious access: Evidence from children's metalinguistic and repair data. *Cognition, 23,* 95–147.

Kearins, J. (1983). A quotient of awareness. *Education News, 18,* 18–22.

Keating, D. P., & Bobbitt, B. L. (1978). Individual and developmental differences in cognitive-processing components of mental ability. *Child Development, 49,* 155–167.

Kintsch, W. (1986). Memory for prose. In F. Klix & H. Hagendorf (Eds.), *Human memory and cognitive capabilities, Part A* (pp. 841–850). Amsterdam: North-Holland.

Kirckpatrick, E. A. (1894). An experimental study of memory. *Psychological Review, 1,* 602–609.

Kliegl, R., Smith, J., & Baltes, P. B. (1986). Testing-the-limits, expertise, and memory in adulthood and old age. In F. Klix & H. Hagendorf (Eds.), *Human memory and cognitive capabilities, Part A* (pp. 395–407). Amsterdam: North-Holland.

Knopf, M., Körkel, J., Schneider, W., & Weinert, F. E. (1988). Human memory as a faculty versus human memory as a set of specific abilities: Evidence from a life-span approach. In F. E. Weinert & M. Perlmutter (Eds.), *Memory development: Universal changes and individual differences* (pp. 334–352). Hillsdale, NJ: Erlbaum.

Körkel, J. (1987). *Die Entwicklung von Gedächtnis- und Metagedächtnisleistungen in Abhängigkeit von bereichsspezifischen Vorkenntnissen.* Frankfurt: Lang.

Kunzinger, E. L. (1985). A short-term longitudinal study of memorial development during early grade school. *Developmental Psychology, 21,* 642–646.

Kurtz, B. E., Schneider, W., Turner, L., & Carr, M. (1986). *Memory performance in German and American children: Differing roles of metacognitive and motivational variables.* Paper presented at the annual meetings of the American Educational Research Association, San Francisco.

Lange, G. (1978). Organization-related processes in children's recall. In P. A. Ornstein (Ed.), *Memory development in children* (pp. 101–128). Hillsdale, NJ: Erlbaum.

Lesgold, A. M. (1984). Acquiring expertise. In J. A. Anderson & S. M. Kosslyn (Eds.), *Tutorials in learning and memory* (pp. 39–60). San Francisco: Freeman.

McGeoch, J. A., & Irion, A. L. (1952). *The psychology of human learning.* New York: Longmans, Green & Co.

Moely, B. E. (1977). Organizational factors in the development of memory. In R. V. Kail & J. W. Hagen (Eds.), *Perspectives on the development of memory and cognition* (pp. 203–236). Hillsdale, NJ: Erlbaum.

Moely, B. E., Hart, S. S., Leal, L., Johnson-Baron, T., Santulli, K. A., & Rao, N. (1986). *An investigation of how teachers establish stable use and generalization of memory strategies through the use of effective training techniques.* Paper presented at the annual meetings of the American Educational Research Association, San Francisco.

Moely, B. E., Leal, L., Pechman, E. M., Johnson, T. D., Santulli, K. A., Rao, N., Hart, S. S., & Burney, L. (1986). *Relationships between teachers' cognitive instruction and children's memory skills.* Paper presented at the biennial meeting of the Southwestern Society for Research in Child Development, San Antonio.

Naus, M. J., & Ornstein, P. A. (1983). Development of memory strategies: Analysis, questions, and issues. In M. T. H. Chi (Ed.), *Trends in memory development research* (Vol. 9, pp. 1–30). Basel: Karger.

Netschajeff, A. (1902). Über Memorieren. *Sammlung von Abhandlungen aus dem Gebiete der Pädagogischen Psychologie und Physiologie, 5,* 293–329.

Offner, M. (1924). *Das Gedächtnis.* Berlin: Reuther & Reichard.

Ornstein, P. A., Baker-Ward, L., & Naus, M. J. (1988). The development of mnemonic skill. In F. E. Weinert & M. Perlmutter (Eds.), *Memory development: Universal changes and individual differences* (pp. 31–50). Hillsdale, NJ: Erlbaum.

Ornstein, P. A., Medlin, R. G., Stone, B. P., & Naus, M. J. (1985) Retrieving for rehearsal: An analysis of active rehearsal in children's memory. *Developmental Psychology, 21,* 633–641.

Ornstein, P. A., & Naus, M. J. (1985). Effects of the knowledge base on children's memory strategies. In H. W. Reese (Ed.), *Advances in child development and behavior* (Vol. 19, pp. 113–148). New York: Academic Press.

Paris, S. G., Lipson, M. Y., & Wixson, K. K. (1983). Becoming a strategic reader. *Contemporary Educational Psychology, 8,* 293–316.

Paris, S. G., Newman, R. S., & Jacobs, J. E. (1985). Social contexts and functions of children's remembering. In M. Pressley & C. J. Brainerd (Eds.), *Cognitive learning and memory in children* (pp. 81–115). New York: Springer-Verlag.

Pressley, M. (1982). Elaboration and memory development. *Child Development, 53,* 296–309.

Pressley, M., Borkowski, J. G., & O'Sullivan, J. (1985). Children's metamemory and the teaching of memory strategies. In D. L. Forrest-Pressley, G. E. MacKinnon, & T. G. Waller (Eds.), *Metacognition, cognition, and human performance* (Vol. 1, pp. 111–153). Orlando: Academic Press.

Pressley, M., Forrest-Pressley, D., & Elliott-Faust, D. J. (1988). What is strategy instructional enrichment and how to study it: Illustrations from research on children's prose memory and comprehension. In F. E. Weinert & M. Perlmutter (Eds.), *Memory development: Universal changes and individual differences* (pp. 101–130). Hillsdale, NJ: Erlbaum.

Pressley, M., Forrest-Pressley, D., Elliott-Faust, D. J., & Miller, G. E. (1985). Children's use of cognitive strategies, how to teach strategies, and what to do if they can't be taught. In M. Pressley & C. J. Brainerd (Eds.), *Cognitive learning and memory in children* (pp. 1–47). New York: Springer-Verlag.

Rabinowitz, M., & Chi, M. T. H. (1987). An interactive model of strategic processing. In S. J. Ceci (Ed.), *Handbook of the cognitive, social, and physiological characteristics of learning disabilities* (Vol. 2, pp. 83–102). Hillsdale, NJ: Erlbaum.

Rabinowitz, M., & Glaser, R. (1985). Cognitive structure and process in highly competent performance. In F. D. Horowitz & M. O'Brien (Eds.), *The gifted and the talented: A developmental perspective.* Washington, DC: American Psychological Association.

Radossawljewitsch, P. R. (1907). Das Behalten und Vergessen bei Kindern und Erwachsenen nach experimentellen Untersuchungen. In E. Meumann (Hrsg.), *Pädagogische Monographien* (Bd. 1, pp. 129–193). Leipzig: Nemnich-Verlag.

Rogoff, B., & Mistry, J. (1985). Memory development in cultural context. In. M. Pressley & C. J. Brainerd (Eds.), *Cognitive learning and memory in children* (pp. 112–142). New York: Springer-Verlag.

Schneider, W. (1985). Developmental trends in the metamemory–memory behavior relationship: An integrative review. In D. L. Forrest-Pressley, G. E. MacKinnon, & T. G. Waller (Eds.), *Metacognition, cognition, and human performance* (Vol. 1, pp. 57–109). Orlando: Academic Press.

Schneider, W. (1986). The role of conceptual knowledge and metamemory in the development of organizational processes in memory. *Journal of Experimental Child Psychology, 42,* 218–236.

Schneider, W. (in press). Problems of longitudinal studies with children: Practical, conceptual and methodological issues. In M. Brambring, F. Lösel, & H. Skowronek (Eds.), *Children at risk: Assessment and longitudinal research.* New York: De Gruijter.

Schneider, W., Borkowski, J. G., Kurtz, B. E., & Kerwin, K. (1986). Metamemory and motivation: A comparison of strategy use and performance in German and American children. *Journal of Cross-Cultural Psychology, 17*, 315–336.

Schneider, W., Körkel, J., & Vogel, K. (1987). Zusammenhänge zwischen Metagedächtnis, strategischem Verhalten und Gedächtnisleistungen im Grundschulalter: Eine entwicklungspsychologische Studie. *Zeitschrift für Entwicklungspsychologie und Pädagogische Psychologie, 19*, 99–115.

Schneider, W., Körkel, J., & Weinert, F. E. (1987a). *The knowledge base and memory performance: A comparison of academically successful and unsuccessful learners.* Paper presented at the annual meetings of the American Educational Research Association, Washington, DC.

Schneider, W., Körkel, J., & Weinert, F. E. (1987b). The effects of intelligence, self-concept, and attributional style on metamemory and memory behaviour. *International Journal of Behavioural Development, 10*, 281–299.

Schneider, W., & Pressley, M. (1988). *Memory development between 2 and 20.* New York: Springer-Verlag.

Siegler, R. S. (1986). *Children's thinking.* Englewood Cliffs, NJ: Prentice-Hall.

Smirnov, A. A., & Zinchenko, P. I. (1969). Problems in the psychology of memory. In M. Cole & N. Maltzman (Eds.), *A handbook of contemporary Soviet psychology* (pp. 452–502). New York: Basic Books.

Sodian, B., Schneider, W., & Perlmutter, M. (1986). Recall, clustering and metamemory in young children. *Journal of Experimental Child Psychology, 41*, 395–410.

Sophian, C. (1984). Developing search skills in infancy and early childhood. In C. Sophian (Ed.), *Origins of cognitive skills* (pp. 27–56). Hillsdale, NJ: Erlbaum.

Strauss, S., & Stavy, R. (Eds.) (1982). *U-shaped behavioral growth.* New York: Academic Press.

Wagner, D. A. (1981). Culture and memory development. In H. C. Triandis & A. Heron (Eds.), *Handbook of cross-cultural psychology* (Vol. 4, pp. 187–232). Boston: Allyn & Bacon.

Waters, H. S., & Andreassen, C. (1983). Children's use of memory strategies under instruction. In M. Pressley & J. R. Levin (Eds.), *Cognitive strategy research: Psychological foundations* (pp. 3–24). New York: Springer Verlag.

Weinert, F. E. (1986). Developmental variations of memory performance and memory-related knowledge across the life-span. In A. Sörensen, F. E. Weinert, & L. R. Sherrod (Eds.), *Human development: Multidisciplinary perspectives* (pp. 535–554). Hillsdale, NJ: Erlbaum.

Weinert, F. E., Knopf, M., Körkel, J., Schneider, W., Vogel, K., & Wetzel, M. (1984). Die Entwicklung einiger Gedächtnisleistungen bei Kindern und älteren Erwachsenen in Abhängigkeit von kognitiven, metakognitiven und motivationalen Einflussfaktoren. In K. E. Grossmann & P. Lütkenhaus (Eds.), *Bericht über die 6. Tagung Entwicklungspsychologie* (pp. 313–326). Regensburg: Universitäts-Druckerei.

Weinert, F. E., & Schneider, W. (Eds.) (1986). *First report on the Munich Longitudinal Study on the Genesis of Individual Competencies (LOGIC).* Munich: Max Planck Institute for Psychological Research.

Weinert, F. E., & Schneider, W. (Eds.) (1987). *The Munich Longitudinal Study on the Genesis of Individual Competencies (LOGIC). Report No. 3: Results of wave one.* Munich: Max Planck Institute for Psychological Research.

Weinert, F. E., Schneider, W., & Knopf, M. (1988). Individual differences in memory development across the life-span. In P. B. Baltes, D. L. Featherman, & R. M. Lerner (Eds.), *Life-span development and behavior* (Vol. 9, pp. 39–85). Hillsdale, NJ: Erlbaum.

Wellman, H. M. (1983). Metamemory revisited. In M. T. H. Chi (Ed.), *Trends in memory development research* (pp. 31–51). Basel: Karger.

Wellman, H. M. (1985). The origins of metacognition. In D. L. Forrest-Pressley, G. E. MacKinnon, & T. G. Waller (Eds.), *Metacognition, cognition, and human performance* (Vol. 1, pp. 1–31). Orlando: Academic Press.

Wohlwill, J. F. (1973). *The study of behavioral development.* New York: Academic Press.

II   Language development

4 The role of social interaction in the transition from communication to language

LUIGIA CAMAIONI

The transition from prelinguistic communication to language acquisition has been a favorite topic in the developmental literature of the past two decades. Research on early communication patterns and their relation with later linguistic patterns has been motivated by a belief in *continuity* more than in discontinuity. In some studies early behaviors were taken to be precursors of later, more complex behavior (cf. Bullowa, 1976; Freedle & Lewis, 1977), whereas in other studies they were taken as the source from which later behaviors emerge, that is, as prerequisites or predictors (cf. Bruner, 1983; Camaioni, De Castro Campos, & De Lemos, 1984). Although we cannot yet ascertain whether early behaviors are necessary and sufficient to account for later behaviors, the answer to one question – Which patterns can justifiably be taken as precursors or predictors of which more advanced behaviors? – is becoming more evident.

In studying the transition from prelinguistic to linguistic development, the crucial problem one confronts is how to define the social and inter-actional measures that are assumed to be significantly related to the later linguistic measures. Moreover, the hypothesis that linguistic patterns derive, at least partially, from early interactive patterns, can be empirically tested only on the basis of longitudinal studies that consider a rather wide age range, from the first half of the first year of life to the middle or end of the second year. Such longitudinal studies should also focus on individual differences, comparing subjects or groups of subjects who differ in some criterial aspects of early language development (e.g., rhythm or rate), possibly derived from different trends or profiles in the development of the prelinguistic interactive patterns taken as precursors.

My aim in this paper is to review and discuss different research approaches to the study of a developmentally continuous transition from sociointeractive to linguistic patterns in the first years of life, and to evaluate their methodological and explanatory implications. The chapter is divided into three major sections. In the first, I consider in more detail the domain of adult–child interaction research, particularly with regard to the influence of parental behavior on the child's communication development and the construction of shared meanings. In the second, I address the theoretical issues concerning the continuity or derivation between language and developmentally prior communication systems. This section also provides empirical evidence favoring the claim of a significant relation between specific adult–child interactive patterns and subsequent linguistic development displayed by the child. The third section will briefly examine the transition from one-word utterances to multiword utterances and the emergence of syntax, in the light of the foregoing theoretical and methodological proposal.

The influence of parental behavior on child's communication development

For the past two decades research into human social development has consisted mainly of an analysis of processes that could be defined as "socialization through interaction" (Newson, 1977). This new approach, which is opposed both to environmentalist positions (social learning theory) and to nativist positions (ethology), may be characterized methodologically as follows:

1. Transition from the study of macrosocial variables – for example, global dimensions of parental behavior (permissiveness, authoritarian-ism, etc.), feeding and toileting practices, or children's personality characteristics (dependence, independence, aggressiveness, etc.) – to the analysis of microbehaviors and microsequences characterizing face-to-face interaction, particularly dyadic interaction;
2. Transition from the use of indirect data collection methods, such as the administration of questionnaires and interviews to parents or teachers, to the use of direct observation and the microanalytic examination of interactive behaviors.

In this approach socialization is based on interaction. "It always involves two (or more) participants, each already equipped with his own set of predispositions, aims, intentions and predilections, and any interaction between them must therefore inevitably involve a negotiating process, as a result of which progressive modification in the behavior of both participants takes place" (Schaffer & Crook, 1978, p. 58).

Within this general framework, which has so far proved to be highly productive in terms of research results and methodological progress, I think two different approaches can be identified. The first, which I define as "interaction as synchronization," emphasizes the importance of the temporal organization underlying the interactive sequences, as a result of which the latter are basically reduced to the former.

According to this trend, the aim of the early mother–child interactions
is to attain an interpersonal synchrony based on the temporal integration
of the two participants' behavior. This synchrony is accomplished on the
basis of two main factors: (a) the infant's spontaneous behavior, temporally organized according to endogenous mechanisms and characterized
by a regular periodicity (usually an activation–pause pattern); (b) the
mother's sensitivity to this periodicity and her desire to respond by
inserting her behaviors into the time patterns governing the child's
microrhythms. The acknowledgment of these two factors implies both
the need to attribute some sort of social preadaptation to the infant –
that is, the availability of endogenous mechanisms (visual apparatus,
auditory apparatus, etc.) that serve to deal with other people – and the
need to recognize some form of innate "compatibility" among the genetic mechanisms by means of which the child is "programmed" to send
certain signals and the adult to respond to them.

Various studies have provided examples of highly synchronized interpersonal exchanges between mother and infant during the early months
of life. These include the brilliant analyses done by Kaye (1977) on
sucking, by Schaffer, Collis, and Parsons (1977) on vocal exchanges, by
Stern (1974) and Collis and Schaffer (1975) on visual interaction.

All these authors stress the presence of common characteristics ensur-
ing the "smoothness" and "harmony" of the early interactions. Because
the different child behaviors (sucking, smiling, crying, vocalizing, visual
attention) are discrete and occur in an on–off pattern, the mother can
fill in the gaps between one activation period and the next and alternate
her behavior with the child's, thereby setting up an *apparent* dialogue.
However, turn taking is not the only possible time pattern that can be
used to insure effective interpersonal synchronization. Also, an overlapping pattern has been described (see Stern, 1977) in which the behaviors of the two participants occur at the same time rather than in
sequence. It can nevertheless be demonstrated that the behavior of one
member of the pair began a very short time *after* the behavior of the
other. The overlapping pattern in any case seems to occur under special
conditions (intense emotional involvement), whereas the alternation pattern is certainly more frequent and characterizes most early interactions.

In sum, parents (especially mothers) often behave as though their
children can take turns during interaction sequences, and thus they treat
young infants (between 2 and 5 months of age) as potentially competent
social partners. Moreover, Western parents generally impute motives,
skills, and intentions to their infant's behaviors, interpreting them not
just as an index of the infant's inner feelings or states but as intentional
attempts to communicate feelings or states. As Schaffer points out,

however, "the fact that parents think children start life as real persons tells us something about parents, not about children" (1984, p. 77). The question that arises at this point is how the child, through being interpreted as exhibiting an intentional and meaningful behavior, becomes able to assign intention and meaning to one's and other's acts.

Schaffer's (1984) answer is that the first exchanges between the child and his or her caretaker are actually "pseudodialogues" – that is, unidirectional sequences that are entirely dependent on the adult's willingness to construct and maintain them. They will become "true" dialogues (i.e., according to Schaffer, bidirectional exchanges in which adult and child assume joint responsibility for the conduct of the interaction) only toward the end of the first year of life, when the child has acquired the notions of "intentionality" and "reciprocity" and can thus actively and intentionally participate in constructing the dialogue. The previous question can indeed be reformulated as follows: How does the child acquire the capacity for intentionality and reciprocity, which will in turn allow him to play a more symmetrical role during child–adult interactive exchanges? How is it possible to explain this transition from the partner's reciprocal involvement to the mutual understanding, in which the child does not simply "react" to the other's behavior but succeeds in "understanding" his partner's intention and aims?

This brings us to the second research approach in which the mother–baby interaction is viewed "as an attempt by the mother to enter into a *meaningful* set of exchanges with her infant" (Newson, 1977, p. 46; emphasis added). In other words, this approach focuses attention on the fact that shared meaning between parent and child, although primitive, is essential to the definition of the dyad as a sociocommunicative system – that is, a system composed of individuals who are capable of mutual understanding and jointly pursue their goals. In this sense, "intersubjectivity involves being able to assume (correctly) that the meaning an object or event has to you will be the meaning it has to your partner. Without that, there can be no real dialogue. Its rudiments can be achieved, however, by either partner making a correct inference from the other's behavior" (Kaye, 1982, p. 150).

Priority is thus given in the investigation to processes leading to the construction of mental entities or shared meanings rather than to the integration of the partners' respective responses. Even though the detailed study of these processes is only at the beginning, the results of the research done in this direction seem to be rather promising. Methodologically speaking, this is a research in which social interaction is not analyzed as such, that is, in its general features (e.g. turn taking, role learning). Rather, specific types of interactive sequences or episodes that conform to a previously introduced definition are selected for the purpose of analysis.

From this perspective, a number of authors have studied "imitation sequences" or "matching episodes," frequently occurring in mother–infant interaction during the first year of life, as an interpersonal activity that contributes to mutual understanding as well as to progress toward the more conventional means of communication achieved later in development (Kaye, 1982; Masur, 1984; Pawlby, 1977; Uzgiris, 1984). This research indicates that the imitation is *reciprocal* – not only does the child imitate the mother but the mother also imitates the child. In all studies, mothers imitated their infants more frequently than infants imitated them during the first year of life. Nevertheless, correlational analyses showed that infants who imitated more of their mothers' acts had mothers who imitated more of their infants' acts, demonstrating the reciprocity inherent in early imitations (Camaioni, 1986; Masur, 1984). In particular, Pawlby (1977) found a positive correlation between the frequency with which mothers imitate children between the ages of 4 and 6 months and the frequency with which children imitate their mothers between the ages of 6 and 10 months. This finding suggests that the mother's previous tendency to imitate may have helped to generate a similar behavior in the child. Indeed, when she imitates a behavior that belongs to the child's spontaneous repertoire, the mother is "marking out" this behavior and drawing the child's attention to it. This increases the likelihood of the child reproducing the same behavior in similar circumstances in order to get the mother to do likewise. The construction of a "shared object" (gesture, movement, vocalization, etc.) may thus begin and becomes part of the communicative code used by the mother–child pair.

Furthermore, the mother does not imitate all the possible actions carried out by the child but *selects* from the child's repertoire those behaviors more likely to take on a communicative meaning and favors communication signals of the more conventional type (pointing, waving, etc.) as a function of the child's growing age.

In Pawlby's (1977) study, between 6 and 10 months of age the imitation of facial expressions declined, whereas the imitation of object-related acts and speech-related vocalizations increased. Consistent with the trend reported by Pawlby, Masur (1984) found that after 10 months of age mothers were particularly likely to imitate infants' vocalizations and words. Finally, in a study based on older children (6 to 18 months of age; Camaioni, 1986), the imitation between mother and child was shown to display the same gradual change from the use of nonstandard signals (sounds, gestures, etc.) to the use of more abstract and conventional signals (gestural and linguistic symbols), which characterizes the child's communicative development as he goes from prelanguage to the onset of language. In particular, after 12 months of age the dyads observed showed a significant decrease in the imitation of sounds and prosodic patterns and an equally significant increase in the imitation of words and referential gestures. No significant differences related to children's age were found for the remaining three types of imitation considered (facial expressions, gestures, actions with objects).

These changes toward greater conventionality may be due to selective matching of infant acts by the mother as well as to selective response to infant matching by the mother or to both. In any case, the results reviewed so far support the claim that imitation exchanges between mother and child in the first year of life have a communicative function and may serve as a stepping stone to the child's achievement of more conventionally meaningful modes of communication, because they focus on actions that are in the process of being developed by the child (i.e., conventional sounds and gestures).

From interaction patterns to language acquisition: the issue of continuity

The concept that the child's repeated and systematic involvement in "structured" interaction formats represents not only the context in which communication can take place but also the *matrix* generating the contents of such communication in the form of shared meanings now seems to have gained the support of several authors (cf. Kaye, 1982; Newson, 1977; Trevarthen, 1977; Uzgiris, 1984) and is based on empirical data. This position is harder to maintain when the term *communication* is replaced by that of *language*. This is because the hypothesis of communication and language being interdependent in terms of generative processes clashes with a consolidated research tradition favoring the partial or complete independence of the sociocommunicative and the linguistic structures acquired by the child.

In the 1970s, the concern with the influence of social interaction on language development was a reaction to the neglect of such factors in the "nativist" theories of language acquisition inspired by Chomsky (1968). Since then, despite several attempts to determine the role that others (especially parents) play in language acquisition, it has proved difficult to demonstrate the specific ways in which children's social context influences their early linguistic development. In a recent review of the literature, Shatz has argued:

With regard to the question of the relation between language and communication development, we have seen an explosion of work that has carefully described early interactive patterns between infants and their caretakers. Yet, any real evidence that patterns of interaction developed in the early months or even the first year of life have any direct bearing on the speed or order of language acquisition skill is lacking. (1983, p. 877)

In particular, two aspects of the social context have attracted the researchers' attention. Numerous observational studies have examined relations between parental speech and the pattern and rate of children's linguistic development. A second line of research has examined the early social games played by mothers and infants as having an important role in assisting the child's transition into language. These two lines of research have, however, very different strengths in establishing causal connections and longitudinal predictions. In studies providing support for an association between features of parental and child speech (cf. Furrow & Nelson, 1984; Gleitman, Newport, & Gleitman, 1984), although A (parental speech) predicts B (child speech) in the future, A does not precede B – that is, B exists part of the time when A is first measured. This leaves the question of the direction of effects: although it is plausible that parental input influences the rate and/or content of the child's speech, an alternative explanation is that the child's own speech influences parental speech. There simply is no way of sorting out the direction, even on the grounds of plausibility.

In studies examining the relation between early "social games" or "standard action formats," played by mothers and infants during the first year of life, and the subsequent language development displayed by the children, it is possible to show that A (social games) not only predicts B (child speech) but precedes it as well. In this case, the longitudinal prediction helps sort out the direction of cause and effect because, if A precedes B, it is not plausible to maintain that B causes A.

"Social games" or "standard action formats" (Bruner, 1983; Camaioni & Laicardi, 1985; Ratner & Bruner, 1978) have been defined as those sequences of child–adult (usually the mother) interaction that are characterized by a set of culturally defined and agreed-upon rules, and also contain unique form–function relationships (e.g., *give* always marks the function of asking for an object and *thank you* that of receiving it in the "give and take" game).

It has been claimed that neither social interaction *per se* nor the mastery of its general properties (e.g., turn taking, role differentiation, etc.) could provide a suitable precursor of later linguistic development, but only those interaction episodes characterized by a conventional structure and by unique form–function relationships. In this direction the work of Bruner and colleagues (Ninio & Bruner, 1978; Ratner & Bruner, 1978) approached the problem of the derivation of linguistic patterns from interactive patterns by focusing on the analysis of social games between adult and child insofar as they are games with a conventional structure. The results show how, in their mutual play, adult and child basically work out a restricted and shared set of "meanings" that could act as referents for gradually more advanced communication signals. The fact that the adult repeatedly produces certain standard action or attention formats allows the child first to interpret the adult's actions and signals starting from the positions (privileges of occurrence) they occupy in the routine sequence; and subsequently to reproduce the same actions and signals inside the sequence, usually moving from the use of nonstandard signals to the use of standard lexical items. As a result, the child's role in play gradually changes from mere spectator to actor; he learns to carry out one or more of the actions involved in the game and also to produce the linguistic marking that accompanies, precedes, or completes these actions.

In accordance with this view, subsequent studies (Bakeman & Adamson, 1986; Camaioni & Laicardi, 1985; Smith, Adamson, & Bakeman, 1986) have documented relationships between maternal use of conventional means of encouraging joint attention to objects or events and infants' language acquisition. In particular, when a mother engages with her child in ritualized games or action formats, she both highlights shared objects using conventional more than literal acts, and uses language to focus on the code itself or on aspects of the context in which communication occurs more than on the addresser–addressee contact.

Within this framework, we carried out a long-term longitudinal study of three mother–child dyads, followed for a 12-month period from the children's ages of 6 to 18 months. The aim of this research was twofold: to analyze developmental changes in the quality of social games played by mothers and children during normal home activities; and to show how the conventional nature of some games and the way mothers use language in them might contribute to the child's early mastery of language (cf. Camaioni & Laicardi, 1985).

Thirty-minute observation sessions were carried out every 20 days on the average during a free-play situation in the family environment. All observation sessions (14 for each dyad) were audiotaped and videotaped. The categories used in coding the data were as follows (see Table 4.1): type of mother–child social game; child's role in social game; and mother and child's linguistic production during social game. Videotapes were segmented into interaction episodes defined as social games, and a

Table 4.1. *Measures used to study early social games and the acquisition of
language*

Type of social games	
A. Non-conventional	
1. Tactile and/or motoric stimulation	
2. Perceptual stimulation (visual and/or acoustic)	
3. Vocal imitation	
4. Gestural imitation	

B. Conventional	
5. Give and take	12. No
6. Peekaboo	13. Point and name
7. Horsie	14. Put on–take off, slip on–off, open–shut
8. Patacake	15. Joint book reading
9. Bye-bye	16. Question–answer
10. Ball	'17. Linguistic imitation
11. Build–knock down	18. Other

Child role in social game
A. Passive
B. Active

Linguistic production in social game
A. Mother
B. Child

Source: Camaioni & Laicardi, 1985.

distinction was made between "unconventional" games (characterized
by the *repetition* of specific behaviors) and "conventional" games (characterized by the presence of invariant *roles*).

In all dyads conventional games increased in significant linear fashion
between 6 and 12 months of age, whereas the frequency of unconventional games over the same age range remained constant. From 6 to 12
months children also became increasingly able to play an active role
during games. However, if the child's active participation was differentiated as a function of game type (conventional versus unconventional), the active role increased significantly only in the case of conventional
games. No significant trend was found for the period from 13 to 18
months either in game type or in the child's role. Besides these similar
developmental trends the three dyads showed a consistent pattern of
differences. First, there were significant interdyad differences in the
proportion of total games accounted for by conventional and unconventional types respectively, and in the distribution of active and passive
roles in conventional games. Second, the dyads differed significantly in

the mother's capacity for linguistically marking the conventional game turns in which the child's participation was active rather than passive. From this pattern of differences Dyad 1 appears to differ markedly from the other two dyads in the following aspects: In conventional games, the role assumed by the child was more frequently active than passive; and the mother chose to mark linguistically the conventional game turns in which the child was active rather than those in which he was passive. On the other hand, Dyads 2 and 3 resembled each other in the same aspects – in both dyads the child tended to participate less actively in the game and the mother chose less frequently to mark linguistically the child's active participation.

As far as children's early linguistic development was concerned, all three subjects (subjects 1, 2, and 3) produced their first one-word utterances *only* within conventional game episodes. Moreover, these "first words" corresponded to the linguistic forms used by the mother to mark certain segments of joint action and/or attention during the same types of games. Subject 1 produced a number of linguistic utterances nearly three times greater than that of the other two children (57 versus 24 and 21 respectively) and displayed also a higher variety of linguistic forms (12 versus 10 and 8 respectively). It seems reasonable to relate this different rate of language acquisition to the previously analyzed pattern of interdyad differences in social games. The linguistically most advanced child (Subject 1) turned out to be the same child whose participation in conventional games was more frequently active than passive and whose mother chose to mark linguistically the child's active participation during conventional games. It was hypothesized that the "contingency" between maternal linguistic production and the child's active participation in conventional game episodes provides the child with the ability to relate specific actions to specific interactive contexts (games) as well as to relate sounds to actions or objects shared within the game.

In a study based on 28 infants, who were videotaped at home playing with their mothers, with peers, and while alone at 9, 12, and 15 months of age, Bakeman and Adamson (1986) obtained some interesting findings. First, playing with mothers and playing with same-age peers promoted different ways of communicating. Peer partners provoked babbling as well as positive affect displays but they seemed to invite no more conventionalized acts than no partner at all. Second, infants produced more conventionalized acts (including both gestures as points, show/offers, ritualized requests, regulative gestures, and words) when mothers gave them their attention than when mothers were inattentive, as they were during the alone and peer conditions. In particular, at 9 and 12 months, it was "joint-object play" with the mother that fostered the infants' use of conventionalized acts, whereas at 15 months "action formats" (including instances of book reading, telephoning, giving–receiving, building–destroying, and puzzle playing) clearly affected the production of embedded referential (but not social-regulative) conventionalized acts, and only when formats and joint-object play overlapped (43% of the total time coded as joint engagement). Moreover, at 15 months, formats and, to a lesser degree, discrete conventionalized acts began to appear frequently in the alone condition. For example, one 15-month-old infant performed the format of book reading complete with pointing to pictures while playing alone. This developmental pattern suggests that conventionalized acts, first facilitated by adult assistance and "scaffolding," become increasingly freed from this support.

In another study based on the same sample, Smith, Adamson, and Bakeman (1986) found that both infants' sharing of an attentional focus with their mothers and mothers' conventional object-marking activity when infants were 15 months old were positively related to the size of infants' productive vocabularies at 18 months. Infants with larger vocabularies spent more time engaged in joint object play with mothers and had mothers who more often used conventional means of directing attention to objects, more often used utterances that focused on language per se, and less often used utterances to regulate social exchanges. Taken together, these four variables account for 40% of the variance in infants' vocabulary size at 18 months, significantly more than is predicted by any of the variables taken alone. However, two of these variables made unique contributions to the variance prediction. The partial correlation between mothers' conventional object-marking and vocabulary size was .49 ($p < .05$), and that between mothers' metalingual utterances rate and infants' vocabulary size was .42 ($p < .05$). Interestingly, the metalingual category consists largely of utterances that encourage infants to speak (e.g., "Say hello"; "Can you say hello?") or give feedback regarding infants' speech production (e.g., "What?"). On the other hand, the partial correlation between mothers' social-regulative utterance rate and infants' vocabulary size was significantly negative ($r = -.43$, $p < .05$), a result that corresponds with Nelson's (1973) finding of similar relationships between infants' language acquisition rates and mothers' use of "directives" and "child references."

In the same direction, Harris, Jones, Brookes, and Grant (1986), comparing maternal speech in two groups of children with normal or slower rates of language development, found that mothers of children with slower language development initiated more changes in conversational topic without providing an appropriate nonverbal context. These mothers also made fewer references to objects to which the child was attending and more references to objects to which the child was not attending. In addition, the mothers used fewer specific object labels and more general terms, such as pronouns and general nouns, when talking to their children. Maternal speech was assessed when the children were approximately 16 months old, a point at which none of the children was producing any stable words; children's speech was assessed at approximately 24 months in terms of mean length of utterance (MLU), length of longest utterances, and total number of different words produced.

The transition to syntax

The approach sketched so far, which implies assigning to the social and linguistic activity the same *constitutive* status assigned by Piaget to the child's actions on a primarily nonsocial world, has proved to be productive also as far as later linguistic development is concerned. This approach helps us to overcome the reification expressed in views that argue that language exists "out there" and is acquired by the child in the form of linguistic knowledge. Furthermore, it stresses the active role that the child plays in interactively shaping his or her language, as opposed to portraying the child as a passive learner of a linguistic rule system.

In the foregoing we have tried to argue that the child's first words cannot be interpreted as nouns in the proper sense (i.e., instantiations of object reference) as far as they appear to be linguistic procedures used to refer to the whole or to aspects of the interactional situations in which they were produced. Moreover, these linguistic procedures are seen to correspond quite often to segments of the adult discourse used in the same interactional situations. This amounts to saying that, in order to analyze and interpret the child's first linguistic utterances (words and sentences) correctly, we should adopt linguistic models whose unit of analysis is not the single utterance or word but the *dialogue* – that is, an interactional unit that takes into account the contribution of at least two interlocutors. Following this proposal, De Lemos (1985) has shown the fundamental role of imitation both in dialogue construction and in the emergence of syntax. Immediate and deferred imitation of the interlocutor's preceding dialogue turn (or part of it) is in fact one of the processes that govern not only the construction of child–adult dialogue but also the construction by the child of his or her early linguistic combinations.

As one can see in Examples A and B (see Table 4.2), the child's linguistic contribution to the dialogue consists in answering by incorpor-

Table 4.2. *Examples of one-word utterances and early multiword utterances in child–adult dialogue*

A. L. (1;7), *at the end of a meal, still sitting on his high chair, turns a bit agitated:*
    M: Do you want to get down? Get down?
    L: *Want* ↓
    M: Do you want to get down?
    L: *Get down* ↓ *Get down* ↓

B. L. (1;7), *again on his high chair, ten minutes after the previous episode:*
    L: *Get down* ↓ *Get down* ↓
    M: Do you want to get down?
    L: *Want* ↓

C. L. (1;9), *sits on the floor near his toys:*
    M: Are you going to play?
    L: *Hum* ↑
    M: Hum?
    L: *Play*
    M: What are you going to play at?
    L: *Play* ↓
    M: Play at what?
    L: *Baby* ↓ *Baby* ↓
    M: Baby? Ahn?
    L: *Baby play* ↓
    M: Baby is going to play?
    L: *Yes* ↓ *Baby play* ↓

Source: De Lemos, 1985

ating different parts of his mother's turns (immediate imitation in Example A) or in starting again the dialogue by means of an utterance that can be seen as the partial uptake of the mother's utterance in the same interactional situation (deferred imitation in Example B). It is worth stressing here, relative to both examples, that such an imitation process accounts not only for the child's utterances but also for the adult's. Indeed, both partners take turns in the dialogue by incorporating – either completely or partly – the interlocutor's preceding utterance, thus creating cohesion and maintaining the dialogue through reciprocal imitation. Furthermore, Example C shows that the first multiword utterance (*baby play*) can be described as resulting from the child's uptake of part of the preceding adult utterance (*play*), a topic to which he adds, as a sort of comment, a linguistic segment (*baby*) whose origin can be explained by the process of deferred imitation mentioned previously.

Along these lines several psycholinguists (Ochs, Schieffelin, & Platt, 1979; Scollon, 1979; Shugar, 1978) have advanced the hypothesis that a "vertical syntax," or interturn constructions (where the utterance is constructed through the contribution of different interlocutor's turns), precedes and determines the emergence of a "horizontal syntax" or intraturn constructions (where the utterance is constructed within the same interlocutor's turn).

In sum, "by incorporating the adult's role and the roles assigned to him or her by the adult's utterance in particular situations, the child gradually becomes able to construct her/himself and the Other as interlocutors, at first at an empirical level, and later at a representational level" (De Lemos, 1985, pp. 26–27). "At a representational level" means that he will no longer rely on actual and/or preceding utterances but rather on presuppositions about his interlocutor's intentions and beliefs in a specific situation.

For example, a young girl (cf. De Castro Campos & De Lemos, 1979) was involved for a long time in dialogues with her mother during meals, which were variations on the following pattern:

M: Finish X (for example, orange juice, milk, etc.).
C: No.
M: Why?
C: Because Y.

Around her fourth year of age, she produced complex utterances such as the following:

C: Mommy, I won't drink my orange juice because when I drink, it burns here (pointing to her throat).

In this example the child is constructing her explicative utterance not only on her mother's previous turn or action but on an implicit or presupposed request. Most of the instances of this type of explicative utterance have as a first clause a *negative sentence*, by which the child states her refusal to comply with an action her mother expected her to do (such as drinking the orange juice), followed by a *because clause* that provides justification the child presupposes the mother would request upon her refusal. Thus, what was previously explicit through four dialogical turns becomes the presuppositional and propositional content of only one complex utterance.

Further evidence for the importance of these interturn constructions leading to intraturn constructions can be found in R. Clark's work on imitation in morphosyntactic development (1977) and in Ochs's work (1977) on what she called repetition in children's as well as in adults' dialogues.

From the previous discussion about the child's incorporation of the adult's role and of the adult's expectations of the child's behavior, De Lemos concludes that "*sharing a linguistic object* is equivalent to integrating and coordinating perspectives on the world" (1985, p. 30). One could say indeed that the meaning of a linguistic unit is not already given or constituted but, as a product of a past interactional history, is open to potential redefinition and redetermination.

Conclusions

In summary, two developmental transitions have been described and discussed in the previous sections. Whereas in the first 6 months of life the topic of parent–child communication is almost exclusively the interaction per se, in the second half of the first year of life infants begin to reference objects and events that lie beyond the boundary of interpersonal involvement. Parallel to this shift from person-focused interchanges toward increasingly object-focused exchanges and "standard action formats" is the child's gradual transition from the sole use of literal acts to the performance of conventional acts (gestures and words).

I have argued, along with several authors, that it is wrong to conceive these phenomena as individual abilities to be attributed to the infant, and that they should instead be seen as *socially constituted*. Furthermore, I have tried to show how a "social constructivist" perspective on the acquisition of meaning and symbolic means of communication by children can be used as a fruitful research strategy in the study of early linguistic combinations and complex utterances.

The hypothesis that the intersubjective processes of constituting "shared objects" – involved in reciprocal imitation, conventional games, and dialogue – play a definite role in the intrasubjective process of building up utterances could be correctly related to Vygotsky's claim (1962) on intrapsychic functioning as derived from interpsychic functioning.

With respect to methodological choices, the approach to the transition from communication to language I have sustained so far calls for the adoption of the following three criteria in research design:

1. use of a longitudinal design, which allows us to trace the development of prelinguistic interactive patterns to the point where they become linguistic exchanges;
2. use of a structured joint activity as a research setting. Such situations may be naturally occurring or may involve the imposition of mild experimental constraints on naturally occurring situations;
3. collection of data from both participants in the selected joint activity and interactive analyses of those data.

REFERENCES

Bakeman, R., & Adamson, L. B. (1986). Infants' conventionalized acts: Gestures and words with mothers and peers. *Infant Behavior and Development, 9*, 215–230.

Bruner, J. S. (1983). *Child's talk: Learning to use language.* Oxford: Oxford University Press.

Bullowa, M. (1976). From non-verbal communication to language. *International Journal of Psycholinguistics, 3*.

Camaioni, L. (1986, April 10–13). *Imitative interactions and communicative development in the first two years of life.* Paper presented at the Fifth Biennial Conference on Infant Studies, Los Angeles.

Camaioni, L., De Castro Campos, M. F. P., & De Lemos, C. T. G. (1984). On the failure of the interactionist paradigm in language acquisition: A reevaluation. In W. Doise & A. Palmonari (Eds.), *Social interaction in individual development* (pp. 93–106). Cambridge: Cambridge University Press.

Camaioni, L., & Laicardi, C. (1985). Early social games and the acquisition of language. *British Journal of Developmental Psychology, 3*, 31–39.

Chomsky, N. (1968). *Language and mind.* New York: Harcourt, Brace & World.

Clark, R. (1977). What's the use of imitation. *Journal of Child Language, 4*, 341–359.

Collis, G. M., & Schaffer, H. R. (1975). Synchronization of visual attention in mother–infant pairs. *Journal of Child Psychology and Psychiatry, 16*, 315–320.

De Castro Campos, M. F., & De Lemos, C. (1979). *Pragmatic routes and the development of causal expressions.* Paper presented at the Child Language Seminar, NIAS, Wassemaar.

De Lemos, C. (1985). On specularity as a constitutive process in dialogue and language acquisition. In L. Camaioni & C. De Lemos (Eds.), *Questions on social explanation: Piagetian themes reconsidered* (pp. 23–31). Amsterdam: John Benjamins.

Freedle, R., & Lewis, M. (1977). Prelinguistic conversation. In M. Lewis & L. Rosenblum (Eds.), *Interaction, conversation and the development of language* (pp. 157–185). New York: Wiley.

Furrow, D., & Nelson, K. (1984). Environmental correlates of individual differences in language acquisition. *Journal of Child Language, 11*, 523–534.

Gleitman, L. R., Newport, E. L., & Gleitman, H. (1984). The current status of motherese hypothesis. *Journal of Child Language, 11*, 43–79.

Harris, M., Jones, D., Brookes, S., & Grant, J. (1986). Relations between the non-verbal context of maternal speech and rate of language development. *British Journal of Developmental Psychology, 4*, 261–268.

Kaye, K. (1977). Toward the origin of dialogue. In H. R. Schaffer (Ed.), *Studies in mother–infant interaction* (pp. 89–117). London: Academic Press.

Kaye, K. (1982). *The mental and social life of babies.* Chicago: University of Chicago Press.

Masur, E. F. (1984). *Imitative interchanges during natural mother–infant interactions.* Poster presented at the Fourth International Conference on Infant Studies, New York.

Nelson, K. (1973). Structure and strategy in learning to talk. *Monographs of the Society for Research in Child Development, 38* (1–2, Serial No. 149).

Newson, J. (1977). An intersubjective approach to the systematic description of mother–infant interaction. In H. R. Schaffer (Ed.), *Studies in mother–infant interaction* (pp. 47–61). London: Academic Press.

Ninio, A., & Bruner, J. S. (1978). The achievement of antecedents of labelling. *Journal of Child Language, 5,* 1–15.

Ochs, E. (1977). Making it last: Repetition in children's discourse. In S. Erwin-Tripp & C. Mitchell Kernan (Eds.), *Child discourse* (pp. 125–138). New York: Academic Press.

Ochs, E., Schieffelin, B. B., & Platt, M. L. (1979). Propositions across utterances and speakers. In E. Ochs & B. B. Schieffelin (Eds.), *Developmental pragmatics* (pp. 251–267). New York: Academic Press.

Pawlby, S. J. (1977). Imitative interaction. In H. R. Schaffer (Ed.), *Studies in mother–infant interaction* (pp. 203–226). London: Academic Press.

Ratner, N., & Bruner, J. S. (1978). Games, social exchange and the acquisition of language. *Journal of Child Language, 5,* 391–402.

Schaffer, H. R. (1984). *The child's entry into a social world.* London: Academic Press.

Schaffer, H. R., Collis, G. M., Parsons, G. (1977). Vocal interchange and visual regard in verbal and preverbal children. In H. R. Schaffer (Ed.), *Studies in mother–infant interaction* (pp. 291–324). London: Academic Press.

Schaffer, H. R., Crook, C. K. (1978). The role of the mother in early social development. In H. McGurk (Ed.), *Issues in childhood social development* (pp. 55–78). Cambridge: Methuen.

Scollon, R. (1979). A real early stage: An unzippered condensation of a dissertation on child language. In E. Ochs & B. B. Schieffelin (Eds.), *Developmental pragmatics* (pp. 215–227). New York: Academic Press.

Shatz, M. (1983). Communication. In J. Flavell & E. Markman (Eds.), *Handbook of child psychology: Vol. 3. Cognitive development* (P. Mussen, Gen. Ed.) (4th ed., pp. 841–883). New York: Wiley.

Shugar, G. (1978). Text analysis as an approach to the study of early linguistic operations. In N. Waterson & C. Snow (Eds.), *The development of communication* (pp. 227–251). New York: Wiley.

Smith, C. B., Adamson, L. B., & Bakeman, R. (1986). *Interactional predictors of early language.* Paper presented at the Fifth Biennial Conference on Infant Studies, Los Angeles.

Stern, D. N. (1974). Mother and infant at play: The dyadic interaction involving facial, vocal and gaze behaviors. In M. Lewis & L. Rosenblum (Eds.), *The effect of the infant on its caregiver.* New York: Wiley.

Stern, D. N. (1977). *The first relationship: Infant and mother.* London: Fontana-Open.

Trevarthen, C. (1977). Descriptive analysis of infant communicative behavior. In H. R. Schaffer (Ed.), *Studies in mother–infant interaction* (pp. 227–270). London: Academic Press.

Uzgiris, I. (1984). Imitation in infancy: Its interpersonal aspects. In M. Perlmutter (Ed.), *The Minnesota Symposium on Child Psychology* (Vol. 17, pp. 1–32). Hillsdale, NJ: Erlbaum.

Vygotsky, L. S. (1962). *Thought and language.* Cambridge: MIT Press.

5 The transition from spoken to written language

PETER BRYANT AND JESUS ALEGRIA

The main purpose of developmental studies is to establish the causes of changes that intervene with age. The main question is why an organism moves from one state to a different one. Answering this question consists of describing in a precise way the causal transitional mechanisms underlying the observed change. Two of the most commonly used methods by researchers in this area are the longitudinal-correlational approach and the training approach. The aim of this essay is essentially methodological. We would like to discuss the strengths and the weaknesses of each of these two methods in the study of causes of development. The conclusion will be that neither one on its own is ever going to be adequate, but a combination of the two methods can produce convincing evidence for a causal explanation of transitions. Although our claim is a general one, we are going to discuss it using a concrete example: the transition from just speaking and understanding the language to reading and writing it as well.

In fact, our scope will be even more restricted than that because we want to confine ourselves to the relationships between the awareness of the sound structure of speech – sometimes called phonological awareness – and the process of learning to read. The term *phonological awareness* is very general. It covers abilities like splitting a word into component syllables, and syllables into segments, as well as recognizing that different words have sounds in common (e.g., that "cat" and "hat" rhyme). Some of these activities are a great deal easier than others, and there could also be differences in their relation to reading. It has been clearly demonstrated that there is a positive correlation between phonological awareness and learning to read – the greater the child's ability to manipulate sublexical units of speech, the better he or she will learn to read. It is not at all surprising that relationships of this sort should exist. After all, the alphabet works by breaking words up into individual sounds that are represented by letters, and it is a fair bet that anyone trying to come to grips with the alphabetic code must in some way understand how words are made up of different sounds. Although there is no controversy about its existence, there is a great deal of disagreement about what is cause and what is effect here. Some psychologists argue that phonological awareness precedes reading and partly determines how well children do read. Others look on this form of awareness as the product of learning to read. Because these are the two possibilities we shall consider throughout this chapter, we will give them names and initials. We shall call the first idea phonological awareness to reading (PA to R) and the second reading to phonological awareness (R to PA).

Let us consider briefly the way in which a longitudinal-correlational approach can help us in understanding the causal structure of the relationship between phonological awareness and reading acquisition. Its strength is that it can establish a definite relationship between the two (or more) variables. Its weakness is that one cannot be sure that the relationship is genuinely causal. However strongly both variables correlate, there is still the possibility that both could be determined by some unknown and therefore unmeasured *tertium quid*. Suppose that we were to find that some measure of awareness of speech sounds were shown to predict children's success in reading. We could not say on the basis of just this result that the former determines the latter. There may be some more general linguistic or cognitive factor that determines both these things. Of course, every attempt should be made to rule out such factors. For example longitudinal studies should all include measures of IQ and control for IQ levels in multiple regressions. Without such controls for IQ, one could not rule out the plausible hypothesis that psychometric intelligence determines both phonological awareness and reading, and that neither of these two specific skills affects the other. Many of the available predictive studies do control for intelligence, and some have controlled for verbal skills as well (Bradley & Bryant, 1983; Lundberg, Olofsson, & Wall, 1980). But one still cannot be sure even here that there is no unknown factor at work.

The second method frequently used by developmental psychologists to explore causal transitional mechanisms involves training studies. This approach is characterized by a quite different combination of strengths and weaknesses. The main strength of a training study is that it does establish a cause. It does so because it involves the experimental method, the main purpose of which is to establish causes by comparing different experimental conditions. If, for example, you train some children in phonological awareness and you add a control group of other children who are given exactly equivalent experiences except that these do not involve phonological teaching, and if you then find that the first group makes more progress in reading, you can be sure that in this case phonological awareness has had an effect on reading. However, there is a weakness here too. Training studies can be artificial. It may be that you get an effect that has no relationship with what happens normally. There is no guarantee that the experimental condition that has produced a change is related to the child's experiences in real life. An example that comes easily to mind is the history of the study of conservation, Piaget's most famous experiment. There have been many successes in training children to succeed in the conservation task, and almost as many different methods. Perhaps there is some common link between them all, but they are so heterogeneous that it seems unlikely. Many of the experimental successes in prompting conservation may have little to do with the experiences that normally lead a child to be able eventually to solve the problem.

We do not describe the weaknesses (as well as the strengths) of these two methods in order to argue that one should not use them. On the contrary, we think that both should be used, but in combination with each other. Our point is that the strengths of each method cancel out the weaknesses of the other. Longitudinal studies can establish relationships that really do exist in real life, and that is exactly what the training study fails to do. The training study shows that a relationship is definitely causal, and thus fills the main gap left by any longitudinal study. Together, the two methods are capable of giving us a really convincing answer to a causal question. We agree that this is the only convincing way to establish causal links.

In the following sections we are first going to examine the empirical evidence collected in a purely correlational perspective. The purpose of these studies was to investigate the development of phonological awareness and its relations with reading acquisition. It is argued that they merely demonstrate the existence of a relation between the two variables. Then we examine the studies done using a training procedure directly designed to test the causal nature of this relation. Finally we discuss the way in which the combination of both methods has helped us to disentangle the problem of the relationships between phonological awareness and reading acquisition, and the more general scope of our methodological claim, which concerns conceiving longitudinal experiments and interpreting their results in causal terms.

Correlational studies

Part of the studies revised in this section were, in a more or less explicit way, set up to test the hypothesis that phonological awareness causes reading acquisition. As noted before, correlational studies cannot on their own establish causes. They can however suggest them and, as we will argue, phonological awareness is probably not a unitary construct but has different aspects and some of them look like causes of reading acquisition whereas others seem to result from it.

To examine phonological awareness in children, researchers have devised numerous experimental situations, their common point being that all of them need to perform explicit operations with sublexical units of speech. The experiments discussed in this section will be grouped as a function of the experimental task.

One-to-one correspondence tasks

Liberman, Shankweiler, Fischer, and Carter (1974) devised the now well-known tapping task. Children aged 4, 5, and 6 years had to segment words by tapping out the segments with a wooden dowel. They had to tap once either for each syllable in a word ("popsicle" = 3 taps), or for each phoneme ("toy" = 3 taps). The children did well in the syllable task. The phoneme task, in contrast, was more difficult for them: only 17% of the 5- and 70% of the 6-year-olds reached criterion and the 4-year-olds could not manage the task. After 1 or 2 years, many of the children were given a standardized test of reading, which showed that those who had most difficulty with the phoneme task had also made least progress in reading. The authors concluded that there was a relationship between phonological awareness and reading. They admit, however, that nothing in the results allowed one to establish the direction of cause and effect. They pointed out that the rapid growth of performance in the phoneme task between 5 and 6 years could be the result of reading instruction, but that it could equally be "a manifestation of some kind of intellectual maturation" (Liberman, Shankweiler, Liberman, Fowler, & Fischer, 1977).

Tunmer and Nesdale (1985) later confirmed the relationship between phoneme-tapping and reading. They asked 6-year-old children to tap out the sounds in words that either contained digraphs or did not. The children's success with digraph words was related to their reading, even after differences in verbal skills (as measured by a vocabulary test) were controlled. In the same study, the authors compared segmentation of words and pseudowords that either contained single-phoneme vowel sounds normally represented by digraphs (e.g., "-ee," "-oo") or did not. If children use spelling knowledge to help them in the phonemic segmentation task, they may make "overshoot errors" (i.e., extra taps) on the vowel digraph words. This was what happened.

In much the same way, Ehri and Wilce (1980) suggested that we should hear the same number of sounds in a word like "pitch" as in a word like "rich," unless we use our knowledge of the words' different spelling patterns. They asked 9- and 10-year-old children who have been taught to read and write to segment pairs of such words ("pitch," "rich," "new," and "do") into phonemes using counters and also to spell the words. The children gave an extra tap in over half of the words with extra letters, and in hardly any of the words without extra letters. Ehri and Wilce showed that much the same pattern occurred in another task in which pseudowords were used and children had been taught to spell these either with or without an extra letter. It seems that children rely on the spelling of words in phonemic segmentation tasks. The procedure used by the children to segment the items was clearly dependent on spelling knowledge, so it has developed necessarily after reading acquisition. This does not imply that the spelling-dependent procedure is the only available one. It could be that it is the most efficient or the easiest for those who have learned to read and write but that kindergartners can use a different one. The attempts to submit the task to children before they can read have been unsuccessful (Liberman et al., 1974). Thus, the tapping task seems to involve a sort of phonological awareness that develops after reading acquisition.

Reversal and transposition tasks

Another way to test these children's awareness of speech sounds is to ask them to put these sounds into a different order than the one presented by the experimenter. Lundberg et al. (1980) in a longitudinal study, asked 6-year-old children to say particular words backward and then tested the children's reading later (it must be said that in Sweden, where the experiment took place, formal reading instruction began at 7 years). The reversal task was a good predictor of reading. Here is evidence of a prereading skill that could be causal. However, one cannot rule out the possibility of both skills being determined by some unknown third factor that accounts for the relation between them.

 Alegria, Pignot, and Morais (1982) used this kind of task with children aged 6 and 7 years, half of whom were taught at school by a phonic method; the other half were taught with the "whole-word method," in which little attention is paid to speech segments. In three different tasks, the children had to reverse the order of two words, of two syllables, and of two phonemes. The children taught by the whole-word method did badly in the phoneme reversal task, and a great deal worse than those taught by phonics. The two groups were at roughly the same level in the syllable reversal task. Like the study of Lundberg et al. this study showed a high correlation between the phoneme reversal task and the teachers' evaluation of reading but in the phonics group only, not in the whole-word group.

The authors conclude that their results support the notion of a "reciprocal relation between reading instruction (in an alphabetic system) and awareness of phones" (p. 454). Both groups were learning to read and so reading on its own cannot explain the difference between the groups in the phoneme task. The results are in accordance with the notion that developing an awareness of phonemes needs some external intervention, like the one given by phonic reading instruction. We shall return to this problem later in the chapter.

Segmentation and blending

Another way of getting at phonological awareness is to ask people either to break words up into their sounds ("cat" to /c-a-t/) or to form words from those sounds (/c-a-t/ to "cat"). Fox and Routh (1975) devised a version of this task that proved suitable for young children. They asked 3- to 7-year-olds to identify the first word in a sentence ("Peter" out of "Peter jumps"), the first syllable in a word ("Pete" in "Peter"), and the first phoneme in a syllable (/pe/ in "Pete"). The first two of these tasks were easy whereas the phoneme task was difficult. However the 3-year-olds were right 25% of the time, and by the age of 6 the children were right all the time. The syllable and phoneme segmentation measures were significantly correlated with reading, but again this tells us nothing about the direction of cause and effect.

The success of the preschool children in Fox and Routh's segmentation task was surprising because its structure was similar to the tapping task, which was almost impossible for them. The results can be explained by the fact that they only had to identify the first part of the experimenter's utterance. Content, Kolinsky, Morais, and Bertelson (1986) have recently shown that it is relatively easy to have preschoolers cut out the final segment of an utterance just by giving them a corrective feedback at each trial. They argue that this can be done using a strategy that does not involve dealing with phonemes.

Share, Jorm, Maclean, and Matthews (1984) studied 543 children who were seen initially at 5 years and who were seen again when they were 6 and 7 years. At 5 they had to divide words into either two segments /c-at/ or into three /c-a-t/. This test turned out to be the strongest predictor of reading skills over the following two years, and even stronger than the vocabulary scores. However, it is not clear from their report whether the relationship between segmentation and reading was still significant after verbal skills (IQ scores were not available) were partialled out.

Lundberg, Olofsson, and Wall (1980) did control for differences both in nonverbal IQ and in language skills. They looked at segmenting and blending in preschool children and then at their reading and spelling in their first and second years at school. The reading scores were best predicted by the children's previous success at phoneme manipulation. The correlation between preschool scores in these tasks and later reading varied between .45 and .55. The correlation between other tasks, such as syllabic manipulation and rhyming and reading, never reached a value greater than .33.

There is also evidence about children who are at school already. Perfetti, Beck, and Hughes (1981) (summarized by Perfetti [1985]) examined the relationship between these skills and reading in children who were taught either by the whole-word method of teaching or by the "phonics method." They measured the children's ability to blend and segment before they began to learn to read, blending by the synthesis of isolated sounds into a word (e.g., /c-a-t/ to "cat") and segmentation by Liberman et al.'s (1974) tapping task, and a phoneme deletion task (e.g., "Cat without the /t/ leaves what?"). The children were given these tests on four different occasions at intervals of two months and their progress in reading was monitored each time as well.

They showed that blending predicted later reading both in children taught phonically and in those taught by the whole-word method. However, the teaching method was relevant to the segmentation scores. For the phonic group early reading predicted segmentation skills, which in turn predicted later reading ability. In contrast, there was no such relationship in the whole-word group. They concluded that blending skills affect reading: "Success at reading depends on it" (p. 45). Segmentation skills, on the other hand, are affected by the experience of learning to read. "It is reading itself . . . that enables the children to be able to analyse words and to manipulate their segments" (p. 46). The relationship between blending and later reading cannot be used to conclude anything about causes because potential *tertium quids* may not have been excluded. However, these differences between children taught with different methods, together with the results of Alegria et al. (1982), demonstrate that we should take into account not only the child's abilities but also the ways in which he or she is being taught to use them.

Deletion task

In deletion and elision tasks, children have to work out how a word would sound if a particular phoneme were removed. Bruce (1964) devised the first deletion task. He gave children with mental ages between 5 to 9 years three tasks. In one (jam-am) they had to delete the first sound, in another (snail-sail) the middle sound, and in the third (fork-for) the last sound. These tasks proved to be extremely difficult. The mean scores out of 30 for the 5- and 6-year-old groups were 0.0 and 1.8 respectively. Even the 7-year-olds only managed 8.75. Later, each child was asked to spell some of the words, but no relation was found between spelling and Bruce's tasks.

Rosner and Simon (1971) independently devised a similar test of phonological awareness. They asked children aged from 5 to 11 to delete either the initial, medial, or final consonants or the initial or medial syllables from words (e.g., man-an, desk-deck, belt-bell, carpet-pet, reproduce-reduce, location-lotion). The test was again extremely difficult and nearly impossible for the youngest group. There was a significant relationship between performance on the test and reading, even when IQ was controlled. However, we cannot be sure what was causing what from this correlation.

Finally, it is worth mentioning that dyslexic children from 6 to 9 years old with normal IQ were extremely poor at deleting the first consonant from an utterance (Morais, Cluytens, & Alegria, 1984). However, once again these data do not allow us to tell cause from effect.

Rhyming

A judgment that two words rhyme or that they begin in the same way is a form of analysis of sounds in words. Many children can make good judgments about rhyme and alliteration long before they know how to read. Children's preschool experiences with rhyme might have a direct effect much later on their reading.

In Lundberg et al.'s study, prereading rhyme scores were related to reading 2 years later. Bradley and Bryant (1983) produced a similar result in a 3- to 4-year longitudinal study of 368 children who were first tested on rhyme and alliteration at 4 or 5 years. At this time none of the children could read. These rhyme and alliteration scores strongly predicted reading and spelling 3 to 4 years later when the children were 8 or 9, even after the factors age, IQ, and memory were partially out. The effect was specific to reading: The same scores did not predict the children's mathematical skills.

Ellis and Large (1987) looked at several metalinguistic tasks, including the Bradley and Bryant rhyming and alliteration tests, and at reading and spelling in 40 children over a 3-year period. The children were first seen at age 5, and then at yearly intervals until age 8. When they were 8, the children were divided into three groups: high IQ but poor reading (Group A), high IQ and good reading (Group B), low IQ and poor reading (Group C). The largest difference between Groups A and B was in the rhyme test. Group B children were significantly better than Group A children, in spite of the fact that the two groups were matched on intelligence. The second largest difference between these groups was in the test of rhyme production. So the most striking difference between good and poor readers was in rhyme. Rhyme scores were strongly related to reading in Groups A and C.

A study that does not show a particularly strong relationship between rhyming and reading was done by Stanovich, Cunningham, and Cramer (1984). They gave 6-year-olds several tests of phonological awareness tasks, including two of rhyme. Most of the correlations between the tests were high, but those between rhyme and the other tasks, though positive, were relatively low. The relation between rhyme and scores in a reading test were low. However, as the authors note, there was a ceiling effect in the rhyme scores, and this was probably the reason for the lack of a connection. The important rhyme scores are probably those taken before children go to school. The same explanation can be proposed for the relatively weak correlations between rhyme and reading obtained by Lundberg et al. (1980). Although their subjects were kindergartners when tested for metalinguistic skills, they were 7-year-olds. The rhyming task was probably already too easy for them at this age.

Thus, rhyme comes before reading and predicts it. This skill might reflect the informal experience children have at home, before they go to school, with nursery rhymes and word games. This is an important question because rhyming seems to be one of the most precocious manifestations of phonological awareness. So it is necessary to consider what its origin is.

As far as we know, there is only one empirical study on this matter. Maclean, Bryant, and Bradley (1987) reported some longitudinal data on 66 children from the time that they were 3 years 4 months until they were 4 years 7 months. During that period, the children were given several tests of rhyme and alliteration detection. At the start of the project, the extent of their knowledge of nursery rhymes was measured. Some final measures were taken at the end of this period of early signs of reading. The results suggest a definite environmental influence on this aspect of phonological awareness. There was a strong relationship between the children's knowledge of nursery rhymes and the subsequent development of phonological awareness as measured by tests of alliteration and rhyme detection. This relationship was significant, even after statistical controls were included for the differences in IQ and in the parents' educational level. There was also a connection between the children's knowledge of nursery rhymes at the start of their project and signs of early reading 15 months later.

Furthermore, there was little sign of a difference between children from different social backgrounds on the measure of knowledge of nursery rhymes (once IQ had been controlled). One of the more interesting results of this project was that very nearly all the children knew at least one nursery rhyme.

This connection with nursery rhymes suggests, although it does not prove, a causal connection between experiences children have – presumably at home with their parents – and the growth of phonological awareness. It seems quite possible that the children's ability at rhyming is at least partly determined by the willingness of their parents to interest them in nursery rhymes and other routines that involve rhyme.

Of course, this is still a speculative hypothesis because it is only correlational and thus does not exclude a *tertium quid*. We will have to await the results of an intervention study (Does an increase in experience with nursery rhymes lead to sharper phonological awareness and eventually to better reading?) to be sure of the causal connection. This study is in progress.

Summary of the correlational studies

The research that we have reviewed so far establishes a clear relationship between phonological awareness and reading. Cause and effect, however, are still not clear. The sort of phonological awareness involved in rhyming sensitivity is a precocious one and shows systematic correlations with reading acquisition: On the one hand, children are able to play rhyme and alliteration games before they learn to read; on the other hand, these abilities predict their progress in reading, even when the effects of differences in intelligence have been removed. It also seems that children's very early experiences at home may lead to this particular form of phonological awareness.

The evidence coming from tasks in which the children really have to manipulate single phonemes suggests that only those who have learned to read can do them. With a very small number of exceptions, prereaders are indeed not able to do them. In this case, as in the previous one, a *tertium quid* cannot be excluded, so causation is not established. At this stage, we can only say that there is a connection that looks like a causal one between PA and R, but we are not sure that it is a genuine causal connection, or whether it runs from PA to R or from R to PA.

Training studies

As said before, the correlational evidence alone does not allow one to establish causal relationships between the terms of the correlation. The critical test for the causal hypothesis is the training procedure. Training experiments should include adequate control groups. Training in phonological awareness inevitably involves experiences with factors that have nothing to do with phonological awareness, such as contact with an adult or experience with pictures and books. Control groups are needed to rule out the influence of these extra factors. Unseen control groups are inadequate. In the case of training a child to read, the method used could be critically related to phonological awareness. The particular orthography is also important: Learning to read Chinese logography or alphabetic writing can obviously produce rather different effects on phonological awareness.

There should also be a clear distinction between the independent and the dependent variable. In the case of the PA to R hypothesis, the training should be in phonological awareness (the independent variable) and should not involve reading directly.

Another requirement is that the outcome measures should be a genuine test of the independent variable, either reading or phonological awareness, depending on the hypothesis under scope. For example, tasks such as deciphering nonsense words or associating visual symbols and sounds might be inadequate because these tasks are related to reading by a theory that might be inadequate. Thus, to evaluate the reading abilities of a child in the present context, ordinary tests aimed at establishing reading comprehension have to be used.

Finally, the evaluation of phonological awareness is not a simple matter either. If a very general, and consequently vague definition of phonological awareness was adopted, it does not matter what kind of speech segmentation test is used to evaluate it. But, as we have shown in the correlational part of this essay, some tasks are easier to do than others. Their relationships with phonological awareness have to be clarified in order to understand the meaning of the effects of reading on phonological awareness. We are now going to look at studies done in the PA to R perspective and, then, those in the opposite direction.

Training studies in the PA to R perspective

As far as we know, there have only been two attempts to train phonological awareness on its own and to use realistic reading measures. One was carried out by Olofsson and Lundberg (1985) with a follow-up by Olofsson (1985). It involved 95 children (mean age, 6:11) who were divided into experimental and control groups. The experimental group was trained in rhyming, segmentation, and blending, whereas the control groups either participated in a "nonverbal auditory training programme" or were given "normal Swedish preschool experiences." A year later, the children were given tests of spelling, of silent reading, and of reading irregular words. The results were disappointing. "Great variances, ceiling effects and group heterogeneity created many difficulties" (p. 21). The control group started at a higher reading level than the experimental group of children. The two groups reached much the same level in the posttests. After adjustments were made for initial reading level, the experimental group was significantly better at spelling and reading irregular words, but there were no differences between the groups in silent reading.

The follow-up study by Olofsson (1985) a year later showed some qualitative effects, but no lasting improvement in reading and spelling. He found that most of the experimental group's spelling errors tended to be "rule governed." Even when they made mistakes, they followed rather sophisticated morphophonological rules. In contrast, the controls produced simpler, phonological spellings.

The other study dealt with the categorization of words by sounds (rhyme and alliteration). Bradley and Bryant (1983) took 65 6-year-old children and divided them into four groups. One was trained over a period of 2 years in sound categorization. A second was trained for 1 year in sound categorization, and for the second year both in sound categorization and in relationships between the sounds and the alphabetic letters. A third group was taught to categorize the same words semantically, and the final group was an unseen control. After a year or more, the children were tested for reading, spelling, and mathematics.

The crucial comparison was between the children trained in sound categorization and those trained in semantic categorization. A difference between these two groups would be evidence for a causal link between phonological awareness and reading. The first group was ahead by 3 to 4 months on all the standardized tests of reading and spelling, but there was much error variance and the difference was not significant.

We cannot yet conclude that training in phonological skills has an effect on reading, although combining such training with experience with alphabetic letters does lead to considerable improvements. Training studies are an essential link in the chain of any argument about cause and effect. As far as the role of phonological awareness is concerned, that link is a weak one.

Training studies in the R to PA perspective

The evidence for this hypothesis is generally indirect. Very little of it falls easily into the longitudinal intervention framework that we have used so far and into which the research on the other hypothesis fits so easily. In fact, we can only think of one longitudinal study that looks directly at the possibility that progress in reading predicts the development in phonological awareness, and that is the research by Perfetti (1985) which we have described already.

Training studies are scarce as well, with one notable exception. Members of the Brussels group have pioneered an extreme form of a natural training experiment, in which they compare groups who have learned to read (the taught group) to illiterate (untaught) groups.

The possibility that performance in tasks involving phonetic manipulation is the product of learning to read was studied by Morais, Cary, Alegria, and Bertelson (1979). They compared a group of Portuguese illiterates and other adults of nearly the same age and of the same social origin called ex-illiterates because they had been illiterate but had learned to read in adult literacy programs. There were two tasks. One was to add a sound to a word ("alha^Go"–"palha^Go"), and the other to subtract a sound from a word ("purso"–"urso"). The illiterate group was much worse at this task than the ex-illiterate one. The authors concluded that the ability to manipulate phonetic segments of speech depends to a great extent on the experience of learning to read.

However, it is not certain that the two groups were equivalent in every way apart from reading. That would imply that pure chance determined which adults took the literacy courses and which ones did not. The second worry is that illiterate performance at adding and deleting phonemes was evaluated with pseudowords. The real difficulty for the illiterate people could be not at phonetic manipulation but at dealing with nonsense material. Concerning this last point, it is interesting to mention more recent data comparing illiterates and ex-illiterates (Morais, Bertelson, Cary, & Alegria, 1986). In this work a greater variety of tests was presented to the subjects. The results confirm the previous ones and add that illiterates reached nonnegligible scores in syllables manipulation and in rhyming tasks, some of which involved nonsense material. This indicates that illiterates have specific problems with phonetic segmentation tasks and that the nonsense hypothesis cannot explain their differences with the control group of ex-illiterates.

The claim made by Morais et al. (1979) has received strong support from Read, Zhang, Nie, and Ding (1986), who compared a group of people taught an alphabetic version of written Chinese (Pinyin) with another group who had learned only the traditional Chinese logographic orthography on tasks that were the exact equivalents of Morais et al.'s (1979) tests. The results were strikingly similar to those of Morais et al. The Pinyin group was better in both tasks, and the difference was more pronounced with pseudowords than with real words (93% and 83% correct for real and pseudowords in the Pinyin group and 37% and 21% correct in the nonalphabetic readers group). The nonalphabetic group reached roughly the same level as the Portuguese illiterate group, and the Pinyin group had results similar to those of the ex-illiterate group. The authors' conclusion was that "while the ability to recognise sameness and difference between phonemes within words appears to be a precondition for alphabetic literacy ... the ability to manipulate (add or delete) phonemes within words appears to be a consequence of it."

However, Pinyin was introduced in Chinese schools in the 1940s, and so the non-Pinyin subjects were on the whole older people who had been to school before this time. The discrepancy in the two groups' ages was quite considerable (mean ages of 49 and 33 years). The only remark that can be proposed against this objection is an indirect one. In the latest study involving illiterates (Morais et al., 1986), the authors examined a possible effect of age on segmentation performance. The age of the illiterates varied between 25 and 60 years. The results are totally negative on this matter. So there is no serious reason to believe that the results reported by Read et al. could be explained by the age differences between the groups.

The results of Read et al. have an indirect consequence on the interpretation of the illiterate data. The hypothesis that illiterate and ex-illiterate subjects could differ at a level that is not limited to literacy sounds less plausible after knowing that, as Bertelson (1986) underlines, "logographic literate Chinese are at the same low level as Portuguese illiterates" (pp. 11–12).

The Portuguese illiterates' data, together with the Chinese logographic readers' data, suggest that phonetic manipulation skills do not develop as a consequence of reading acquisition but, more specifically, in the context of alphabetic reading. This is also in agreement with the experiment described before, which compared first graders from classes using whole-word methods to teach reading and classes using phonic ones. The first group conforms to the definition of nonalphabetic readers, whereas the second is a classical alphabetic one. The results showed an important difference between groups at phonetic manipulation. The performance of the whole-word Belgian first graders was in this task comparable with that of illiterates and nonalphabetic Chinese readers. More recent data obtained with whole-word first graders using a wider range of tasks – phonetic and syllabic counting and deleting and rhyming – confirms the previous results (Alegria, Morais, & d'Alimonte, 1987).

It is interesting to add in this context the results obtained by Mann

(1986) with primary school Japanese children. She submitted them to a series of tasks including phonetic counting and phonetic deleting. The prediction that can be derived from the data just reviewed is that these subjects' ability to deal with phonetic segments must be as poor as that showed by illiterates and nonalphabetic readers. The results partially confirm the prediction: First graders were indeed rather poor at phonetic counting and deleting but they reached a relatively high level of perform-ance by the fourth grade. The reason for this is not clear. We can speculate that the Kana syllabary has diacritics that permit readers to distinguish voiced and unvoiced stops. Kana also includes separate characters for some phonetic sounds – vowels and one nasal consonant. Bertelson (1986) has suggested that "the critical experience for reaching segmentation into phonemic units would be exposure to a submorphemic orthography" (instead of phonological orthography). This interpretation is at the present moment ad hoc. It is interesting, however, to mention that in a longitudinal study with whole-word first graders we have also found some modest (but significant) improvement at phonetic deleting and counting tasks (Alegria et al., 1987). Strictly speaking, the chil-dren have not been exposed to an alphabetic writing system – their teacher has not mentioned the existence of phonemes and the class exercises they did consisted of manipulation of words and syllables – but they do face a submorphemic orthography. The fact that they met it in a learning-to-read context, as was the case in the Japanese group tested by Mann, could be critical.

Conclusion

The main aim of the present work was methodological. We have re-viewed some recent work in the area of reading acquisition in order to make a general claim concerning developmental research designed to look for causes of transition. The rationale of our proposition has been exposed in the introduction and it is not necessary to repeat it here. Its basic message is that correlational research (usually but not necessarily longitudinal) is a good way to search for potential factors that determine the transition from one particular state to another one. It cannot, how-ever, demonstrate that the putative factors are really the cause of the transition.

The literature presented in the chapter concerning the correlational evidence gives some good examples. The strong correlations demon-strated between rhyming ability at 4 or 5 years and subsequent success at reading and writing cannot be taken as causal evidence: A unique different factor could indeed determine both abilities, rhyming at 4 and reading some years later. The results showing that only those children who have learned to read are able to perform tasks involving the explicit manipulation of phonetic segments – for example, deleting the initial consonant from an utterance or counting its phonetic elements – do not logically lead to a causal interpretation either. A *tertium quid* could be that both tasks, phonetic segmentation and reading, are difficult tasks requiring a great deal of "psychological maturity," which is ordinarily absent at 5 and present at 7.

The conclusion is that the suggestions from correlational data must be tested by using experimental methods. The presumed cause will become a genuine one if, when experimentally manipulated, it shows the expected influence on the presumed effect. So our general claim would be that the study of transitional mechanisms in psychology, as long as we are concerned by the establishment of causal links, must combine the correlational approach with a training one.

What happens if we apply our methodological proposition to the study of the relationships between phonological awareness and reading? If a confused picture emerges from the analysis, this could be seen as unfavorable for our methodological point. The first thing that emerges from the data examined is that the different ways used to explore phonological awareness in children produce very different results. Some tasks are relatively easy and prereaders were able to deal with them. Others are rather difficult for prereaders. A single phonological ability to manipulate sublexical speech units appears to be too global to be adequate. As a consequence, we cannot expect to find causal links between a concept so widely defined and reading, which is also a complex combination of abilities. As Bertelson (1986) has stated, "only by analyzing both processes into simpler episodes can one hope to reach a level of description at which unidirectional (causal) influences would be found" (p. 11). One of the merits of the approach proposed here is that it has helped to make clear that a deeper, more theoretically motivated analysis is necessary and it points toward some possible paths (e.g., Morais et al., 1987, for a recent attempt in this direction).

A straightforward conclusion from the training studies we have reviewed establishes that the particular form of phonological awareness involved in rhyme precedes and influences a child's progress in the initial stages of learning to read. The kind of phonological awareness involved in tasks asking for the isolation of single phonemes seems to develop after children begin to learn to read in an alphabetic system, and is at least partly dependent on that learning.

It is easy to see a possible reason for the second of these two connections. Learning to read in an alphabetic system involves understanding how letters map into words. This constitutes a great pressure for the child to analyze speech into phonetic or phonemic elements. The connection between rhyming and reading is harder to understand. Rhymes do not deal with single phonemes. To know that "cat" and "mat" rhyme, one has to isolate the "at" sound, which of course involves two phonemes. This raises an awkward question for those who think that rhyme prepares a child for learning about the alphabet. Alphabetic letters represent phonemes, and thus deal with smaller units of sound than those on which rhymes are based. Why then should there be a causal relationship between a preschool child's sensibility to rhyme and reading later on? A possible answer could be that reading, in addition to its phonetic analysis requirements, also involves categorizing words that have the same spelling patterns and the same (rhyming) sounds – like "at" in "cat" and "hat," "aus" in "house" and "mouse," and so forth. It is quite clear that this sort of categorization plays an important part in learning to read, and recent evidence (Goswami, 1986) shows that even children who are only just beginning to learn to read take advantage of these categories by generalizing what they have learned about the spelling pattern of one word to that of another.

So our tentative conclusions about this particular transition are that children acquire one form of phonological awareness – categorizing by rhyme before learning to read; that this helps them come to grips with reading by making it possible for them to build up orderly categories of words that share common spelling patterns; and that the experience of learning about the alphabet makes them aware of single phonemes in words. None of these conclusions would have been possible without the combination of longitudinal and training results, which we consider to be essential in any research on causal mechanisms in development.

REFERENCES

Alegria, J., Morais, J., & D'Alimonte, G. (1987). The development of speech segmentation abilities and reading acquisition in a whole word setting. Unpublished manuscript.

Alegria, J., Pignot, E., & Morais, J. (1982). Phonetic analysis of speech and memory codes in beginning readers. *Memory and Cognition*, *10*, 451–456.

Bertelson, P. The onset of literacy: Liminal remarks. *Cognition*, 1986, *24*, 1–30.

Bradley, L., & Bryant, P. E. (1983). Categorising sounds and learning to read – a causal connection. *Nature*, *301*, 419–421.

Bruce, D. J. (1964). The analysis of word sounds. *British Journal of Educational Psychology*, *34*, 158–170.

Content, A., Kolinsky, R., Morais, J., & Bertelson, P. (1986). Phonemic segmentation in pre-readers. *Journal of Experimental Child Psychology, 42,* 49–72.

Ehri, L. C., & Wilce, L. S. (1980). The influence of orthography on readers' conceptualisation of the phonemic structure of words. *Applied Psycholinguistics, 1,* 371–385.

Ellis, N., & Large, B. (1987). The development of reading: As you seek so shall you find. *British Journal of Psychology, 78,* 1–28.

Fox, B., & Routh, D. K. (1975). Analyzing spoken language into words, syllables and phonemes: A developmental study. *Journal of Psycholinguistic Research, 4,* 331–342.

Goswami, U. (1986). Children's use of analogy in learning to read: A developmental study. *Journal of Experimental Child Psychology, 42,* 73–83.

Liberman, I. Y., Shankweiler, D., Fischer, F. W., & Carter, B. (1974). Explicit syllable and phoneme segmentation in the young child. *Journal of Experimental Child Psychology, 18,* 201–212.

Liberman, I. Y., Shankweiler, D., Liberman, A. M., Fowler, C., & Fischer, F. W. (1977). Phonetic segmentation and recoding in the beginning reader. In A. S. Reber & D. L. Scarborough (Eds.), *Toward a psychology of reading.* New York: Lawrence Erlbaum.

Lundberg, I., Olofsson, A., & Wall, S. (1980). Reading and spelling skills in the first school years predicted from phonemic awareness skills in kindergarten. *Scandinavian Journal of Psychology, 21,* 159–173.

Maclean, M., Bryant, P., & Bradley, L. (1978). Rhymes, nursery rhymes, and reading in early childhood. *Merrill-Palmer Quarterly, 33,* 255–281.

Mann, V. (1986). Phonological awareness: The role of reading experience. *Cognition, 24,* 65–92.

Morais, J., Alegria, J., & Content, A. (1987). The relationships between segmental analysis and alphabetic literacy: An interactive view. *Cahiers de Psychologie Cognitive – European Bulletin of Cognitive Psychology, 7,* 415–438.

Morais, J., Bertelson, P., Cary, L., & Alegria, J. (1986). Literacy training and speech segmentation. *Cognition, 24,* 45–64.

Morais, J., Cary, L., Alegria, J., & Bertelson, P. (1979). Does awareness of speech as a sequence of phones arise spontaneously? *Cognition, 7,* 323–331.

Morais, J., Cluytens, M., & Alegria, J. (1984). Segmentation abilities of dyslexics and normal readers. *Perceptual and Motor Skills, 58,* 221–222.

Olofsson, A. (1985). Effects of phoneme awareness training in kindergarten on the use of spelling-sound rules in Grade 2. In *Phonemic awareness and learning to read: A longitudinal and quasi-experimental study.* Unpublished doctoral dissertation, University of Umeå, Sweden.

Olofsson, A., & Lundberg, I. (1985). Evaluation of long term effects of phonemic awareness training in kindergarten: Illustrations of some methodological problems in evaluation research. *Scandinavian Journal of Psychology, 26,* 21–34.

Perfetti, C. A. (1985). *Reading ability.* Oxford: Oxford University Press.

Perfetti, C., Beck, I., & Hughes, C. (1981, March). *Phonemic knowledge and learning to read.* Paper presented at the meeting of the Society for Research in Child Development, Boston.

Read, C., Zhang, Y., Nie, H., & Ding, B. (1986). The ability to manipulate speech sounds depends on knowing alphabetic reading. *Cognition, 24,* 31–44.

Rosner, J., & Simon, D. P. (1971). *The auditory analysis test: An initial report.*

Pittsburgh: University of Pittsburgh, Learning Research and Development Center.

Share, D. L., Jorm, A. R., Maclean, R., & Matthews, R. (1984). Sources of individual differences in reading acquisition. *Journal of Educational Psychology*, *76*, 1309–1324.

Stanovich, K. E., Cunningham, A. E., & Cramer, B. R. (1984). Assessing phonological awareness in kindergarten children: Issues of task comparability. *Journal of Experimental Child Psychology*, *38*, 175–190.

Tunmer, W. E., & Nesdale, A. R. (1985). Phonemic segmentation skill and beginning reading. *Journal of Educational Psychology*, *77*, 417–427.

III Social and emotional development

6 Social transition in adolescence: a biosocial perspective

HÅKAN STATTIN AND DAVID MAGNUSSON

Introduction

Adolescence is a phase in the life cycle that is associated with reaching sexual and social maturation. At its lower end some measure of puberty can mark the entry into this period, but no definite end point can be established. During this period dramatic shifts occur in different areas: endocrine, bodily, emotional, cognitive, moral, social, and interpersonal. As a primarily social marker of development, adolescence is associated with a number of developmental tasks, such as acquiring an appropriate sex role and identifying oneself as a mature member of society. The person should factually and emotionally establish independence from parents and achieve a sense of autonomy and individuation. New reference groups are formed, mainly through interaction and identification with peers. During this period most teenagers establish their first contacts with the opposite sex.

In psychosocial terms, the period of adolescence can be grossly characterized as a progression from uniform to more differentiated socialization practices and from other- to self-directed action. In the early adolescent years, parents' standards of behavior regarding limit setting, discipline, and privileges are quite similar from one family to another (cf. Frank & Cohen, 1979). Parents primarily exercise a type of authority that requires unidirected respect for and conformity to their standards. Over time, adolescents demand from their parents and are granted more freedom to handle things on their own and to establish a more self-reliant way of living. The disengagement from the dependence on the family normally speeds up in midadolescence.

Age-graded influences

The psychosocial functioning of adolescents is commonly interpreted, directly or indirectly, against the background of "the developmental tasks" that the teenagers encounter or are about to encounter and the

147

factual socializing conditions that prevail at different times in adolescence. Social norms, roles, and social expectancies are intimately connected with chronological age. People behave differently at different ages, and seem quite conscious of whether they are "early," "on time," or "late" with respect to major social life events in the life cycle (Foner, 1975; Jessor & Jessor, 1975; Neugarten & Datan, 1973; Riley, Johnson, & Foner, 1972). Age has been said to be as much a regulator of time as of social behavior. The assumption of a unitary psychosocial development suggests that to each chronological age point there is connected a "social clock" (Neugarten & Datan, 1973) or certain expected developmental tasks and associated social behavior.

Some of these age-related social roles and attached behaviors are formalized in society, expressed as prescribed minimum ages. If the reader were a Swedish citizen, this formalization would constitute a social timetable into adulthood. One starts school when one is 7 and stays there 9 obligatory years. Together with most of one's 16-year-old peers one goes on to the gymnasium and stays there an additional two or three years. Then, if the possibilities are available, one progresses to the university by the age of 18 or 19 at the earliest. A person is treated as a "minor" by society until the age of 15. After 15, the situation changes rapidly. Fifteen years is the age of criminal responsibility. At the age of 15 one is also given the formal right to one's own sexual life. Moreover, the individual, for the first time, is allowed to have an employment, to see action movies and thrillers, to enter some discotheques and dances, and to drive a moped. Family allowances, which have been sent monthly to the adolescent's parents, stop by the age of 16. At the age of 18 one is treated as an adult citizen by the law and is allowed to vote in general elections, enter adult dances, and see "adult movies." At the age of 18 one may also take driving lessons in order to apply for a driver's license.

Most social behaviors are not of this formal type, in terms of being legally endorsed or otherwise regulated. They are of a more informal nature. To take an example from our own research, in a free-response task we asked the girls in our research group, when they were between 14 and 15 years, what benefits, if any, they saw in becoming older. Almost unanimously they looked forward to becoming older. It was obvious that the girls at this age thought being older meant having more legal rights and, generally, more freedom from restrictions. Most of the girls looked forward to gaining entry to age-limited discotheques, to attending cinemas, to driving a moped, to acquiring a driver's license, and to the possibility of earning their own money. Besides, being older meant handling one's own affairs, having more freedom to do as one liked, having more to say about daily routines, and being accepted as an independent person in control of her own fate. Some girls wrote that they wanted to be older because their circle of friends were older, and they wanted to be on equal terms with them. A substantial proportion of the girls mentioned that if they were older, they would be spared their parents' admonitions and be accepted as they were. Finally, a few girls answered that to be older, for them, meant being allowed to have their own children.

The general theoretical consensus is that adolescent transition behavior cannot be disassociated from age-prescribed and age-normative social behaviors at different points in time during adolescence: for example, how society has arranged social activities at different ages, what behavior and transition tasks are typical, what characterizes parent–child relations and peer relations, what conditions prevail for boy–girl contacts. In fact, this view is the common "normal developmental" approach to problem behavior among teenagers. Nevertheless, chronological age, connected with age-appropriate social behavior patterns, is not the only time scale for dealing with the emergence of transition behaviors in normal adolescent development. Research on physical maturity has demonstrated conclusively that the assumption of an age-homogeneous development does not always hold true; hence, chronological age cannot be used as the only meaningful reference scale for development (Goldstein, 1979; Magnusson, 1983; Peskin, 1967; Petersen & Taylor, 1980; Young, 1963). The age-related perspective, which appears to posit a unitary progression through which teenagers change in a similar way across time, might well disguise the existence of quite different developmental paths for subgroups of persons, which would become evident if social transitions were viewed from a maturational timing perspective.

A biosocial approach

The question of how problem behavior arises among teenagers and how these new social behaviors are linked with a "maturity" or a normal developmental view has concerned us for some time (Magnusson, 1988; Magnusson & Stattin, 1982; Magnusson, Stattin, & Allen, 1985; 1986; Stattin & Magnusson, 1988). In view of the empirical findings of quite different gender-linked connections between physical growth and psychosocial functioning, and because our own research up to the present time mainly has dealt with this issue for female development, the following discussion will be limited to the impact of maturational timing on social behavior in adolescent females.

The basic assumption. The major starting point of our research is that physical development is accompanied by changes in social life, such that early biological maturation corresponds to an earlier display of social behaviors that originate in adolescence (Davies, 1977; Dornbusch, Carlsmith, Gross, Martin, Jennings, Rosenberg, & Duke, 1981; Goldberg, Blumberg, & Krieger, 1982; Kiernan, 1977; More, 1953). Consequently, at a given time, individual variations in the adopting of "typical" teenage behaviors can be understood from the point of view of differential biological maturation. Interindividual differences in the engagement in social behaviors to a certain extent indicate that persons enter the normal process of transition into new social patterns at different times.

In another context (Magnusson et al., 1986; Stattin & Magnusson, 1988), we have argued that a match or fit between the social time and the biological time offers the most useful conceptual frame within which to analyze the impact of maturational timing on psychosocial adjustment. The linking of the social life patterns that prevail at different ages to biological maturation provides the frame for understanding *why* differences between early and late maturing girls appear, as well as *which* differences are most likely to occur.

When examining the consequences of the timing of physical growth, the usual period of investigation has been the early teenage years, around ages 12 and 13. A quite reasonable position holds that these years are the time when major psychosocial effects are to be expected, due to the interindividual differences in timing of physical growth that are maximal between early and late developers during these years. For example, between 10 and 13 years the greatest variation occurs in weight among girls, while the ages around 12 and 13 yield the greatest variation in height. Additionally, during the age period, the menarcheal variable is most closely connected with other growth parameters such as breast size and pubic hair (Petersen, 1979). Later, these other growth indicators become increasingly more disconnected with the time of the menarche. There are other reasons, as well, for expecting the major impact of maturity timing in these years. Substantial shifts in intrapsychic organization and gender-linked activities have been attributed to the menarcheal event. Because the early teens is the time when girls normally attain menarche, and the time of the optimal cutting point for differentiating between girls who have passed and girls who have not yet attained menarche, it seems quite reasonable that investigations have been concentrated on these early teenage years.

From the outlook that the consequences of being early versus late maturing vary as a function of age-specific social expectancies, roles, and norms, we arrive at some other conclusions that seldom have been explicated in research on physical growth in females. Acknowledging the fact that there will be changes in self-perceptions of one's maturity status induced by physical maturity in a wide sense in the early teens, and by the menarche in a more narrow perspective, the prospect of transforming changes in self-conception into behavior will vary with the character of the response by the environment.

Uniform social conditions accross families in the early teenage years set limits for the expression of an early physically maturing girl's adult image of herself. If the conditions are similar from one family to another with regard to regulations at home (time to be in at evenings, bedtime, spending money, choices of clothes, etc.), the early developed girl has few possibilities to translate her more physically matured status into more independent forms of activity. More options appear later on when parents generally are prepared to grant their daughters more freedom to handle their daily lives on their own. Then, the early maturing girl may derive advantage from her advanced physical development and may create opportunities to channel her self-conceptions into behavior.

In short, it can be expected that individual differences in the timing of physical maturation have comparatively little impact on social behavior until a certain degree of environmental responsiveness to a girl's physical maturation is at hand. This responsiveness will tend to emerge in mid-adolescence where independence and autonomy, intensive and intimate peer contacts, and the establishment of heterosexual contacts constitute central parts of the daily life of the adolescent girl. Rather than to say that the major behavioral consequences of physical maturity appear when the physical differences among growing girls are at their maximum, at 12 to 13 years of age, the present view suggests that the most differentiation should be sought when the differences among girls, with respect to adopting "teenage-typical" social behaviors and completing major transition tasks of adolescence, are at their maximum in mid-adolescence, not in early adolescence.

A mediating model

So far, the expectancies with regard to the new social behavior that girls establish in midadolescence suggest an association with the biological maturity in girls, such behavior being more prevalent among early physically matured girls than among late matured girls.

However, the empirical evidence of a relationship between the timing of physical growth and acquisition of new social behavior does not necessarily imply a cause–effect relationship, and models attempting to explain the relation between biological change and social development have to go beyond the simple association and reveal the factors that mediate this relationship (Brooks-Gunn & Petersen, 1984; Petersen &

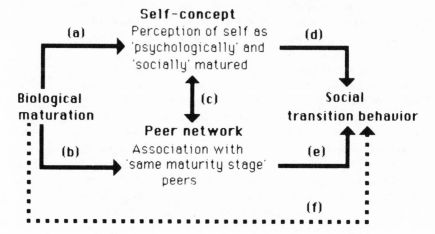

Figure 6.1. A path model for the influence of biological maturation on social transition.

Taylor, 1980; Rossi, 1980). It implies drawing more specific hypotheses regarding the conditions under which the relationship is likely to be manifested and under what conditions its emergence will be less likely.

In concurrence with Petersen and Taylor (1980), we do not think it likely that the direct link between bodily or hormonal changes in girls and social behavior is the principal relationship in development. Rather, the effects of the timing of physical maturity are most likely to be mediated as a consequence of internal and external changes affecting the girl. Elsewhere (Stattin & Magnusson, 1988), we have proposed a general model that delineates changes in four systems: (a) the biological (changes in endocrine and hormonal systems; changes in body shape, height and weight; maturation of reproductive organs); (b) the psychological (perception of self as "psychologically," "socially," and "reproductively" mature; gender identity, sex-role; adult image; concern about autonomy and emancipation; interest in adult-type activities and roles; heterosexual interests); (c) the interpersonal (loosening ties with and less dependence on parents; establishment of heterosexual relations; association with "same maturity stage" peers); and (d) the behavioral (social and emotional adaptation).

The major factors within these four systems, which are thought to be linked to interindividual differences in social behavior among girls in midadolescence, are presented in a path diagram in Figure 6.1. What should be observed is the role supposed to be played by the interpersonal network. In agreement with earlier research emphasizing the role of the interpersonal component in female social identity (Marcia, 1980), it is assumed that peer relations are a critical mediating factor responsible for the association between physical maturity and social behavior. In contrast to popular views that the interpersonal factor works to inhibit problem behavior (Miller, 1979), the model partly suggests the opposite – namely, that the interpersonal relations under certain conditions might act to facilitate breaches of norms.

A comment should be inserted with respect to the paths presented in Figure 6.1. The model proposed should not be considered as a direct, causal, biological model with interindividual differences in social transition being primarily determined by differential physical growth in development. What the model outlines is that, to the extent physical growth is involved in the process of reaching adult status, its role for behavior is seldom direct, but rather indirect. Note that physical growth itself, even though it follows a more or less predetermined course once its onset occurs in individuals, is not independent of experiential factors. *When* pubescence enters is not randomly based. It is connected with general cultural environmental conditions, factors such as nutrition, living standard, and health, as well as with genetic determinants, and specific individual experiences. For example, birth order and the number of siblings have been found to be associated with age of menarche, malnutrition (as evidenced in anorexia nervosa), illness, and intensive athletic activity have been found to delay the entry of puberty. Stress in a wide sense can lower the age at which the puberty sequence starts. Effects of eating habits and sleeping problems at age 8 on the point in time of menarche have been reported. Among nonexercising females, those who reach menarche early are, at the average, heavier than those who reach menarche late. Among exercising females on the elite level, the amount of exercising seems to be a vital factor for when puberty occurs. Studies have been performed investigating the correspondence of menarcheal age between girls and their mothers, as well as between girls and their sisters. Menarcheal age has been studied for monozygotic twins, dizygotic twins, and nonrelated subjects. These studies show that menarcheal age is under genetic influences. There are also seasonal variations with proportionally more girls attaining menarche in spring and summer.

The path in Figure 6.1 is initiated by changes in the biological system. Interindividual differences in the timing of physical maturity are thought to have consequences primarily for (a) the self-system: resulting in differences in perceiving oneself as "psychologically," "socially," and "reproductively" mature; and (b) social network constellations: associations with peers who are congruent with one's biological stage of maturity. The end result of change in these respects is the adopting of behavior

patterns common in these peer networks. Self-perceptions and peer constellations are proposed to connect individual differences in biological
maturation with the individual differences in psychosocial functioning
observed at a certain time in midadolescence. No direct effect of biological maturation on behavior is assumed. Rather, the impact of biological maturation on behavior is indirect, operating through self-perceived
maturity and the peer network.

Self-conceived maturity. Physical maturation has generally been thought to
be connected to changes in self-conceptions. The menarche, concentrated in a discrete point in time, is believed by many to be the critical
event instilling lasting changes in self-definition: a confirmation of self as
a female and as an adult (Deutsch, 1944; Kestenberg, 1961; 1967; 1968;
Koff, Rierdan, & Silverstone, 1978). According to a psychodynamic
position, menarche brings order and consolidation to the feminine identity, a more realistic body image, and better perceptual organization
(Blos, 1962; Hart & Sarnoff, 1971; Kestenberg, 1961; 1967; 1968).

The changes in self-concept that occur at the time of the menarche
should not divert our attention from the changes in self-perceptions that
are linked to physical growth in the broader perspective. Just a cursory
glance at a school age class of teenage girls shows great variations in
physical maturity, with a range of 5 to 6 years between the earliest and
the latest developed girl.

From the point of view of the girl, it is not primarily the fact of being
early or late maturing that determines self-perceptions of maturity.
Reaching puberty at a time when none of one's same-age peers, some of
the peers, or most of the peers have reached this developmental point
means very different things. Accordingly, any attempt to understand the
psychological reaction of a girl to her physical change, as well as its
wider meaning potential, must acknowledge the developmental level of
the peer group at the time the person enters the physical growth acceleration. In essence, the role of physical growth in changes of self-
conceptions has to be conceptualized as a social comparison issue
(Faust, 1960; Weatherley, 1964). The girl compares her physical growth
status against the mainstream of same-age peers, and it is this comparison, by herself and by her peers, that determines changes in perceptions
of the self as female and as a potential grown-up. Brooks-Gunn and
Petersen (1984) have suggested that the perception of pubertal timing
relative to peers might be more influential on psychosocial functioning
than the actual physical developmental status of the girls.

This view implies that the primary instigating factor for a girl's
perception of her "social" and "psychological" maturity relative to the

mainstream of peers is directly related to her pubertal timing. In other words, a positive correlation between actual pubertal age and girls' self-perceptions of their psychosocial maturity is assumed.

Peer networks. From our point of view, social behaviors among teenage girls and the understanding of how the factor of biological maturity enters the process have to be approached from the factual patterns of social behavior that exist in the interpersonal ecology of the girls. From this perspective, biological maturation makes for differential opportunity to experience new social behaviors in the peer group.

The most common friend of a teenage girl is another girl at the same age, who attends the same class or the same grade level in the school. That friendship mainly occurs between girls of the same age in the same school environment has led researchers to believe that same-age–same-school friends cover the important peer reference group. Kandel and Lesser (1972), for example, drew the conclusion that "since all but a small minority of friendships among both American and Danish adolescents are with schoolmates, a description of friendships and peer influences within the school serves adequately as a description of all adolescent friendship groups" (p. 171). The frequent use of class-based measures in sociometric investigations illustrates the same belief: Peer interaction within the class is a valid microcosm of peer interaction generally among teenagers.

However, empirical results from our own research indicate that the same-age–same-school friends of girls do not adequately cover the total or necessarily the most important circle of friends of adolescent girls. A general hypothesis suggesting that girls in the midadolescent years tended to associate with peers who matched their physical developmental stage was posited. For girls who developed physically at a normative rate, the friends within the same-sex–same-school sphere would constitute the "expected" circle of friends. For the early and the late physically developing girls, a somewhat different peer constellation would be discovered.

The early developed girls would seek out and be sought out by others who were congruent with their more advanced stage of biological maturity. Partly, the sense of feeling psychologically and socially more mature than other girls would be a determining factor behind the association and identification with older peers. These peers, chronologically older than the girls themselves, would not necessarily be school pupils. Some of them might have quit school and started to work. In effect, a substantial part of the circle of friends of the early developed girls would be outside the "expected habitat" of the average developed teenage girls.

Finally, the earlier reproductive maturity among the early physically developed girls would make them establish stable relations with members of the opposite sex to a greater extent than did the other, later physically developed girls.

In the association with these peer groups, being more "unconventional" than the friends of the average developers, the early matured girls would encounter the more advanced and more tolerant attitudes toward normbreaking that characterize boys and older groups of teenagers. Through association with them, the early matured girl would adopt the more advanced social life patterns that are common in these peer circles. In short, the advanced social behaviors in these peer groups would have the effect that social behavior originating in adolescence would start earlier among the early developed girls than among later developed girls who had fewer unconventional peers in their circles of friends. Furthermore, the adaptation to social behavior patterns exhibited by older peer groups, at a time when these peers are passing through their most normbreaking intensive period in adolescence, would have as a consequence more frequent involvement in such behaviors generally among early developers than among late.

Finally, the later developers would be less apt than earlier developed girls to acquire sophisticated social life patterns in midadolescence. In the midadolescent years they would be less sought out as friends among older peer groups and be met with more indifferent attitudes among boys. Their less mature status would have the consequence of higher association with chronologically younger peers whose childish social life would function as a retarding factor for engaging in more socially matured forms of activities.

An empirical illustration

As a case of social behavior in which the general model for social transitions among females can be tested empirically, we have chosen to focus on drinking habits. The study of the development of drinking habits among teenagers can serve, in several respects, as a focal point for the study of social transition problems generally. Of particular significance is that alcohol drinking is associated with several, often contrary, cultural messages, with social maturation as well as with social maladaptation. Thus, the study of alcohol drinking offers the opportunity to study a transition behavior that is connected with positive as well as with negative social connotations.

In its normal course adolescent drinking, if not prescribed by society, is a social custom connected with approaching a more mature social life pattern and is generally a component of the "natural" growing-up process. On the other hand, that alcohol use among adolescents is not harmless, but is connected with earlier, concurrent, and later social maladaptation, has much empirical support in the literature. Results have been presented indicating that the adult alcoholic starts drinking at an earlier age than others and drinks more frequently during adolescence than do teenagers in general (Cahalan, Cicin, & Crossley, 1969; Helgasson & Asmundsson, 1975). Furthermore, the heavy drinker and the antisocial teenager tend to be one and the same person (Donovan & Jessor, 1978; Rydelius, 1983; Wechsler & Thum, 1973; Zucker & de Voe, 1975). Aggressive acting out behavior often characterizes the person who abuses alcohol (Andersson & Magnusson, 1985; Jones, 1968; McCord & McCord, 1960; Pulkkinen, 1983). In addition, at least among early adult alcoholics, a history of different kinds of criminal offenses is not uncommon (Helgasson & Asmundsson, 1975; Rydelius, 1983). Besides, the path toward excessive alcohol use is akin to the path toward delinquency (Nylander, 1979).

The following summary points may serve as a basis for testing the biosocial model, which defines the effect of the rate of biological maturation on alcohol use among teenage girls:

First, the basic assumption is that differences in the prevalence and the intensity of drinking among midadolescent girls are partly attributable to the maturity timing of the girls. The ealier the girl is developed physically, the more established alcohol habits she will have in the midadolescent years.

Second, the role of biological maturation in alcohol use among teenage girls is assumed to be mediated through *the girl's perception of her own maturity relative to that of others* – early physically developed girls perceive themselves as more mature and are therefore more prone to engage in a behavior reserved for grown-up persons – and through *the girl's circle of friends*. Girls seek and are sought out as friends by those who match them with respect to physical maturity. Early maturing girls associate more often with older peers and/or working peers and have more established relations with the opposite sex than do the later developing girls. These friends exhibit more advanced social behaviors, including alcohol drinking, than do the more "conventional" friends of the other girls.

To the extent that the proposed developmental path for the effects on alcohol drinking of biological maturation is valid, by the testing of the model, the following assumptions can be formulated:

   a. Biological maturation and self-concept. Compared with late matured girls, early developed girls perceive themselves as more mature than others.

b. Biological maturation and peer network. Early matured girls engage more often with older peers and working peers, and they have established boyfriend relations to a greater extent than other girls.

c. Self-concept and peer network. Girls who perceive themselves as more mature than their classmates associate more often with older peers, working peers, and with boyfriends, and less with younger peers, than do girls who perceive themselves as less mature.

d. Self-concept and social transition. Girls who perceive themselves as more mature than others have more advanced alcohol habits in midadolescence than do girls who perceive themselves as less mature.

e. Peer network and social transition. Girls who engage with older peers, working peers, and with boys have more advanced alcohol habits in midadolescence than girls who lack these peer contacts.

f. Biological maturation and social transition. If the model is valid, little direct effect of biological maturation on social transition behavior should be at hand. The relationship between biological maturation and alcohol drinking is indirect and mediated, operating through the self-concept (Path d) and the properties of the peer network (Path e).

For illustrative purposes, three studies will be presented and discussed. The first study elucidates the connection between biological maturation and individual differences among girls with regard to alcohol habits during adolescence, and the role of peers and girls' self-conceived maturity as mediators. The second study focuses on the role of the socialization agents as norm transmitters for drinking among adolescent girls. Finally, in the third study, a closer investigation is made of the "risk" aspect – the long-term effects on alcohol habits of differential timing of maturation among females.

Subjects and data

The subjects in the present study belong to a cohort that has been followed by repeated data collection from their early school years until adulthood in the longitudinal program "Individual Development and Adjustment (IDA)." They belong to a complete school-grade cohort of girls: all those pupils who in 1970, at the age of 15 years, attended the eighth grade in the elementary schools in a mid-Swedish town of about 100,000 inhabitants.

All types of schooling within the ordinary school system in 1970 were represented. Thus, a very wide range of social and psychological upbringing conditions are included. Studies within the project have shown the group of children to be fairly representative of pupils in the comprehensive school system in Sweden in important variables (Bergman, 1973; Magnusson, Dunér, & Zetterblom, 1975; Stattin, Magnusson, & Reichel, 1986).

The study is based on data for those girls for whom complete data on menarcheal age were obtained through a self-report instrument at the age of 14:10 years (14 years 10 months). To control for factual chronological age, the 466 girls who were born in 1955 were selected. All had moved up to the next class in the ordinary manner from the first grade. An empirical calculation indicated that there were virtually no differences in average chronological age among the 466 girls grouped according to menarcheal age.

Menarcheal age

Age at menarche was measured by an item in a questionnaire, the Adjustment Screening Test. The median age for the self-reported menarche was 12.86 years, which corresponds closely to national figures for the age cohort in question (see Lindgren, 1976). The results presented here are based on a grouping of girls into four menarcheal groups: menarche before the age 'of 11; menarche between 11 and 12 years; menarche between 12 and 13 years; and menarche after age 13. This implies, among other things, that variations in early maturation are better discriminated than variations in late maturation.

No significant correlations with intelligence or socioeconomic status were obtained for the menarcheal variable. This is interesting in itself and it is important for the interpretations of other results presented here.

Perceived maturity

In a pupils' questionnaire at the average age of 14:10 years, the following question was given: "Do you feel more or less mature than your classmates?" The questionnaire included mainly questions concerning peer and parental relations, and no mention was made of physical growth or physical maturity. Again, at the average age of 15:10 years, the same question was asked in a pupils' questionnaire in the ninth grade.

Interpersonal relations

To be able to examine the characteristics of the circle of peers, a specific instrument was developed. It was administered at the average age of 14:6 years. The logic behind the instrument can be described as follows. First, the girls were asked to state the total number of close friends in their peer group. Next, they were asked how many of these friends are younger, the same age, or older than themselves. Finally, they were asked how many of the total number of friends are attending school and how many are employed. Thus, the girls partitioned the total number of friends according to both chronological age and social characteristics.

One question in the Adjustment Screening Test administered at 14:10 years dealt with the girls' present and past relations to boys: "Have you now or have you ever had a steady relationship with a boy?"

Alcohol drinking

Data on alcohol use, in the present case the frequency of drunkenness, were obtained on three occasions in the midadolescent years: at the average age of 14:5 years, at 14:10 years, and at 15:10 years. They were collected from a norm instrument and from the Adjustment Screening Test in the eighth grade and from a pupils' questionnaire in the ninth grade. Subjects' answers were analyzed for how many times they had been drunk on respective occasions. The answers were given on five-point Likert scales with the alternatives: (1) never; (2) once; (3) 2–3 times; (4) 4–10 times; and (5) more than 10 times.

The physical maturity–alcohol pathway

Biological maturation and social transition

Are early established alcohol habits associated with a girl's timing of biological maturation? Figure 6.2 shows the prevalence of drunkenness among girls in the four menarcheal groups at age 14:5 years and the percentage figures for frequent drunkenness (4 times or more). The results show a clear-cut association between the age of biological maturation and having been drunk at least once at 14:5 years. The prevalence of drunkenness was considerably higher among early matured girls than among later matured. More than twice as many girls among the earliest matured had had such experiences than among the girls in the latest developed group of girls. The test of differences in drunkenness among the four menarcheal groups was highly significant ($F = 6.80$; $df = 3,431$; $p < .001$).

The differences among the menarcheal groups of girls were even more marked for frequent drunkenness. The percentage of girls with frequent drunkenness experiences were more than five times higher among the earliest matured girls than among the latest matured. Again, the relationship was statistically significant at a high level ($F = 12.13$; $df = 3,431$; $p < .001$).

An established relationship between the maturational timing of girls and early established alcohol habits raises questions about the sub-

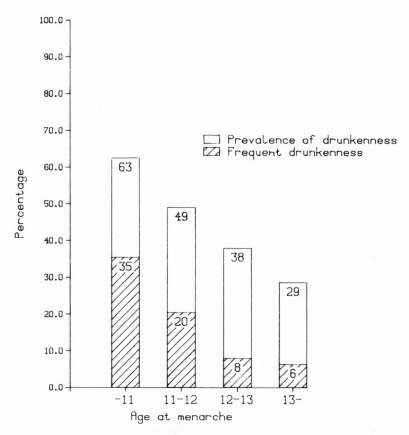

Figure 6.2. Experiences of drunkenness and frequent drunkenness at 14:5 years among girls in four menarcheal groups.

sequent developmental course in the midadolescent years for alcohol use. Therefore, this relationship between biological maturation and alcohol use was compared at the three ages. The prevalence of drunkenness and frequent drunkenness at the respective ages among girls in the four menarcheal groups is presented in Figures 6.3a and b.

In general, there is a steady increase in the prevalence of drunkenness over time. Of particular interest is the inspection of the increase with the passage of time for the four menarcheal groups of girls. For the early developers we witness a ceiling effect. Of the latest developed girls, there was a higher net increase over time for these girls compared with the earlier matured. The "spurt" or the catch-up for the later matured girls is reflected in the statistical tests of significance in drunkenness experi-

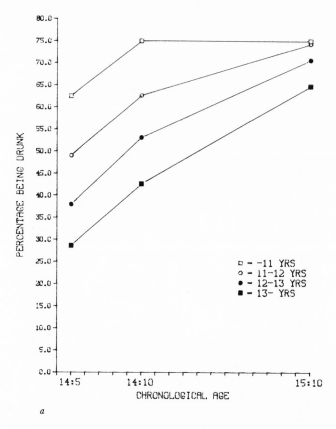

a

Figures 6.3*a* and *b*. The development of alcohol habits in midadolescence among girls in four menarcheal groups.

ences among the four menarcheal groups of girls. At age 14:5 and at age 14:10 years, this difference was significant at the promille level (14:5 years: $\chi^2 = 19.37$, $df = 3$, $p < .001$; 14:10 years: $\chi^2 = 20.75$, $df = 3$, $p < .001$). However, at 15:10 years no statistically significant difference was obtained among the four menarcheal groups of girls ($\chi^2 = 3.26$, $df = 3$, n.s.).

The influence of biological maturation on alcohol habits as determined by the prevalence of drunkenness at the three ages in midadolescence seems to be temporary and restricted to a relatively short period. As a complement to the prevalence figures, data also were analyzed for frequency of drunkenness over the same ages. The catch-up effect among the late developers, observed for drunkenness per se, was not apparent in these analyses. As is depicted in Figure 6.3b, there were clear-cut differ-

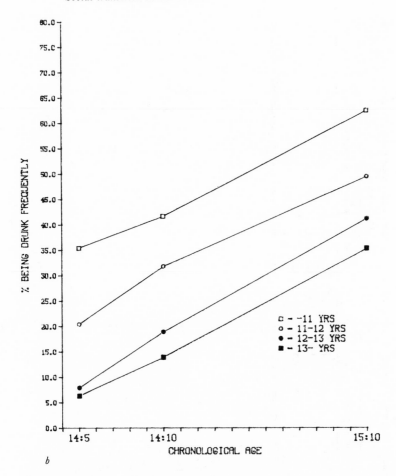

b

ences among the four menarcheal groups of girls at all three age points ($p < .001$ at all age points). The net increase in absolute figures over time was about the same for the four menarcheal groups of girls, implying that the lead that the early matured girls had at 14:5 years was not reduced over time.

Biological maturation and self-concept (Path a)

If physical growth is a quality around which perceived maturity status is organized, and if this self-conception is comparatively based, then we would expect the early developed girls to feel more and the late developed girls to feel less mature than same-age peers in general. This assumption of an intimate link between actual pubertal timing and a

Table 6.1. *Percentage of girls in four menarcheal groups responding to the question "Do you feel yourself more or less mature than your classmate?"*

Age of menarche	Age 14:5 yrs[a]			Age 15:10 yrs[b]		
	More mature	About as mature	Less mature	More mature	About as mature	Less mature
–11	41.7	53.6	2.1	51.3	48.7	0.0
11–12	37.1	60.8	2.1	34.3	62.7	2.9
12–13	20.9	75.7	3.4	20.2	76.3	3.5
13–	16.1	64.3	19.6	16.8	76.5	6.7

[a] χ^2 (6, $N = 434$) = 52.08, $p < .001$.
[b] χ^2 (6, $N = 433$) = 27.91, $p < .001$.

girl's perceived maturity relative to her peers was tested at 14:5 years, and again 17 months later, at 15:10 years. The cross-tabulations of the menarcheal grouping and the perceived maturity measure at these ages are given in Table 6.1.

At 14:5 years, 42% of the earliest matured girls felt themselves to be more mature than their classmates, and only 2% stated that they felt less mature. The situation was quite different among the latest developed girls. Only 16% considered themselves as more mature, and nearly 20% thought of themselves as less mature. The overall relationship between age at menarche and perceived maturity at this age was significant at the .001 level ($\chi^2 = 52.08$; $df = 6$; $p < .001$).

The results of the cross-tabulation at 15:10 years was similar to the connection between menarcheal age and perceived maturity 17 months earlier, and the relationship was significant at a high level of confidence ($\chi^2 = 27.91$; $df = 6$; $p < .001$). They differed in two important respects from the same data at 14:5 years. As might be expected, a lower proportion of the late developed girls rated themselves as less matured at 15:10 years compared with 14:10 years (6.7% vs. 19.6%). This illustrates a catch-up effect among the late developers over time. More unexpected was the finding that an even higher proportion of the earliest developed girls rated themselves as more mature than classmates at 15:10 years (51.3%) than at age 14:5 years (41.7%). From an expected equalization over time, the reversed situation would be the expected.

The data presented in Table 6.1 clearly indicate that girls' conception of their maturity in midadolescence is connected to their physical developmental timing. The apparent differences in perceived maturity are quite noteworthy. At the time the assessment of experienced maturity was made, most of the girls had long since passed their menarche, and most of them had almost reached adult physical status. At the age of 15:10 years just a small percentage of the girls in the research group had not yet had their first menstruation. Thus, the findings presented cannot be attributed to having attained versus not having attained menarche.

Biological maturation and peer network (Path b)

A comparison among the four menarcheal groups of girls, with respect to the character of their peer network, is reported in Tables 6.2 and 6.3. Table 6.2 presents the mean number of friends of different types reported by girls in the four menarcheal groups, and Table 6.3 gives an account of the percentage of girls in respective menarcheal groups who associated with such peers. As can be seen in the first columns in Tables 6.2 and 6.3, almost all the girls stated that they had at least one friend. There is

Table 6.2. *Mean number of friends of various types reported by girls in four menarcheal groups*

Age of menarche	Social characterization			Age of peers		
	Friends total	Friends at school	Employed friends	Younger friends	Same-age friends	Older friends
-11	5.45	3.79	1.36	0.05	2.29	3.05
11–12	4.56	4.18	0.38	0.11	2.89	1.54
12–13	4.76	4.28	0.34	0.30	2.95	1.50
13–	4.25	3.86	0.30	0.23	3.03	0.96
F	2.54	1.17	14.34	2.70	1.89	11.9
p	$< .10$	n.s.	$< .001$	$< .05$	n.s.	$< .001$

Table 6.3. Percentage of girls in four menarcheal groups reporting friends of various types

| Age of menarche | Social characterization | | | Age of peers | | |
	Friends total	Friends at school	Employed friends	Younger friends	Same-age friends	Older friends
–11	100.0	97.6	45.2	4.8	92.9	73.8
11–12	98.9	98.9	21.5	7.5	95.7	55.9
12–13	100.0	98.8	19.5	18.9	96.5	51.5
13–	99.1	99.1	20.4	13.3	94.7	38.9

a tendency, though not significant, that early matured girls reported the highest number of friends and the latest matured group reported the least.

Social characterization. Almost all girls had at least one friend at school, and there were no significant differences among the girls in the four menarcheal groups with respect to the number of schoolmates. A weak curvilinear tendency with the earliest and the latest developed girls reporting fewer school friends could be detected.

Strong significant differences among the menarcheal groups of girls were obtained for employed friends. Twice as many girls among the earliest matured reported that they had working peers as among the other groups of girls. On the average, the earliest matured girls reported that they had four times as many employed friends as did the other girls.

Age of peers. As was expected, most of the friends with whom the girls engaged were same-age peers. Next common were older peers, and more seldom did the girls associate with younger friends. Younger peers in a girl's circle of friends were significantly ($p < .05$) more common among the late developed girls than among the early matured. Of the girls in the two latest developed groups, 16.7% had at least one younger friend, in comparison with 6.7% of the girls in the two earliest developed groups.

No significant differences among the menarcheal groups were obtained with respect to association with same-age peers. A tendency for the earliest developed girls to have a more restricted same-age peer association could be discerned.

In accordance with the hypothesis, there were marked differences among the four menarcheal groups of girls with respect to friendships with chronologically older peers. Almost twice as many of the earliest as compared with the latest matured girls reported that they had at least one older friend, and the number of older friends was three times as many among the earliest matured as among the latest matured girls. It should be observed that the mean number of older peers among the earliest developed girls was *higher* than the mean number of same-age peers, but that the mean number of older friends among other girls was about half the figure for same-age peers.

Opposite sex relations. A detailed account of the girls' steady relations with boys is presented in Table 6.4. Of the latest developed girls, almost half had never had a steady relationship with a boy, and slightly more than 1 of 10 had such a relationship precisely at the time the question was

Table 6.4. *Percentage of girls in four menarcheal groups who have been going steady at the age of 14:5*

Age of menarche	Going steady[a]		
	No	Have been	Are now
−11	17.0	44.7	38.3
11–12	28.6	39.0	32.4
12–13	37.6	41.1	21.0
13–	47.9	40.5	11.6
N	164	186	104
%	36.1	41.0	22.9

[a] χ^2 (6, $N = 454$) = 27.5, $p < .001$.

administered. By contrast, almost 8 of 10 of the earliest matured girls had gone steady with a boy, and close to 4 of 10 had had an established boy–girl relationship when the question was asked at 14:10 years. Steady relationships were not altogether concentrated in the most developed girls. There was a step-by-step increase of such relationships from the latest to the earliest developed girls.

Comments. The data presented in this section show, in a very decisive way, the importance of taking into account the characterization of a girl's peer group when drawing conclusions regarding aspects connected with the peer network between early and late developed girls. When the peers were amalgamated in one heterogeneous group, few differences were obtained between the early and the late matured girls. However, the more fine-grained subsequent analyses revealed marked differences among the girls in the four menarcheal groups, with respect to the type of peers with whom they associated. In accordance with the hypotheses, late matured girls more often associated with younger peers. The early developers were more often engaged with older peers and peers who were already in the labor market. They also had more established relationships with boys than did their late developed counterparts.

Self-concept and peer network (Path c)

As outlined in Table 6.5, girls' concepts of their maturity status were connected with the types of peers in their circles of friends. The girls who felt more mature than others engaged more often with older peers and with working peers, and a higher proportion of these girls had stable

Table 6.5. *Percentage of girls grouped by self-perception of maturity reporting different types of peers in midadolescence*

Perceived maturity	Characteristics of peers			
	Younger peers	Older peers	Working peers	Heterosexual relation
More mature	7.1	69.7	35.4	30.3
About as mature	15.1	46.4	18.1	21.6
Less mature	3.8	34.6	23.1	9.7
χ^2	6.15	18.84	12.16	6.71
df	2	2	2	2
p	< .05	< .001	< .01	< .05

Table 6.6. *Frequency of drunkenness related to perceived maturity among teenage girls*

Experienced maturity	Age 14:5 yrs		Age 15:10 yrs	
	At least once	Frequent	At least once	Frequent
More mature	59.9	28.2	81.9	55.5
About as mature	37.0	10.5	68.4	39.9
Less mature	43.2	5.4	60.0	40.0
χ^2	21.77	28.44	10.76	10.56
df	2	2	2	2
p	< .001	< .001	< .01	< .01

heterosexual relations than did the girls who felt less mature. About twice as many girls who reported that they felt more mature than their classmates had older friends and three times as many of these girls had stable relationships with boys at this age compared with the girls who felt themselves less mature than other girls. Contrary to expectations, however, it was not the girls who conceived of themselves as less mature who associated particularly often with younger peers, but the girls who thought themselves about as mature as their classmates.

Self-concept and social transition (Path d)

That girls' alcohol habits in midadolescence are related to their conceptions of maturity is shown in Table 6.6. The table presents the frequency of drunkenness at 14:4 years of those girls who felt themselves less mature, about as mature, and more mature than their classmates at this age. For comparison, a similar relationship using data collected at 15:10 years is shown.

Girls who felt themselves more mature than girls at 14:5 years engaged more often in alcohol drinking, as measured by the frequency of drunkenness, than did girls who thought themselves about as mature than others or less mature. There was a step-by-step increase in prevalence rate, as well as in frequency of drunkenness, the more mature the girl felt. More than five times as many girls among the girls who declared themselves as more mature had been frequently drunk than had the girls who stated that they felt less mature than other girls.

Also at 15:10 years, girls who reported themselves as more mature engaged more often in alcohol drinking than other girls. At this age, however, few differences in drunkenness frequency appeared between girls who felt themselves about as mature as other classmates and girls

Table 6.7. *Prevalence of drunkenness and frequent drunkenness among girls in midadolescence who associated with or did not associate with peers of different types*

Peer association	Being drunk at least once		Frequent drunkenness	
	%	p	%	p
Older peers				
Yes	50.5	.001	17.5	.01
No	29.8		7.9	
Working peers				
Yes	57.3	.001	22.5	.01
No	35.4		9.9	
Heterosexual relations				
Yes	62.9	.001	28.9	.001
No	34.9		9.2	
Younger peers				
Yes	16.3	.001	2.0	0.5
No	43.9		14.3	

who felt less mature. This finding contributes to the weaker, but still significant, association between perceived maturity and drunkenness at this age, compared with the association 17 months before. Overall, the data attest to more advanced alcohol habits among girls in midadolescence who felt more mature than their classmates in general.

Peer network and social transition (Path e)

Are drinking habits among midadolescent girls related to the type of peers with whom they associate? Table 6.7 gives an account of the frequency of drunkenness among the girls who associated or did not associate with older peers, working peers, and younger peers, respectively, as well as had stable relationships or did not have stable relationships with boys at the time the question on heterosexual contacts was asked.

To engage with older peers and working peers and to have stable heterosexual relations were connected with higher prevalence rates of drunkenness, as well as more frequent alcohol experiences among the research group of girls. Two to three times as many girls who associated with older peers or working peers or were going steady with a boy had been frequently drunk, compared with girls who lacked such peer contacts. By contrast, to associate with younger peers was connected with less experience of alcohol use. The results support the hypothesis of more advanced social behaviors among girls whose circles of friends include "unconventional" peers, and they also support the assumption that association with younger peers functions as a protective factor for engaging in such behaviors.

The mediating model: self-concept and peer network as mediating factors in social transition (Path f)

What remains now is to apply a systematic design for examining the issue of the role of perceived maturity and the peer network as mediators for the association of biological maturation to alcohol drinking. If the hypothesis is correct, that perceived maturity and peer contacts are the principal operating factors mediating the association between biological maturation and drinking behavior in midadolescence, the original differences in frequency of drunkenness among the menarcheal groups of girls should disappear or decrease considerably once these mediating factors are corrected for.

Two questions arise. First, does there remain any significant effect of menarcheal age on frequency of drunkenness once the variation in the dependent variable due to the proposed mediators is eliminated? This is analogous to asking whether there is a hypothesized nonsignificant Path f in Figure 6.1. Our expectations are that much of the original effects of biological maturation on drunkenness frequency in midadolescence should be reduced once corrections have been made for the self-concept and the peer-type measures.

Second, which of the self-concept and the peer-type variables are the potent mediators for the relationship of menarcheal age to frequency of drunkenness?

The issue is one of separating out the influence of menarcheal age on the dependent variable drunkenness going through self-perceived maturity and the peer-type variables, so as to compare the original effect of menarcheal age with the same effect after these intervening factors are brought under control. This general question of how to remove extraneous variance of some variables from the association between the independent and the dependent variable is a difficult one. As has been repeatedly emphasized in statistics textbooks, there are no ideal techniques available for controlling for preexisting differences between groups. Results from such analyses always have to be interpreted with caution.

Given the nonlinear relationships, an analysis of covariance was adopted as the most appropriate method for conducting the control of perceived maturity and the peer-type variables. The specific calculations were performed in the following way:

1. An ordinary ANOVA was initially computed for the subjects with menarcheal age as the independent variable, and frequency of drunkenness as the dependent variable. These calculations were done for the subjects in the research group with *complete* data for self-perceived maturity and the four peer-type variables. They were performed in order to have all calculations to refer to the same individuals so as to have a basis for comparing the F-values in the subsequent covariance analyses.

2. Next, an ANCOVA was computed. It tested if menarcheal age had a statistically significant effect on the drunkenness variable after adjustments had been made for the covariates self-perceived maturity variable and the peer-type variables.

The first issue to be examined is to what extent the original effect of the menarcheal age variable on the drunkenness variable decreased after adjusting for group differences in perceived maturity and associating with the four peer types.

The original differences among the menarcheal groups of girls, which were originally significant at the promille level ($F = 12.56$; $p < .001$), decreased considerably after the introduction of the covariate terms. It was still significant after correcting for the covariates, but now on a much lower magnitude ($F = 2.85$; $p < .05$). So, the present results indicate that the mediation model fits the data quite well as far as drunkenness in midadolescence among teenage girls is concerned.

The model proposed has heretofore been investigated as it relates to the total effect of the self-conception and peer network variables as mediators. All covariates were entered simultaneously into the equation. We now turn to the second question raised: Which of the covariate terms were the most effective ones as mediators for the drunkenness measure? Each one of the five covariates was introduced separately into the equation, with menarcheal age as the independent variable. To identify the covariate that had the greatest mediating potency, we picked out the covariate that, after its effect was separated out, yielded the lowest F-value for the effect of menarcheal age on the dependent variable.

The factor heterosexual relations was the strongest mediator between menarcheal age and drunkenness frequency. If not having its roots precisely in male alcohol habits, female alcohol use seems to be closely connected with associations with the opposite sex. After the single covariate heterosexual relations was introduced, there was a marked reduction in the original effect of menarcheal age ($F = 6.73$; $p < .001$). The result implies that relations to boys in midadolescence explain a large part of the influence of menarcheal age on alcohol drinking.

The reference groups as norm transmitters

A premise in the earlier analyses has been that the differences between early and late developed girls with respect to alcohol drinking have to be viewed in the light of the more advanced social behaviors and leisure-time activities among the friends of the earlier developed girls relative to their later developed counterparts. Against the background of the empirical support for this differential association with peers based upon a girl's biological stage of maturity, it then becomes important to try to illuminate the normative dimensions through which the peer influence is operating. This analysis will not be limited only to peers as norm transmitters. It will also involve an examination of the parental support for alcohol use.

Whether drunkenness among adolescent girls, which is generally recognized as a "problem behavior" and viewed negatively by the adults, can be said to be encouraged by the parents themselves, is an intriguing question. However, the results presented by Stone and Barker (1937; 1939) suggest that girls, through their physical appearance, may change the attitudes of their parents toward greater tolerance for such social behaviors.

The Stone and Barker (1939) data from the "family adjustment" domain support a mutual-reinforcement interpretation of differences in social behavior between pre- and postmenarcheal 12- to 15-year-old girls. The parents gave the postmenarcheal girls more freedom and autonomy to develop their own personal identity and style than did the parents of the premenarcheal girls, who were not allowed as much freedom in deciding on everyday life activities. A greater proportion of the postmenarcheal than of the premenarcheal girls answered affirmatively that they were allowed to stay up late in the evenings, go to parties, have dates and boyfriends, use their spending money as they wished, wear the clothes they liked, wear their hair in the way they wanted, and so forth. On the other hand, the postmenarcheal girls also had more responsibilities, and they reported more often that they had to do more housework than they liked. Indications of parental conflicts occurred more frequently among the early developers. More postmenarcheal than premenarcheal girls felt themselves as a burden to their family and declared more often that they would like to leave home. They complained that their parents teased them about their boyfriends, and they felt embarrassed when their parents bragged about them to other people. They admitted more often than the premenarcheal girls that they concealed their worries and troubles from their parents, had secrets they did not wish adults to know about, and were bothered if their parents wanted to know details of what had happened at parties. Finally, they claimed more freedom.

The premenarcheal girls, by contrast, seemed to have a more sincere and trusting relationship with their parents. A greater proportion of these girls than of the postmenarcheal answered affirmatively that their mother understood them well enough so that they could talk about their problems. Although they were not given as much freedom as the post-menarcheal girls, this did not seem to concern the premenarcheal girls greatly, as they answered more often than their postmenarcheal counterparts that they did not want more freedom and agreed that girls their age should obey their parents.

Together, these results clearly demonstrate that we cannot treat the parents of the early and the late developed girls as a homogeneous group with equal support for the new social behavior patterns that emerge in adolescence. To the extent that we can talk about a faster social development among the early matured girls, we have to acknowledge the possibilities of an analogous "codevelopment" among the parents of the early developed girls.

The literature on adolescent development and problem behavior has until recently been heavily biased toward recognizing the conflicts between networks, such as the generation gap and parent versus peer orientation, to the neglect of the correspondences. Over time the insight has deepened that many of the developmental processes that girls go through in the adolescent years have their counterparts in changes in their immediate environments. Parental permissiveness and privilege giving and the girl's own striving toward adaptation and adoption of new social behavior are often complementary processes over time, rather than solely a source of strife (Bandura, 1972; Steinberg, 1985). Initially, the emancipation on the part of the girl leads to her stumbling; her parents respond by alternatively giving the girl greater privileges and withdrawing them in the fear that the girl is not mature enough to handle her new freedom effectively. The fragile equilibrium proceeds toward greater permissiveness and greater autonomy with the passage of time.

Viewed from this perspective of supporting reference groups, an investigation was designed to examine what feature of peers and parents, as norm transmitters, were involved in the acquisition of alcohol habits among the early and the late developed girls. In the present case, both the perceived *evaluation* of getting drunk among parents and peers and the perceived *sanctions* that the girls expect would emanate from parents and peers, if they found out about the behavior, were investigated. In addition, a closer investigation was made of the *expectancies* the parents were thought to have regarding the girls' alcohol drinking.

The evaluative element of norm transmission concerns the general opinion of the girl getting drunk – whether it is positively or negatively viewed. It reflects the general opinion of drunkenness rather independent of the particular motive forces that appear in concrete everyday life situations. As a distal factor relative to situational behavior, we expected that few differences would appear for this norm transmitter component among the reference groups of the early and the late developed girls. The parents and the peers, respectively, of the early developed girls would hold about the same evaluative opinions with respect to getting drunk as would the parents and the peers of the late developed girls.

The sanctioning of getting drunk would be a normative component that more probably would differentiate the early and the late developed girls, with the parents and the peers of the early developers being more tolerant and reacting less harshly than the parents and the peers of the late developed girls.

Finally, it was assumed that the expectancies the parents had of their daughter's behavior would be another normative component that would differentiate between the early and the late matured girls. With more experiences of advanced social behavior among their daughters, the parents of the early matured girls were hypothesized to expect more alcohol drinking than were the parents of the late developed girls.

The important aspects for the developmental course of the peers' and parents' evaluations, sanctions, and expectations about behavior concern how they are perceived by the girl. These aspects, based on the girl's perception, were assessed in the following way. Data consisted of questions given in the Norm Inventory administered at 14:5 years. The girls were asked how their parents and how their peers evaluated the behavior "getting drunk" ("Here you shall say what your parents [peers] think about getting drunk"), what sanctions they expected from parents and peers ("How do you think your parents [peers] would react, if they found out that you had been drunk?"), and the parental expectations ("What do you think your parents think you would do in a situation like this?").

The testings of differences in norm transmitter components among girls in the four menarcheal groups were performed using one-way analysis of variance. A complementary analysis was made with the response alternatives dichotomized into accepting versus nonaccepting evaluations, sanctions versus no sanctions, and positive expectations versus negative expectations. Table 6.8 presents the results of the comparison among the four menarcheal groups of girls.

The assumptions that few differences between the reference groups of girls in the four menarcheal groups would emerge with respect to evalua-

Table 6.8. *Testings of differences with respect to evaluations, sanctions, and expectations among the parents and the peers of girls in four menarcheal groups*

	Evaluations		Sanctions		Expectations
	Parents	Peers	Parents	Peers	Parents
Consequences of getting drunk	— (—)[a]	< .05 (< .01)	< .05 (< .10)	< .05 (< .001)	< .001 (< .001)

[a] Figures within parentheses refer to dichotomized scores.

tion of normbreaking were partly supported. The parents of the early matured girls did not accept alcohol drinking in their daughters more than did the parents of the late matured girls. However, the acceptance for this behavior among the peers of the early developed girls was higher than the acceptance rate among the peers of the late matured.

As to parents' and peers' sanctioning of getting drunk, the early developed girls reported that their parents and their peers reacted less harshly to this type of behavior than did the parents and the peers of the late matured girls.

The last column in Table 6.8 refers to the parental expectations of the girls. As judged by the significance level of the testings of differences in parental expectations among the menarcheal groups, the early matured girls reported that their parents were considerably more likely to expect them to get drunk than were the parents of the late developed girls.

Thus, alcohol use tended to be bound by close ties to the norm climate both among parents and among peers. Although parents of the early and the late developed girls were equal in their negative evaluations of alcohol use among their daughters, the parents of the early developed girls sanctioned this type of behavior less severely than did the parents of the late matured girls, and the parents of the early matured girls expected their daughters to engage in this behavior more than did the parents of the late developers. The peers of the early developed girls were more accepting of alcohol drinking and they were less sanctioning than were the peers of the late developed girls. Altogether, the more advanced alcohol habits among the early matured girls, reported in earlier sections, had its counterpart in higher tolerance for engaging in this behavior among the parents, and more social support for it among the peers. Thus, the physical growth perspective taken here, suggesting greater involvement in alcohol drinking in midadolescence among early relative to late developers, is also clearly associated with a reinforcement of this behavior among the two important reference groups in the interpersonal ecology of girls.

The long-term effects

As elaborated in earlier studies (Magnusson et al., 1985; 1986), two hypotheses concerning the long-term consequences of biological maturation can be formulated. One hypothesis refers to a *general* maturational impact. It suggests that physical maturation has a general effect on alcohol habits when girls attain some point or phase in their puberty sequence. When they reach this point, they tend to acquire more regular drinking habits. Hence, the fact that we can observe interindividual differences in alcohol drinking among females at some time in adolescence is due to the circumstance that some girls have already passed this point in their puberty sequence whereas others still have not come as far. Because all girls ultimately will pass the pubertal point and subsequently acquire experiences involving alcohol, we should not expect any persistent or long-term consequences. Consequently, physical maturation has an impact on alcohol drinking, but the variations among girls in maturity timing will only affect the point in time when the girls start to drink. From this interpretation we would assume that the late developed girls would catch up with the early developers with the passage of time. Thus, the relationship between maturational timing and alcohol drinking would be attenuated over time.

Some features in our data support this interpretation. Consider alcohol drinking per se. As reported earlier, the marked differences in the percentage of subjects among the early developers relative to the percentage of the late developed girls at 14:5 years tended to decrease over time due to a "catch-up" among the late developed girls. Extrapolating this tendency, no differences between the early and the late developed girls with regard to having at least some drunkenness experiences would appear in late adolescence. This pattern is consistent with a timing interpretation of alcohol use among girls.

Another interpretation, a *differential* maturational impact hypothesis, is also possible. One might claim that early developed girls encounter more or less unique reactions and experiences in the midadolescent years, reactions that will not pertain later on for the late matured girls. For example, early developed girls' association with certain type of peers, at a time when the problem proneness among these peers is at its maximum, will not be duplicated by the late matured girls in late adolescence. Such an interpretation does not specify that girls' social behavior generally will be affected, sooner or later, by the biological growth factor. Rather, it suggests that a subgroup of girls, the early developers more or less exclusively, will be surrounded by a peer constellation that heightens these girls' alcohol drinking in the midadolescent years. The unique coexistence of the early developed girls' interest in mature behavior and a peer reference group that strongly reinforces such behavior contributes to a rapid acceleration into advanced drinking habits among these girls relative to others.

Empirical data indicate that the early developed girls were a group of girls with particularly high alcohol consumption in the adolescent years. No attenuation of the differences between the early and the late developers with respect to *frequent drunkenness* was observed. At all three ages, between age 14 and age 16, there were highly significant differences

Table 6.9. *Alcohol consumption at age 25:10 for girls in four menarcheal groups*

Age of menarche	Frequency of alcohol consumption[a]		
	Never	Sometimes	At least weekly
−11	5.7	82.9	11.4
11–12	7.1	79.8	13.1
12–13	9.0	75.2	15.9
13–	11.2	77.5	11.2
N	31	274	48
%	8.8	77.6	13.6

[a] χ^2 (6, $N = 353$) = 2.58, n.s.

among the four menarcheal groups of girls, with the early developers having had such experiences most frequently.

The differential effects model is the one that is of particular interest from the point of view of the researcher looking for long-term effects of maturational timing. If, indeed, some girls, due to their pubertal timing, have distinct experiences and will perceive different reactions from their interpersonal environment than do other girls, distinctly different forms of personality and social functioning may evolve from these girls both in a temporary and in a more lasting way. The finding that the early developed girls were a subgroup of girls with excessive alcohol habits in adolescence may indicate that they are at particular risk for alcohol problems in adulthood.

In connection with a follow-up assessment at adult age, when the women in this research group were on average 25:10 years old, data on alcohol consumption were collected by a mailed questionnaire answered by 90% of all the women who had ever participated earlier in data collection. The two questions that concerned alcohol habits involved how often the subject drank alcohol and how much was consumed on occasions when they drank the most. No systematic relationship between menarcheal age and answers to these questions were discerned. Table 6.9 presents the self-reported data at adult age for frequency of alcohol consumption as related to age of menarche. It illustrates that those who drank most frequently at 25:10 years came as often from the early as from the late developed groups of girls. An analysis including the relationship between pubertal timing and the amount of alcohol consumed at 25:10 years similarly showed no relationship with menarcheal age.

Data on registered alcohol abuse up to adult age were also examined among the four menarcheal groups of girls (Magnusson, 1988). Information was obtained from the police (drunkenness, drunk driving), the social authorities (measures taken in accordance with the Temperance Law; information on treatment at institutions for alcoholics), and open and closed psychiatric services (patient journals). This information on alcohol abuse covers the period from 14 up to 26 years of age. In line with the results obtained for self-reported data, no significant differences in registered alcohol abuse were found among the four menarcheal groups of girls. Only 15 of the 458 girls with complete register data were registered by the age of 26. Of the four groups, 4.3% of the girls who attained menarche before age 11 were registered by the police, by social welfare authorities, or by psychiatrists for alcohol problems; 5.6% of the girls who had menarche between ages 11 and 12; 0.5% of the girls with menarche between 12 and 13; and 5.0% of the latest developed group of girls were registered.

In this context, it might be relevant to mention the results of a broader analysis of the issue of the persistence of norm breaking, an analysis performed by Magnusson, Stattin, and Allen (1986). They compared early and late matured girls with respect to registered crime up to age 26. There was a slight tendency for the early developers to be overrepresented among the girls with criminal records. Nevertheless, in general the results failed to provide strong evidence for the argument that menarcheal age is connected with more persistent antisocial behavior.

Thus, with respect to the long-term effects on alcohol drinking of interindividual differences in biological maturation, the results do not support a differential impact model having subsequent consequences for alcohol use in adult life.

Summary and discussion

The present analysis of social transition among adolescents was undertaken from a somewhat different perspective than the usual age-related psychosocial approach. It departed from a maturational outlook, investigating from the perspective of normal biological development one type of transition behavior among females: alcohol drinking, a social behavior that is viewed both as a normal maturational and as a problem behavior in terms of the norms of the conventional society. A hypothesis was advanced suggesting that early alcohol habits and drinking frequency in midadolescence were related to a girl's maturational timing, such that the earlier developed a girl is, the earlier she engages in this type of behavior and the more advanced is her alcohol habit in the midadolescent period, which generally is the most norm-violating age among females.

From this general outlook more precise paths were delineated. Early developed girls were assumed to have a sense of being psychologically and socially more mature than later developed girls. This self-concept would have the consequence that they would be more ready to adopt grown-up types of behaviors and seek out the company of peers who matched them with respect to maturity status. In the association with chronologically older peers, some of whom were already working, and with older boys, the early developed girls were assumed to encounter more advanced and "mature" leisure-time activities, and the more tolerant attitudes toward breaking conventional rules that characterize older peers. For the more average developed girls, the physical maturity component would not be as salient as for the early developers, and their circles of friends would characteristically involve mainly same-age peers in the same class or in the same school. The late developed girls would be less apt to seek and be sought out as friends by older peers and boys. They would more often seek as friends peers who matched them in their late maturity status – that is, chronologically younger peers. In the association with these younger peers, they would encounter more childish social life patterns and more conventional attitudes toward norm breaking. In effect, girls' perception of their own maturity and the types of peers with whom they are engaged were assumed to form the mediating factors operating for the association between biological maturation and alcohol drinking in midadolescence.

It was empirically supported that early developed girls had more advanced alcohol habits in midadolescence than did late developed girls, that they felt themselves as more mature than their classmates, and that their circles of peers more often involved older peers, employed peers, and boyfriends. Girls' perceived maturity and the types of peers with whom they associated turned out to be important mediators for the demonstrated relationship between maturational timing and alcohol drinking. When the differences in self-conceived maturity, associating with older, working, younger peers, and having heterosexual relations were controlled, much of the difference in alcohol use observed between early and late matured girls was eliminated.

Steady relations with boys was the mediating variable that explained most of the differences in alcohol drinking between the early and the late developers. Girls with established relationships with boys, an over-represented condition for the early developers, engaged more frequently in alcohol use than did girls lacking such relationships.

Similar results, with problem behavior positively related to a girl's popularity with the opposite sex, were reported by Simmons, Carlton-Ford, and Blyth (1987). Support for the finding that engaging in norm breaking is connected with relations to the opposite sex was also reported by Jessor and Jessor (1975). They compared 16- to 18-year-old adolescent girls who had sexual experiences with a comparable group of girls who lacked such experiences for a range of social behaviors commonly occurring in the adolescent years. Their theoretical position made them attend to features in the girls that departed from the expected age-appropriate pattern: "Not only sexual intercourse but other behaviors that mark transitions during the course of development – beginning to drink, for example, or taking a full-time job – are normatively age-graded. . . . Engaging in such behavior at earlier stages constitutes a departure from regulatory norms, and it is precisely in this context that a social psychology of deviance or problem behavior has its logical applicability" (p. 474). Engaging in sexual behavior at an earlier age than the socially normative, they argued, is exactly the type of behavior that denotes a transition "toward a more mature status." Thus, the comparison between girls who had sexual experiences with boys and girls who lacked such experiences would isolate girls who generally engaged in behaviors that departed from age-normative social expectancies from the girls who mainly engaged in social behaviors that followed the conventional age-appropriate pattern.

With longitudinal data, Jessor and Jessor (1975) confirmed these theoretically derived hypotheses. The nonvirgins reported lower value on achievement than virgin females; they expressed lower expectations for achievement and higher expectations for independence, a more tolerant attitude toward deviance, lower religiosity, more peer orientation, less church attendance, and higher general deviance. Whereas 89% of the nonvirgin high school females had started to drink alcohol, the similar percentage for the virgins was 62%.

The theoretical framework of Jessor and Jessor (1975) shares much of the same perspective found in our research. In common is the outlook that deviance proneness among girls in adolescence has to be viewed against what is the normative, socially expected behavior at a particular age. We also agree that an earlier display of person features that characterize a more mature status implies a higher risk for engaging in problem-type behaviors. Moreover, we share the viewpoint that relations to the opposite sex are involved in the process toward maturity.

Jessor and Jessor (1975), however, make sexual behavior their starting point, and one is left to guess what made some but not other girls engage in sexual intercourse with boys. From our point of view, sexual intercourse is intimately connected with physical maturity, and it is another way of stating that some girls, by virtue of an earlier biological maturation, are within the influence circle of more unconventional peers than are later physically developed girls. Social deviance does not occur as a function of becoming nonvirgin. It occurs as a consequence of entering peer circles where the prevalence of problem behavior is higher than among the usual same-age–same-sex–same-class friends of other girls.

The finding in the present study of a match between early physical status and having peers who share the same advanced maturity characteristics, as well as having relationships with boys, was complemented by results showing greater involvement with younger peers among girls who were later developed. The association with younger peer groups among the late developers and the establishment of younger peers as a mediating factor for the relationship between biological maturation and alcohol drinking support the idea that younger peer contacts function as a protective factor against social maladjustment in the midadolescent years.

In the second section of the present article, we examined the tolerance and support for alcohol drinking among the two reference groups of the girls – among parents and among peers. Although the parents of the early and the late developed girls had similar evaluative opinions of alcohol drinking among their daughters, the parents of the early developers sanctioned this behavior less severely than did the parents of the late developed girls. The parents of the early developed girls also expected that their daughters should be involved in such behavior to a higher extent than did the parents of the late developed girls. With respect to peer support, the peers of the early developers had less negative evaluations of getting drunk than did the peers of the late developed girls, and they reacted less critically to this type of behavior than did the peers of the late developed girls. In short, the more frequent alcohol use among the early matured girls had correspondences in more tolerance for this behavior among both their parents and their peers than was the case with the late developed girls. The finding of more approval for alcohol use among the socialization agents of the girls who matured early biologically supports the argument that alcohol drinking is a social facet of a normal biological maturational process.

It is commonly found that the *earlier* the *onset* of problem behavior in adolescence, the *more frequent* the involvement, and the *more contexts* in which it is expressed, relative to peers, the greater is the risk that the behavior will take on a negative future social prognosis (Loeber & Dishion, 1983). The early developed girls presented a picture of drinking habits in adolescence that is connected with a future risk prognosis: They started to drink earlier than other girls, and they drank more frequently. In spite of this, their alcohol consumption at adult age did not differ from that of other girls, and the proportion of girls among the early developers who were registered alcohol abuse cases was not greater than among the other girls. Other data on social maladaptation at adult age – for example, registered crime (Magnusson et al., 1986) – agree with these alcohol data in showing little risk for adult social problems. What remains is the existence of a group of girls who, within a limited period of time in the adolescent years, are more socially deviant than girls in general. From the point of view of normal biological development, connected with adaptation to the social behavior among groups of peers who are, for the girls' age, advanced socially, the resultant problem behavior among the early developed girls is understandable. Chronologically speaking, these girls are expected to show the social behavior patterns that prevail among their same-age peers. Biologically, however, they are more similar to older teenagers, and in comparison with them, they do not stand out socially. Consequently, what is interpreted negatively and with a deviant connotation by the adult world may be, from the perspective of these girls, no more than a change of social behavior in the direction toward the habits and leisure-time activities more common among older peers, working peers, and boys. The acquisition of new social behavior is facilitated by a self-concept of greater maturity and a willingness to engage in behaviors that signify a more mature status.

This example demonstrates how biological factors, through self-perception and interpersonal relations factors, are transformed into differences among girls, with respect to a social transition behavior operating during a limited period in the adolescent years. It illustrates the importance of taking an interactional perspective on development (Magnusson & Allen, 1983) – investigating how the individual, through perceptions, physiological processes, and behavior, functions and develops as a totality in relation to the environment. Attempts are clearly needed to pinpoint how the subsystems of perceptions, thoughts, physiology, and action develop in interplay with each other over time. This design of process or path models, mapping the various types of influences – within the person and the environment – that influence behavior at different ages is clearly needed. The present research, which attempted to analyze systematically one type of social transition behavior in adolescence from a biological viewpoint, represents such an interactive hypothesis-testing model.

With reference to the topic of this volume, two main conclusions can be drawn from our presentation. First, the empirical results, obtained in the frame of a biosocial model for social transition, illustrate the necessity of investigating social transition during adolescence by following the same individuals across time – that is, by performing longitudinal studies, in order to understand and explain the transition process as well as the factors that are operating in that process. Because longitudinal research has become fashionable, we must also emphasize what the presented results demonstrate: First, the investigation must cover a considerable age period in order to avoid false conclusions. Second, the differences in long-term outcomes for different aspects of individual functioning illuminate the importance of studying a broad spectrum of factors in order to avoid generalizations regarding the social transition process and its outcomes, which can be based on single variable studies.

In this chapter, data for alcohol habits have been used as an empirical illustration of a biosocial model for social transitions. The results concerning that specific aspect of social behavior are clear-cut. However, they cannot without consideration be generalized to hold for other aspects. Only by studying individuals across considerable time in longitudinal research, through incorporation of a broad set of data, can we hope to elucidate the complex social transition process during adolescence (see Stattin & Magnusson, 1988).

NOTE

This paper was prepared in the longitudinal project Individual Development and Adjustment at the Department of Psychology, University of Stockholm. It was supported from funds from the Swedish Council for Social Research.

REFERENCES

Andersson, T., & Magnusson, D. (1985). Aggressiveness in middle childhood and registered alcohol abuse in early adulthood (Report No. 639). Stockholm: The University of Stockholm, Department of Psychology.

Bandura, A. (1972). The stormy decade: Fact or fiction. In D. Rogers (Ed.), *Issues in adolescent psychology* (2nd ed., pp. 91–97). New York: Appleton-Century Crofts.

Bergman, L. R. (1973). Parents' education and mean change in intelligence. *Scandinavian Journal of Psychology, 14*, 273–281.

Blos, P. (1962). *On adolescence: A psychoanalytic interpretation*. New York: Free Press.

Brooks-Gunn, J., & Petersen, A. C. (1984). Problems in studying and defining pubertal events. *Journal of Youth and Adolescence, 13*, 181–196.

Cahalan, B., Cicin, I. H., & Crossley, H. M. (1969). *American drinking practices* (Rutgers Center of Alcohol Studies). New Brunswick: College and University Press.

Davies, B. L. (1977). Attitudes towards school among early and late-maturing adolescent girls. *Journal of Genetic Psychology, 131*, 261–266.

Deutsch, H. (1944). *Psychology of women* (Vol. 1). New York: Grune & Stratton.

Donovan, J. E., & Jessor, R. (1978). Adolescent problem drinking: Psychosocial correlates in a national sample study. *Journal of Studies on Alcohol, 9,* 1506–1524.

Dornbusch, S. M., Carlsmith, J. M., Gross, R. T., Martin, J. A., Jennings, D., Rosenberg, A., & Duke, P. (1981). Sexual development, age, and dating: A comparison of biological and social influences upon one set of behaviors. *Child Development, 52,* 179–185.

Faust, M. S. (1960). Developmental maturity as a determinant in prestige of adolescent girls. *Child Development, 31,* 173–184.

Foner, A. (1975). Age in society: Structure and change. *American Behavioral Scientist, 19,* 144–165.

Frank, R. A., & Cohen, D. J. (1979). Psychosocial concomitants of biological maturation in preadolescence. *American Journal of Psychiatry, 136,* 1518–1524.

Goldberg, S., Blumberg, S. L., & Krieger, A. (1982). Menarche and interest in infants: Biological and social influences. *Child Development, 53,* 1544–1550.

Goldstein, H. (1979). *The design and analysis of longitudinal studies.* New York: Academic Press.

Hart, M., & Sarnoff, C. A. (1971). The impact of the menarche: A study of two stages of organization. *Journal of the American Academy of Child Psychiatry, 10,* 257–271.

Helgasson, T., & Asmundsson, G. (1975). Behavior and social characteristics of young asocial alcohol abusers. *Neuropsychobiology, 1,* 109–120.

Jessor, S. L., & Jessor, R. (1975). Transitions from virginity to nonvirginity among youth: A social-psychological study over time. *Developmental Psychology, 11,* 473–484.

Jones, M. G. (1968). Personality correlates and antecedents of drinking patterns in adult males. *Journal of Consulting and Clinical Psychology, 32,* 2–12.

Kandel, D., & Lesser, G. (1972). *Youth in two worlds.* San Fransisco: Jossey-Bass.

Kestenberg, J. S. (1961). Menarche. In S. Lorand & S. Schneer (Eds.), *Adolescents: Psychoanalytic approach to problems and therapy* (pp. 19–50). New York: Hoeber.

Kestenberg, J. S. (1967). Phases of adolescence, part II. *Journal of the American Academy of Child Psychiatry, 6,* 577–614.

Kestenberg, J. S. (1968). Phases of adolescence, part III. *Journal of the American Academy of Child Psychiatry, 7,* 108–151.

Kiernan, K. E. (1977). Age at puberty in relation to age at marriage and parenthood: A national longitudinal study. *Annals of Human Biology, 4,* 301–308.

Koff, E., Rierdan, J., & Silverstone, E. (1978). Changes in representation of body image as a function of menarcheal status. *Developmental Psychology, 14,* 635–642.

Lindgren, G. (1976). Height, weight, and menarche in Swedish urban school children in relation to socio-economic and regional factors. *Annals of Human Biology, 3,* 501–528.

Loeber, R., & Dishion, T. (1983). Early predictors of male delinquency: A review. *Psychological Bulletin, 94,* 68–99.

Magnusson, D. (1983). Implication of an interactional paradigm for research on human development (Reports from the Department of Psychology, Suppl. 59). Stockholm: University of Stockholm.

Magnusson, D. (1988). *Individual development from an interactional perspective: A longitudinal study.* Hillsdale, NJ: Erlbaum.

Magnusson, D., & Allen, V. L. (1983). *Human development: An interactional perspective.* New York: Academic Press.

Magnusson, D., Dunér, A., & Zetterblom, G. (1975). *Adjustment: A longitudinal study.* Stockholm: Almqvist & Wiksell.

Magnusson, D., & Stattin, H. (1982). Biological age, environment, and behavior in interaction: A methodological problem (Reports from the Department of Psychology, No. 587). Stockholm: University of Stockholm.

Magnusson, D., Stattin, H., & Allen, V. L. (1985). Biological maturation and social development: A longitudinal study of some adjustment processes from mid-adolescence to adulthood. *Journal of Youth and Adolescence, 14*, 267–283.

Magnusson, D., Stattin, H., & Allen, V. L. (1986). Differential maturation among girls and its relation to social adjustment: A longitudinal perspective. In P. B. Baltes, D. L. Featherman, & R. M. Lerner (Eds.), *Life-span development and behavior* (Vol. 7, pp. 135–172). New York: Academic Press.

Marcia, J. E. (1980). Identity in adolescence. In J. Adelson (Ed.), *Handbook of adolescent psychology* (pp. 159–187). New York: Wiley.

McCord, W., & McCord, J. (1960). *Origins of alcoholism.* Stanford, CA: Stanford University Press.

Miller, P. Y. (1979). Female delinquency: Fact and fiction. In M. Sugar (Ed.), *Female adolescent development* (pp. 115–140). New York: Brunner/Mazel.

More, D. M. (1953). Developmental concordance and disconcordance during puberty and early adolescence. *Monographs of the Society for Research in Child Development, 18*, no. 1.

Neugarten, B. L., & Datan, N. (1973). Sociological perspectives on the life cycle. In P. Baltes & K. W. Schaie (Eds.), *Life-span developmental psychology: Personality and socialization.* New York: Academic Press.

Nylander, I. (1979). A 20-year prospective follow-up study of 2164 cases at the child guidance clinics in Stockholm. *Acta Paediatrica Scandinavica,* Suppl. 276.

Peskin, H. (1967). Pubertal onset and ego functioning. *Journal of Abnormal Psychology, 72*, 1–15.

Petersen, A. C. (1979). Female pubertal development. In M. Sugar (Ed.), *Female adolescent development* (pp. 23–46). New York: Brunner/Mazel.

Petersen, A. C., & Taylor, B. (1980). The biological approach to adolescence: Biological change and psychological adaptation. In J. Adelson (Ed.), *Handbook of adolescent psychology* (pp. 117–155). New York: Wiley.

Pulkkinen, L. (1983). The search for alternatives to aggression. In A. P. Goldstein & M. H. Segall (Eds.), *Aggression in global perspectives.* New York: Pergamon Press.

Riley, W., Johnson, M., & Foner, A. (1972). *Aging and society.* New York: Russell Sage.

Rossi, A. S. (1980). Life-span theories in women's lives. *Signs, 6*, 4–32.

Rydelius, P.-A. (1983). Alcohol-abusing teenage boys. *Acta Psychiatrica Scandinavica, 68*, 368–380.

Simmons, R. G., Carlton-Ford, S. L., & Blyth, D. A. (1987). Predicting how a child will cope with the transition to junior high school. In R. M. Lerner & T. T. Foch (Eds.), *Biological-psychological interaction in early adolescence.* Hillsdale, NJ: Erlbaum.

Stattin, H., & Magnusson, D. (1988.). Early biological maturation and female development. Unpublished manuscript.

Stattin, H., Magnusson, D., & Reichel, H. (1986). Criminality from childhood to adulthood: A longitudinal study of the development of criminal behavior. Part 1. Criminal activity at different ages (Reports from the longitudinal project Individual Development and Adjustment [IDA], No. 63). Stockholm: University of Stockholm.

Steinberg, L. (1985, March). *The ABCs of transformations in the family at adolescence.* Paper presented at the Third Biennial Conference on Adolescence Research, Tucson, AZ.

Stone, C. P., & Barker, R. G. (1937). Aspects of personality and intelligence in postmenarcheal and premenarcheal girls of the same chronological age. *Journal of Comparative Psychology, 23,* 439–455.

Stone, C. P., & Barker, R. G. (1939). The attitudes and interests of premenarcheal and postmenarcheal girls. *Journal of Genetic Psychology, 54,* 27–71.

Weatherley, D. (1964). Self-perceived rate of physical maturation and personality in late adolescence. *Child Development, 35,* 1197–1210.

Wechsler, H., & Thum, D. (1973). Teenage drinking, drug use, and social correlates. *Quarterly Journal of Studies in Alcohol, 34,* 1220–1227.

Young, L. B. (1963). Aging adolescence. *Developmental Medicine and Child Neurology, 451*–460.

Zucker, R. A., & de Voe, C. I. (1975). Life history characteristics associated with problem drinking and antisocial behavior in adolescent girls: A comparison with male findings. In R. D. Wirth, G. Winokur, & M. Roff (Eds.), *Life history research in psychopathology.* Minneapolis: University of Minnesota Press.

7 Developmental change in children's understanding of mixed and masked emotions

PAUL L. HARRIS

How should we study emotional development in the child? Recent reviews of research on emotional development (e.g., Campos, Barrett, Lamb, Goldsmith, & Stenberg, 1983) have concentrated on the facial expression of emotion in early infancy and on the development of an attachment between infant and caretaker. By concentrating on the emotional behavior that is overtly displayed by the infant, such research avoids many of the pitfalls associated with research on the subjective experience of emotion. When we turn to the study of emotional development in the older child, we face an obvious difficulty. The emotional reactions of older children are much less obvious. As compared with infants, they can conceal and control their emotional reactions to a much greater extent, even to the point where they may not be visible to another person. With adults, we can usually ask them to tell us about their subjective experience, a technique employed in some of the classic experiments on the psychology of emotion (Schacter & Singer, 1962). With children, on the other hand, it is not clear whether our questions will be understood or, if our questions are understood, whether children are capable of accurately reporting their emotions.

Such doubts raise an important research question, in its own right. How does the self-knowledge of the adult with respect to his or her emotional experience develop, however incomplete that self-knowledge might ultimately be? In this chapter, I describe recent research that examines the emergence of such knowledge. In doing so, I make use of research on infants and young children in order to point to the gap between the complexity of children's emotional reactions and the limited self-knowledge that is manifest even in middle childhood. In the concluding section, I underline the similarities between the child's developing understanding of emotion and the child's psychological insight in other domains.

I shall concentrate on two aspects of emotional development: the fact that the same situation or person can elicit, either concurrently or in

191

quick succession, conflicting or ambivalent feelings in the child, and the fact that the emotion that a child displays may conflict with the emotion that is really felt, as indexed by other, less direct measures. For each of these two aspects, a transition occurs in the course of development: In the initial period, the child exhibits the emotional behavior in question but does not show much insight; in the second period, which may extend over several years, the child gradually becomes more aware that such behavior is displayed.

The expression of ambivalence

When do children start to show mixed or conflicting feelings toward the same target? Students of the baby's attachment to its caretaker have long made use of the so-called strange situation, in the course of which the baby is separated from and reunited with his or her caretaker (usually, but not always, the mother). The idea behind the strange situation is that by taxing the baby, the way in which he or she seeks and maintains contact with a caretaker can be brought under the microscope when the attachment system is aroused. For my purposes, and for attachment theory as well, the crucial episode of the strange situation is when baby and caretaker are reunited. It is at this point that a minority of babies exhibit ambivalence in the sense that they seek out contact with the mother by approaching her, but also resist that contact by struggling to be released when they are picked up and cuddled. By contrast, the majority of babies (the so-called securely attached group) both seek and maintain contact with the mother – they show little or no resistance to bodily contact with her. Finally, a third group, and again this is typically a minority reaction in most but not all samples, show more or less steady avoidance of the mother; they do not seek her out when she reappears but busy themselves with other objects in the room (Ainsworth, Blehar, Waters, & Wall, 1978; IJzendoorn & Kroonenberg, in press).

Although the origins and predictive validity of these patterns of behavior are considered controversial by some authors (Lamb, Thompson, Gardner, Charnov, & Estes, 1984), other authors have pointed to impressive stabilities from the first year (Grossman, Grossman, Spangler, Suess, & Unzner, 1985) to 6 years, for the children as well as for the mothers (Grossman, Fremmer-Bombik, Rudolph, & Grossman, 1988; Main, Kaplan, & Cassidy, 1985; Ricks, 1985). Moreover, the ambivalent pattern (whatever its origins and whatever it augurs) is widely documented. For example, in Israel (Sagi, Lamb, Lewkowicz, Shoham, Dvir, & Estes, 1985) and in Japan (Miyake, Chen, & Campos, 1985), the ambivalent pattern is displayed by about one-third of the sample.

Thus, research in attachment suggests that by the age of 12 months, a minority of babies exhibit ambivalent reactions to a central person in their lives, namely their primary caretaker.

What triggers the ambivalent reaction? Attachment theorists doubt that it reflects anything distinctive about the emotional constitution of the baby. For example, they deny that the different emotional patterns that occur upon reunion reflect inherited variations in temperament. Instead, they claim that on the basis of past experience with a particular caretaker, the baby builds up a set of expectations, a so-called working model, of how comforting the caretaker will be (Bretherton, 1985). An inconsistent response by the caretaker, a vacillation between solace and passivity or neglect, will mean that the baby will come to expect such inconsistency, and the ambivalent pattern will be triggered. In support of these claims, the same baby may be consistent from 12 months to 18 months in its ambivalent reaction to reunion with one caretaker, but it may still show a secure reaction upon reunion with another caretaker. Even recent evidence showing that there may be some modest stability in the baby's reaction to different caretakers still indicates that the same baby is often securely attached to one caretaker but ambivalently attached to another (Belsky & Rovine, 1987). Thus, it is reasonable to conclude that although the ambivalent reaction is shown by only a minority of infants, it could in principle be exhibited by many more infants were they exposed to inconsistent handling.

Given such early displays of ambivalence in dyadic contexts, one might reasonably expect that young children would rapidly become capable of acknowledging the existence of ambivalence. Thus, having experienced mixed feelings in their own lives, they should readily recall situations in which such feelings have occurred or recognize that certain situations would elicit them. In fact, recent research suggests that this expectation is wrong. The acknowledgment of ambivalence takes several years. Indeed, it is not until about 9 or 10 years that children systematically admit that the same situation or person can elicit both positive and negative feelings.

The acknowledgment of ambivalence

Harter (1977) noticed that children that she saw in the course of her clinical work had difficulty in acknowledging that, for example, they both loved and felt angry toward an absent parent or relative. To check whether such difficulties were especially characteristic of emotionally disturbed children Harter (1983) asked normal children aged 4 to 10 years to describe situations in which they had experienced both a positive and a negative feeling. Several stages were identified. The youngest children (around 4 to 5 years) denied that such mixed feelings were possible at all. Somewhat older children (around 6 to 8 years) did describe situations that would elicit both positive and negative feelings, but their examples typically involved two successive events. For example: "I was cross when my brother messed up my toys, but happy when he tidied them up later." Only at about 8 to 12 years of age did children describe situations that would elicit positive and negative feelings concurrently. A follow-up study (Harter & Buddin, 1987) has confirmed these results and has shown, in addition, that when children start to acknowledge ambivalence, they initially describe two distinct but concurrent situations (e.g., "I was sitting in school feeling worried about all the responsibilities of a new pet, but I was happy that I got straight A's on my report card"). Subsequently, they describe single situations that might elicit ambivalence (e.g., "I was happy that I got a present but mad that it wasn't what I wanted").

These results suggest that there is a long time interval of several years between the expression of ambivalence and its acknowledgment. Whereas the 1-year-old is capable of *expressing* ambivalence toward a given target, it is only at about 9 or 10 years that children can *describe* a single target that will elicit ambivalence. One might argue that this discrepancy between expression and acknowledgment reflects the fact that the 1-year-olds did not have to invent or recall a situation; they were confronted with it. By contrast, the children tested by Harter did have to invent or recall a situation. Maybe children would admit to mixed feelings much earlier if they were confronted with verbally presented situations rather than being asked to invent them. To test this idea, I presented 6- and 10-year-olds with stories containing situations likely to elicit ambivalence (Harris, 1983). For example, the story might describe a lost pet who is found but injured. The children were asked to say whether the protagonist would experience each of four basic emotions: happiness, sadness, anger, fear. The younger group typically acknowledged that the protagonist would feel a positive emotion or a negative emotion but not both. Thus, they might claim that the character would feel happy about the recovery of the lost pet, or sad about the pet's injury, but not both. The older children were more willing to acknowledge that the protagonist would experience both feelings at the same time. This age change could not be explained in terms of differential memory for the stories. Children in both age groups typically recalled the critical events in the story. Thus, a younger child who insisted that the protagonist would only feel happy on recovering the pet, despite the pet's injury, had not forgotten that the pet had been injured.

These results reinforce Harter's conclusion that children take a long time to be able to acknowledge mixed feelings. Still, one could object that both the results that I have just described and those obtained by Harter pertain to hypothetical or recollected events. Perhaps children would acknowledge ambivalence if they were questioned at the moment when they are actually confronted by a situation that leads to mixed feelings. To examine this possibility, we questioned 8- and 13-year-olds who had just been sent away from home to start life at a new boarding school. This situation is one that attachment theorists might well expect to elicit ambivalence: The novel environment of the school is likely to provoke excitement and curiosity, but the separation from parents is likely to intensify feelings of attachment. One might expect children to feel a mixture of excitement and sadness, or excitement and anxiety. Indeed, we did find that the majority of the children at 8 and 13 years of age did admit to such mixed feelings or said that someone in their situation could feel such ambivalence. Nevertheless, we still found the age-associated change that Harter and Buddin (1987) describe for this period. The 8-year-olds tended to explain their mixed feelings in terms of two separate or potentially separate situations that happened to be concurrent. Thus, they felt excited about all the new things that there were to do in the school but worried because, given that it was a boarding school and they were away from home, they missed their mother. The 13-year-olds, on the other hand, tended to explain their mixed feelings in terms of a single situation that could be appraised from two different viewpoints. For example, they felt excited about the new lessons that they would be doing at school but worried about whether they could cope with the new material (Harris & Lipian, 1989).

Two questions arise about these findings. First, we can ask what makes it so difficult for the child to acknowledge mixed feelings, especially when they are expressed so early? Second, are there stable individual differences in the speed with which children arrive at this acknowledgment?

Two modes of appraisal

My answer to the first question is that children engage in two different types of situational appraisal: a rapidly developing and relatively exhaustive mode of appraisal that immediately translates itself into emotional behavior, and a more slowly developing system of conscious appraisal, whereby causal links between particular situations and particular emotions are identified in a sequential and nonexhaustive fashion, at least among younger children. I will explain each of these two types of appraisal in more detail.

The first type of appraisal can explain the behavior of ambivalent infants upon reunion with their mother. Thus, according to attachment theory, the mother's return is appraised, more or less simultaneously, in two distinct and eventually contradictory ways: On the one hand, her return signals the possibility that security can be regained by approaching her and contacting her: on the other hand, as the infant approaches her and seeks comfort, the infant is also reminded of past dissatisfactions, of occasions when comfort has been sought but not gained. We may suppose that the appraisal system automatically delivers instructions to the emotional response system. Thus, the dual appraisal delivers two conflicting instructions, one leading the infant to seek to maintain contact, and the other leading the infant to resist that contact. Note that in this appraisal system, the infant need not register or evaluate its own emotional responses in any way. These responses are guided by the appraisal system but the emotional responses themselves need not be fed back into the appraisal system. In other words, the infant has no awareness of its own emotional reactions.

The second type of appraisal is different in two respects. First, children become self-reflective in the sense that they appraise not only the situation that arouses a particular emotion, they also register the emotion that they express as a result. Recent research shows that even 2-year-olds can identify such links between situations and emotions, and report on them (Bretherton, Fritz, Zahn-Waxler, & Ridgeway, 1986). Indeed, by 4 or 5 years children know enough about the situations that elicit emotions to be able to predict, on the one hand, the emotion that will be provoked by a particular situation, and on the other to think of situations that would elicit a particular emotion (Harris, 1985). Thus, in contrast to the first type of appraisal, the second allows children to identify their own emotional reaction to a given situation.

The second type of appraisal is also different in that it operates in a sequential nonexhaustive fashion. Thus, a particular situation is encountered or described and the child examines it for components that are stored in his or her knowledge base of situations that elicit either a positive or a negative emotion. Once such a component is identified, the child can report the emotion that is linked to it, but at that point appraisal ceases. For the most part, situations contain only one emotionally charged component and can be easily identified as leading to a positive or negative emotion. Thus, a given situation such as a gift or a loss is typically associated with either positive feelings or negative feelings but not both; the child can accurately pick out whichever feelings are appropriate to the situation. Some situations, however, contain more than one component and the child's nonexhaustive appraisal of those components leads to an admission of one emotion but a denial of any other.

What would prompt a child to engage in a more exhaustive analysis? There are two different possibilities: The change might be brought about by processes internal to the child; or it might be encouraged by the child's day-to-day social experience. If, as I have suggested, there is a system of appraisal that leads to ambivalent behavior from an early age, we must suppose that children will sometimes find themselves in situations that elicit mixed feelings, feelings that they express nonverbally and with appropriate behavior, although they explicitly acknowledge only one feeling. Under such circumstances, other people may nevertheless react (verbally or nonverbally) to the emotion that they fail to acknowledge. Such socially marked reactions might well trigger a further mental search for an appropriate elicitor. For example, a sibling who is the target of the child's angry resistance may complain or an observing adult might ask what is wrong. The success of the ensuing search is likely to depend on the extent to which the eliciting component can be easily identified. This will depend, in turn, on its distinctiveness from the component that gave rise to the single emotion that is acknowledged, just as the results of Harter and Buddin (1987) would suggest. As we shall see, attachment theory offers further clues concerning the extent to which particular emotional reactions will or will not be socially marked.

Individual differences

Turning to the second question – Are there individual differences in the age at which children acknowledge mixed feelings? – current research suggests a positive answer (Harter & Buddin, 1987). However, the research that has been carried out hitherto has all been cross-sectional in design. For example, both Harris (1983) and Harter and Buddin (1987) studied children of different ages on a single occasion and found marked individual differences. Thus, among the 10-year-olds that Harris tested, there were some that failed to acknowledge mixed feelings for any of the three stories that they heard, but there were also some who acknowledged mixed feelings for all of the three stories. Similarly, in the study carried out by Harter and Buddin (1987) some children in the age range from 9 to 11 years denied that mixed feelings could be experienced concurrently; some acknowledged that they might be provoked by two distinct situations; and some acknowledged that they might be provoked by a single dual-faceted situation.

The obvious question that arises from these individual differences is whether they are stable across development. To answer this question we obviously need a longitudinal design to establish, for example, whether a child who is precocious in acknowledging ambivalence for successive events is also precocious in doing so for distinct, simultaneous events and also for single events.

A longitudinal study might also indicate whether such individual differences can be linked to an individual's early attachment history. From the perspective of attachment theory, one might expect securely attached individuals to be better able to articulate their mixed feelings. Although they may experience ambivalent feelings toward attachment figures less often, they will be more likely to express overtly the hurt or disappointment that they do sometimes feel toward such figures. This prediction is plausible if we suppose that securely attached individuals will be confident that the open expression of their feelings will not threaten the relationship and will elicit some comfort or solace from the parent. Accordingly, one might expect children who have a history of secure attachment to talk more openly about the conflicting feelings that they may experience upon reunion or during disciplinary encounters with a caretaker. Some support for this prediction is reported by Main et al. (1985). A group of 6-year-olds, whose attachment status to their mother and father had been assessed in infancy, were interviewed about reactions to a hypothetical separation. They were shown a series of six photographs of children undergoing separation from their parents. The separations ranged in severity from mild (the parent saying goodnight to the child) to severe (the parents leaving for a two-week vacation). Children were asked what the child in the picture would feel and do. Replies were scored for emotional openness. Emotionally open children readily imagined the pictured child as sad, lonely, fearful, or angry during the separation, whereas emotionally closed children remained silent or passive or insisted that the child would feel fine or feel nothing. There proved to be a strong relationship between this measure and earlier attachment to the mother. Secure infants were more emotionally open at 6 years, whereas insecure infants were more closed.

Especially interesting from the standpoint of attachment theory are those children with a history of ambivalent attachment. Such children will presumably often express conflicting feelings toward their caretaker. In principle, one might expect the frequent experience and expression of ambivalence in infancy to encourage its acknowledgment in later childhood. However, in line with the speculation earlier, it may be important for children to receive some explicit acknowledgment of their ambivalent feelings if they are to acknowledge them fully. Children with a history of ambivalent attachment may rarely receive that explicit acknowledgment from a parent and therefore have a general difficulty or retardation in exhibiting mixed feelings. Their difficulties might, however, prove more subtle. They might admit to conflicting feelings but encounter difficulties in their integration. Recall that Harter and Buddin (1987) found that children find it easier to admit to mixed feelings if each feeling can be linked to a distinct target; the appreciation that such feelings can arise in relation to a single target was especially difficult. Likewise, as noted earlier in the chapter, we found that 8- and 13-year-olds differed in their willingness to trace ambivalent feelings back to two facets of the same situation. Thus, it is feasible that children with a history of ambivalent attachment will be ready to acknowledge the oscillation of their feelings, while at the same time insisting that the caretaker precipitates such lability by behaving inconsistently across time. For example, they may insist that the caretaker is cheerful and loving at certain times but irritable and rejecting at others, or loving and available when they are at home but distant and unavailable during separations. By contrast, the securely attached child will be capable of admitting, for example, that feelings of trust and resentment can be concurrently aroused by a parent who combines warmth and firmness.

A longitudinal study would also allow us to raise an important but neglected question in development. How exactly does the child construct and reconstruct a mental picture of the past, and in particular how does the child construct a picture of his or her emotional reaction to past events? For example, consider a typical 6-year-old who has difficulty in acknowledging ambivalent reactions. How will that same child, questioned later about his or her emotional reactions to an earlier emotionally charged event, recount his or her reactions? Will the child reinterpret the initial reaction and now admit to an ambivalent reaction? Alternatively, will the child reiterate the initial univalent acknowledgment?

This question is essentially similar to the question raised by Piaget about memory for more neutral inputs such as seriated arrays (Liben, 1977). Piaget presented young children with various arrays that were difficult for them to remember accurately. For example, they might be presented with an array of sticks arranged from left to right by height, but they would reproduce them as two groups, a group of short sticks and a group of long sticks. However, when the children were questioned later about what they had seen, a more accurate seriated array could be produced. Piaget's intriguing interpretation is that the earlier experience is reinterpreted in the light of intervening cognitive development. We may ask a similar question about the child's emotional experiences. Specifically, in examining the past does the child reinterpret it in the light of current cognitive structures, or is earlier emotional input taken in, stored, and retrieved in a frozen, unyielding form?

This specific question points to a more general issue in emotional development. Hitherto, much work in attachment theory has been aimed at the identification of continuities in emotional development. At the same time, work with adults strongly suggests that early relationships with a parent are reflected upon and reevaluated (Main et al., 1985). The complementary perspectives of attachment theory and cognitive-developmental theory may be especially useful in thinking about these different outcomes. It seems reasonable to suppose that a good deal of reinterpretation comes about in the wake of cognitive development. At the same time, the continuities that do exist indicate, as attachment theory would suggest, that there may be important restrictions to the possible reevaluation that can occur.

Display rules

In the course of development, children gradually come to exert control over the expression of emotion. For example, most cultures expect children to mask their disappointment, their disgust, and even their pride in particular situations. How children come to exercise control over the expression of emotion has only recently become a topic for research but already there are sufficient data to sketch a developmental story. In certain respects we see the same type of developmental change as we saw with respect to ambivalence. Specifically, children first adopt display rules at the behavioral level but with little acknowledgment of the discrepancy that is thereby created between their actual feelings and the emotion that they convey to others. Only later do they acknowledge the discrepancy between real and apparent emotion and its misleading impact.

A good place to start the developmental story is a recent study by Cole (1986) in which she refined and extended an earlier experiment of Saarni (1984). The children were first shown some toys and asked to rank them from the one that they liked most to the one that they liked least. After then looking at some pictures with the experimenter, the children were rewarded with a present that consisted of one of the toys that they had rated as their favorite. The children's facial expressions were filmed for half a minute following receipt of the toy. This procedure was repeated a second time except that they were given their least favorite toy on the second occasion. The crucial question was how the children would react to the disappointing gift: Would they smile as they typically did on being given their favorite toy or would they openly express their disappointment? Cole found that boys and girls reacted differently. The boys tended to express their disappointment overtly. They rarely smiled and tended to show various negative facial expressions. The reaction of the girls was more complex. Although, like the boys, they exhibited various negative expressions, they also smiled despite their disappointment. Indeed, they smiled as often in response to the disappointing gift as they had done to the preferred gift.

Thus, the girls but not the boys appeared to mask their disappointment. They were not entirely successful in doing this because they still expressed some of the facial movements associated with disappointment, but they did manage to smile. Moreover, the youngest girls aged 4 years were just at good at this masking strategy as the oldest girls aged 8 years.

To check whether the girls really were deliberately controlling their facial expression, Cole carried out a follow-up study with a group of 3- to 4-year-old girls. In this study, half the children examined the disappointing gift in the presence of the experimenter, but the other subjects were given the gift and left to examine it alone. Cole's reasoning was that when examining the gift alone, children's spontaneous disappointment should be visible on their faces. Conversely, when examining the gift in front of the experimenter, children might be expected to control their facial expression deliberately.

The results bore out these expectations. Specifically, when they examined the gift alone, the children rarely smiled, and often produced expressions of disgust or disappointment. When they opened the gift in the presence of the experimenter, on the other hand, children were more likely to smile and exhibited less disappointment. Afterward, the majority of children in both groups explained that they had been hoping for a different gift and when they were actually given the opportunity to exchange the gift, they all did so. Thus, there was clear evidence that irrespective of whether they attempted to conceal their disappointment, all the children had actually been disappointed.

In a later interview, the children were questioned by a familiar adult. To encourage the children to be as candid as possible, this person was always different from the person who had given them the disappointing gift. The children were asked how they had felt when they received the disappointing gift and also whether the person who gave it to them knew how they felt. With probing, the majority of children acknowledged that they had been disappointed. Nevertheless, no child made any reference to having controlled their facial expression and only one child indicated that the experimenter would know how they felt on the basis of their facial expression. In explaining why the experimenter might or might not know how they felt, they focused on whether they had *told* the experimenter. Thus, the interview revealed no systematic awareness by the children that one's emotion can be revealed or concealed by one's facial expression.

The children's lack of explicit awareness concerning the use of display rules was confirmed in a second task. They were told stories that involved a disappointment for the main character, such as a disappointing birthday gift, and they were asked to say how the story character would feel, how he or she would look on her face and why. The preschool children almost invariably claimed that the story character would not only feel sad but also look sad. Thus, Cole's results suggest that although 3- to 4-year-olds may deliberately control their facial expression, they have little explicit awareness of the discrepancy that is thereby created between real and apparent emotion or of the impact that such a misleading display can have on an observer.

When do children start acknowledging the existence of such display rules? An important pioneering study was carried out by Saarni (1979). She presented 6-, 8- and 10-year-olds with stories in which it would be appropriate for the protagonist to experience one emotion but display another. For example, in one story, a situation similar to that used by Cole (1986) was described. The story protagonist is given a gift and upon opening it in front of the donor finds a disappointing toy inside. Subjects were asked to describe the look on the story character's face and to give a rationale. The results indicated that the 6- and 8-year-olds rarely invoked a display rule or gave an appropriate rationale. They typically claimed that the protagonist would look the way that he or she really felt. Thus, for the disappointing gift story, they claimed that the protagonist would look sad. Even when given a prompt by the experimenter ("Could the story character look a different way on his or her face?"), the younger subjects rarely invoked a display rule. Ten-year-olds, on the other hand, were more adept at the task. They often claimed that story characters would not express their real emotion and they gave an appropriate rationale.

We have taken a further look at children's understanding of display rules in an effort to uncover any minimal understanding that might be present. We suspected that part of the difficulty facing the younger children might be to work out just when it is appropriate to hide one's feelings. Accordingly, we used stories in which the protagonist's reason for hiding his or her feelings was explicitly stated. In other respects, the stories were similar to those used by Saarni (1979). After listening to each story, children were asked to say how the protagonist really felt, what emotion was apparent on his or her face, and in later experiments to say what emotion other story characters would attribute to the protagonist. Across several studies (Gardner, Harris, Ohmoto, & Hamazaki, 1988; Gross & Harris, 1988; Harris, Donnelly, Guz, & Pitt-Watson, 1986; Harris & Gross, 1988), a clear developmental story has emerged.

At 4 years of age, the insight that real and expressed emotion need not coincide is fragile or nonexistent. Only a minority of 4-year-olds show any signs of systematic understanding. Most typically claim that the expressed emotion will coincide with the real emotion. By 6 years of age, a sharp improvement has taken place. The majority of 6-year-olds appreciate the relationship between apparent, real, and attributed emotion. Specifically, they appreciate that the expressed emotion need not coincide with the real emotion and that, when it does not coincide, other story characters will be misled and mistakenly attribute the expressed emotion to the protagonist rather than the actual emotion.

Pulling together the results of these various studies, it appears that development proceeds through three stages. In the first stage, at about 4 years, children can express an emotion that is discrepant from their real emotion. Although this facial mask is adopted in the appropriate social circumstances (e.g., in the presence of someone who has offered a gift), 4-year-olds show little insight into the discrepancy between appearance and reality that they themselves can create. Instead, they typically assume that expressed emotion and real emotion coincide. In the second stage at about 6 years of age, children who are given explicit information about someone's reason for concealing their emotion can work out the person's real emotion; they can also appreciate that the person will express a different emotion on their face; and, finally, they understand that an observer will be misled by the person's outward display and take that emotion to correspond to what they really feel. If, however, the reasons for hiding emotion are not made explicit, the 6-year-old will also typically fall back on the default option, and conclude that real and apparent emotion coincide. Finally, in the third stage at about 10 years children appear to realize spontaneously that real and apparent emotion may not coincide. Even if they are not alerted to such discrepancies between reality and appearance by the explicit mention of reasons for concealment, 10-year-olds are likely to invoke such display rules in predicting the expressed as distinct from the real emotion.

How do children come to appreciate that real feelings and apparent feelings need not coincide? Certain initially plausible hypotheses do not stand up under scrutiny. For example, it is tempting to suggest that the child observes other people displaying a facial expression that does not coincide with their real feeling, and works out on the basis of several examples that reality and appearance need not coincide. For example, the child might see an older sister graciously smiling at a tedious aunt, or an older brother smiling despite having fallen over. Taken in isolation, however, such episodes cannot be very instructive because there is no way for the child to decide whether the smile is or is not genuine in each case. Because the difference between a fake smile and a genuine smile is subtle, it seems unlikely that young children could spot the difference, let alone work out the fact that the fake smile has been deliberately displayed so as to conceal a genuine emotion. Indeed, when young children are given the task of distinguishing between genuine displays of emotion and deliberately deceptive displays, they perform very poorly (DePaulo & Jordan, 1982; DePaulo, Jordan, Irvine, & Laser, 1985).

A second possibility, particularly in light of the early emergence of children's ability to control their facial expression deliberately, is that adults explicitly call attention to the fact that certain facial expressions are impolite or unacceptable even when the child feels the emotion associated with them. Such adult prescriptions might well lead children to attempt to control their facial expression, but they seem unlikely to alert children to the fact that such control can be used to *mislead* other people. In the first place, the adult who prescribes the display rule will obviously not be misled by it. In the second place, although an adult may encourage the child to express an appropriate emotion to other people in order not to hurt their feelings ("You should look pleased when Grandma gives you a present"), they are unlikely to instruct the child that such a display rule can be used to mislead other people about their genuine emotion. Yet our results indicate that insight into the misleading impact of display rules is well established by 6 years.

How then do children come to be aware that they may express an emotion that does not fully coincide with their real feelings? My guess is that children learn from two contradictory sources of information, one that is socially marked, the other being self-consciously monitored. The simplest way to illustrate this idea is to return, once again, to the example of the disappointing gift. Let us suppose that the child has, by dint of adult prescription, learned to smile upon receipt of a gift or to attenuate deliberately any negative expression, particularly in front of the gift giver. From the results of Cole (1986) we know that this is possible by 3 to 4 years of age, at least for girls. We may suppose that the child is aware, despite the fake expression, of his or her real feelings. The child presumably feels disappointed and knows it because of the various thoughts and subjective feelings that are provoked by the gift. Note that this assertion is not uncontroversial. Since the time of William James, a good deal of ink has been spilled on variants of the claim that we infer how we feel from various nonverbal indexes of emotion. This type of inference strikes me as the exception rather than the rule. It implies, for example, that the children would be inclined to infer that they were happy with the disappointing gift if they managed to look positive in front of the experimenter who gave it to them. Yet, it will be recalled that the majority of children in Cole's second study acknowledged with prompting that they were sad or cross about the drab gift that they had been given. Moreover, even the few children who insisted that they were happy were probably doing so out of politeness rather than any genuine confusion concerning how they felt about the gift because all of the children traded in the drab gift when they were eventually given the opportunity and most (80%) explained that they had been hoping for a different toy.

We may further suppose that at first the child can voluntarily control his or her facial expression, without monitoring the outcome and its impact on other people. Similarly, there are various motor patterns that we can execute with little explicit awareness of the nature or sequence of the movements that we produce.[1] Thus, the child may be more aware of the real emotion that is provoked by the situation and its accompanying thoughts than the facial expression that he or she has composed. Other people, by contrast, having less access to the child's thoughts and subjective feelings may be more sensitive to the emotion that the child is expressing facially and react accordingly. Seeing the child smile, they may respond as if the child were really happy with the gift, thereby drawing the child's attention to their mistaken belief. This argument implies that children discover that they can conceal their emotions by being simultaneously confronted by two conflicting sources of information: their own subjective experience and the reactions that other people have to their apparent emotion. Note that for this argument to be valid, it is not necessary for the children's expression to mislead in every instance. Observers may sometimes guess the child's real emotion from the situation or from the fact that the display rule is ineptly executed. Nevertheless, even with such cues it is likely that display rules will sometimes have a misleading impact and other people's misapprehension will alert the child who adopts them to that misleading impact.

This analysis implies that children will be especially likely to discover and understand the use of display rules that serve to protect other people's feelings because they will be encouraged to adopt such display rules and thereby discover their impact. For example, they will be expected to display gratitude to someone who offers them a gift, but not to boast when they beat a rival. Displays that are self-serving – for example, not looking embarrassed after stealing a cookie or after an act of clumsiness – should be understood later because children will have to discover such displays for themselves. Support for this prediction was obtained by Gnepp and Hess (1986). Children from 6 to 15 years of age consistently reported more display rules for situations in which the motive was prosocial rather than self-protective.

The study of children's understanding and use of display rules has only begun in the past few years, despite the fact that one of the most striking differences between babies and adults is the uninhibited spontaneity of the baby and the more strategic self-control of the adult. If the previous analysis is correct, we again might be able to learn from a short longitudinal study of children between the ages of 2 and 6. Such a study might be especially informative if it were combined with an evaluation of the emotional climate in the home, such as that offered by the PACES scale (Saarni, 1987). This scale measures the extent to which parents adopt an accepting or permissive response versus a controlling or restrictive response to the emotional-expressive behavior displayed by the child. The analysis that I have suggested predicts that both the adoption and understanding of display rules will be influenced by that climate. Specifically, in homes where there is a restrictive or controlling attitude, we would expect children both to adopt and to understand display rules at a somewhat earlier age than children living in more permissive homes. However, it would be expected that such differences should only occur for prosocial rules. Whatever the home atmosphere, children should be able to discover that some display rules can serve a self-protective function. Preliminary support for this prediction was obtained in a study comparing emotionally disturbed and normal children, who were equated for intelligence and socioeconomic background (Adlam-Hill & Harris, 1988). The emotionally disturbed children showed a less systematic understanding of display rules than the normal children. More detailed analysis showed, however, that the emotionally disturbed children did not exhibit a pervasive lag. They were especially likely to ignore the possible use of display rules that served prosocial ends. When the situation called for self-protection, on the other hand, the emotionally disturbed children were just as likely as the normal children to acknowledge the likelihood of a discrepancy between the emotion felt and the emotion displayed. Moreover, although they rarely couched their explanation for the adoption of a display rule in prosocial terms, they often gave an egocentric rationale, reversing the pattern observed among the normal children and the pattern observed by Gnepp and Hess (1986).

Conclusions

In this chapter, I have tried to show that the child's understanding of his or her emotional behavior may emerge some years after the behavior in question. In the case of ambivalence, there is evidence that even infants exhibit a vacillatory pattern of approach and avoidance toward the same person, but such ambivalent feelings are not acknowledged for several years. In the case of display rules, 3- and 4-year-olds can display one facial expression when they are being observed and another, different expression when they are alone, one that is more in keeping with what they actually feel and the choices and explanations that they subsequently make. Yet they do not explicitly acknowledge the distinction between real and apparent emotion until around 6 years of age. In each of these two examples, the child exhibits a behavioral differentiation that is not explicitly acknowledged when the child is interviewed. Thus, the preschooler asserts that he or she has only one feeling toward another person, not two conflicting feelings. Similarly, the preschooler answers as if the expressed emotion and the real emotion were equivalent to one another, with no conflict between the two.

Is this pattern peculiar to emotional development? One might be tempted to argue that the emotional repertoire of the infant and preschooler is quite complex and sophisticated so that such a lag is only to be expected, whereas in other domains a similar lag will not be found. In this concluding section, I shall argue, on the contrary, that there are helpful parallels to be drawn between emotional and cognitive development.

For the purposes of illustration, I shall focus on one interesting example, namely comprehension monitoring: the ability to identify utterances or passages of text that are hard to understand or anomalous in relation to what has been stated earlier. Young children tend to be overly optimistic about their comprehension in such cases and deny having encountered any anomalies or inconsistencies. Older children, by contrast, are more likely to acknowledge having encountered a sentence or proposition of which they cannot make sense.

One early interpretation of this age change was that there is an increase with age in so-called constructive processing (Bransford, Barclay, & Franks, 1972). In listening to or reading a text, young children might be less active in building a mental model of what they have just heard that is continuously updated in the light of later input (Kintsch & van Dijk, 1978). Effectively, they do not actively try to integrate later parts of a text with what has gone before, so they fail to notice when inconsistencies arise (Markman, 1977; 1979). Subsequent research, however, has indicated that this line of explanation is probably wrong. There is no clear evidence that young children are deficient in constructive processing. Indeed, when younger (aged 8 to 9 years) and older children (aged 11 to 12 years) are asked to read a text, and the speed with which they read each sentence or proposition is assessed, both age groups pause when they encounter an anomaly, providing clear evidence that the anomaly has been detected, presumably because it cannot be readily integrated with the mental model that has been constructed on the basis of what has gone before (Harris, Kruithof, Meerum Terwogt, & Visser, 1981; Zabrucky & Ratner, 1986). Nevertheless, despite this similarity in constructive processing, the older children are much more systematic in acknowledging their comprehension difficulties. Thus, they are likely both to admit that part of the text did not fit in with the rest of the story and also to remember words or phrases from the anomalous segment, whereas the younger children deny having encountered anything problematic and, even when given the story to reexamine, fail to pick out the anomaly (Harris et al., 1981).

This phenomenon is strikingly similar to those I have described with respect to emotion. At the behavioral level, younger children exhibit a differentiated response in the sense that they adjust their reading speed, by slowing down or pausing if the text that is currently being processed does not fit with what has gone before. Yet in subsequent interviews that differentiation is not made; the younger children do not distinguish the anomalous segment from other parts of the text.

How should we explain the difficulties encountered by the younger subjects? We may consider two plausible but ultimately inadequate explanations. First, with respect to both comprehension monitoring and the understanding of emotion, it is possible to argue that the differentiation exhibited by younger children is at the behavioral level, and that difficulties arise only when they are asked to articulate verbally the nature of their response – for example, by explicitly acknowledging mixed feelings, or the discrepancy between real and apparent emotion or between their comprehension of one part of a text and another. This interpretation, however, lacks explanatory force. In all the experiments described, a simplification of the verbal requirements of the task leads to no observable improvement. For example, in one experiment on children's understanding of mixed feelings, they were presented with a list of emotions and asked to say yes or no to each (Harris, 1983). The 6-year-olds were more likely than the 10-year-olds to say yes to a single emotion from the list. In the studies of children's understanding of real and apparent emotion, they were asked to choose one of three response options (happy, sad, OK); 4-year-olds were more likely than 6- and 10-year-olds to make the same choice for the real and apparent emotion (Harris & Gross, 1988). In the study of comprehension monitoring, children were asked to say whether or not everything made sense, and also (if they had not spontaneously identified it) to point to an anomalous line in the text (Harris et al., 1981). In each study, therefore, the verbal response to be made was very simple, and sometimes it could be replaced by a nonverbal response. Thus, the hypothesis that the age change can be explained in terms of verbalization difficulties on the part of the younger children seems weak at best. This is not to deny that younger children have difficulties in making a differentiation at the verbal level that they do make at the behavioral level, but it is to deny that difficulties in verbalization per se have much explanatory value.

A second approach can be borrowed from social psychology. Nisbett and Wilson (1977) have argued that adults rarely, if ever, have access to the mental processes that intervene between stimulus and response, so that their explanations of their behavior are often inaccurate, and rarely more accurate than those that might be offered by an observer having recourse to a priori cultural theories about psychological causation. Similarly, one might argue that younger and older children alike lack any introspective access to their mental processes, but older children, having acquired a more elaborate version of the folk psychology adopted by adults, offer retrospective accounts that are more acceptable by adult standards. Yet a closer scrutiny reveals that this interpretation is based on a bad analogy. Nisbett and Wilson (1977) have argued that adults are poor at identifying the stimuli and the ensuing mental processes that cause a particular response. My argument has not been that younger children differ from older children in their inaccurate diagnosis of the stimuli or intervening mental processes that cause their actions, but rather that they fail to acknowledge the behavioral differentiation that they exhibit. Thus, the developmental task facing the child is to develop a more accurate representation of his or her behavior.

How is this more accurate representation achieved? It is tempting to argue that in each of the three examples I have discussed, the child eventually gains access to a behavioral program that is initially run off automatically or unconsciously (Gelman & Gallistel, 1978; Rozin, 1976). Thus, the child must gain access to the program that governs the expression of emotion, or to the program that governs reading speed. This type of metaphor implies that the child becomes self-conscious by either penetrating down into some hitherto inaccessible program or by copying that program into a new format where it can be reworked (Karmiloff-Smith, 1987). Such metaphors have a computational ring to them: A computer does indeed allow us to make a copy of a file from a subdirectory that may be reworked without compromising the original file. Yet, it is by no means clear what would trigger such accessing operations in the child's mind. The child's mind may have computational properties, but we have no obvious candidate for the operator who would normally take responsibility for putting those computational properties to work in accessing and copying files.

For this reason, I prefer the metaphor of amplification to that of access. My hypothesis is not that children become self-conscious by penetrating inward or downward. Instead, they produce variation in behavior that goes unnoticed unless it is amplified in some way by an environmental correlate. Such amplification can be achieved in various ways. For example, biofeedback experiments provide subjects with an artificial amplification of fluctuations in autonomic behavior of which they would normally be unaware (Miller, 1983). Nursery rhymes provide an amplification of the rhyming word play that preschoolers sometimes produce and they appear to increase their awareness of words that do and do not rhyme; the phonetic alphabet (in contrast to the syllabary or the logograph) provides an environmental correlate of phonetic regularities that exist across words and exposure to such an alphabet increases phoneme detection (Bryant & Alegria, this volume).

With respect to emotion and text comprehension, the amplification is likely to be offered by the social environment. Variation in behavior is correlated with particular social consequences, and this social amplification gradually alerts children to regularities in their behavior that would otherwise go unremarked. Thus, in the case of ambivalent reactions, the mixed emotional response that children produce has an impact on other people who respond to both the positive and the negative emotion that is displayed. This social feedback encourages children to carry out a more exhaustive analysis of the situation rather than stopping as soon as a single emotion of one given valence has been identified. Similarly, the social feedback that follows the use of a display rule can alert children to the fact that the emotion that they are conveying to other people by means of their facial expression does not correspond to the emotion that they actually feel. Finally, the questions that children encounter in the course of reading – the type of questions that will be posed by a good teacher – can facilitate comprehension monitoring. Such questions can be posed before (Markman & Gorin, 1981) or after (Brown, 1987; pp. 103–5) the reading of a given text. In either case, the questions serve to amplify for children the variation in ease of reading that they can already manifest.

NOTES

I gratefully acknowledge the helpful advice and acute comments of Klaus Grossman, who encouraged my efforts to find links between research on attachment and on the child's understanding of emotion.

1 Even among adults, there is good evidence that they may assume a facial expression with no conscious awareness of the particular expression that they have produced. Thus, in order to manipulate mood, Laird, Wagenar, Halal, and Szegda (1982) asked adults to move their facial muscles successively so as

to compose their face into a given facial expression. Few adults realized what emotion their face expressed although for some subjects their mood moved into line with that expressed emotion.

REFERENCES

Adlam-Hill, S., & Harris, P. L. (1988). *Understanding of display rules by emotionally disturbed and normal children.* Unpublished manuscript, University of Oxford, Department of Experimental Psychology, Oxford.

Ainsworth, M. D. S., Blehar, M. C., Waters, E., & Wall, S. (1978). *Patterns of attachment: A psychological study of the strange situation.* Hillsdale, NJ: Erlbaum.

Belsky, J., & Rovine, M. (1987). Temperament and security in the strange situation: An empirical rapprochement. *Child Development, 58,* 787–795.

Bransford, J. D., Barclay, J. B., & Franks, J. J. (1972). Sentence memory: A constructive versus interpretive approach. *Cognitive Psychology, 3,* 193–209.

Bretherton, I. (1985). Attachment theory: Retrospect and prospect. In I. Bretherton & E. Waters (Eds.), Growing points of attachment theory and research. *Monographs of the Society for Research in Child Development, 50,* 3–35.

Bretherton, I., Fritz, J., Zahn-Waxler, C., & Ridgeway, D. (1986). Learning to talk about emotions: A functionalist perspective. *Child Development, 57,* 529–548.

Brown, A. (1987). Metacognition, executive control, self-regulation, and other more mysterious mechanisms. In F. E. Weinert & R. H. Kluwe (Eds.), *Metacognition, motivation and understanding.* Hillsdale, NJ: Erlbaum.

Campos, J. J., Barrett, K. C., Lamb, M. E., Goldsmith, H. H., & Stenberg, C. (1983). Socioemotional development. In M. M. Haith & J. J. Campos (Eds.), *Handbook of child psychology: vol. 2. Infancy and developmental psychobiology* (P. Mussen, Gen. Ed.) (pp. 783–915). New York: Wiley.

Cole, P. M. (1986). Children's spontaneous control of facial expression. *Child Development, 57,* 1309–1321.

DePaulo, B. M., & Jordan, A. (1982). Age changes in deceiving and detecting deceit. In R. S. Feldman (Ed.), *Development of nonverbal behavior in children* (pp. 151–180). New York: Springer-Verlag.

DePaulo, B. M., Jordan, A., Irvine, A., & Laser, P. S. (1985). Age changes in the detection of deception. *Child Development, 53,* 701–709.

Gardner, D., Harris, P. L., Ohmoto, M., & Hamazaki, T. (1988). Japanese children's understanding of the distinction between real and apparent emotion. *International Journal of Behavioral Development, 11,* 203–218.

Gelman, R., & Gallistel, C. R. (1978). *The child's understanding of number.* Cambridge: Harvard University Press.

Gnepp, J., & Hess, D. L. R. (1986). Children's understanding of verbal and facial display rules. *Developmental Psychology, 22,* 103–108.

Gross, D., & Harris, P. L. (1988). Understanding false beliefs about emotion. *International Journal of Behavioral Development, 11.*

Grossman, K., Fremmer-Bombik, E., Rudolph, J., & Grossman, K. E. (1988). Maternal attachment representations as related to patterns of infant–mother attachment and maternal care during the first year. In R. A. Hinde & J. Stevenson-Hinde (Eds.), *Relationships within families* (pp. 241–260). Oxford: Oxford University Press.

Grossman, K., Grossman, K. E., Spangler, G., Suess, G., & Unzner, L. (1985). Maternal sensitivity and newborns' orientation responses as related to quality of attachment in Northern Germany. In I. Bretherton and E. Waters (Eds.), Growing points of attachment theory and research. *Monographs of the Society for Research in Child Development, 50*, 233–256.

Harris, P. L. (1983). Children's understanding of the link between situation and emotion. *Journal of Experimental Child Psychology, 36*, 490–509.

Harris, P. L. (1985). What children know about the situations that provoke emotion. In M. Lewis & C. Saarni (Eds.), *The socialization of emotions*. New York: Plenum Press.

Harris, P. L., Donnelly, K., Guz, G. R., & Pitt-Watson, R. (1986). Children's understanding of the distinction between real and apparent emotion. *Child Development, 57*, 895–909.

Harris, P. L., & Gross, D. (1988). Children's understanding of real and apparent emotion. In J. W. Astington, P. L. Harris, & D. R. Olson (Eds.), *Developing theories of mind* (pp. 295–314). Cambridge: Cambridge University Press.

Harris, P. L., Kruithof, A., Meerum Terwogt, M., & Visser, T. (1981). Children's detection and awareness of textual anomaly. *Journal of Experimental Child Psychology, 31*, 212–230.

Harris, P. L., & Lipian, M. S. (1989). Understanding emotion and experiencing emotion. In C. Saarni & P. L. Harris (Eds.), *Children's understanding of emotion*. Cambridge: Cambridge University Press.

Harter, S. (1977). A cognitive-developmental approach to children's expression of conflicting feelings and a technique to facilitate such expression in play therapy. *Journal of Consulting and Clinical Psychology, 45*, 417–432.

Harter, S. (1983). Children's understanding of multiple emotions: A cognitive-developmental approach. In W. F. Overton (Ed.), *The relationship between social and cognitive development* (pp. 147–194). Hillsdale, NJ: Erlbaum.

Harter, S., & Buddin, B. (1987). Children's understanding of the simultaneity of two emotions: A five-stage developmental acquisition sequence. *Developmental Psychology, 23*, 388–399.

IJzendoorn, M. H. van, & Kroonenberg, P. M. (1988). Cross-cultural patterns of attachment: A meta-analysis of the strange situation. *Child Development, 59*, 147–156.

Karmiloff-Smith, A. (1987). *Constraints on representational change*. Paper presented at the Workshop on the Production of Drawings: Developmental Trends and Neurological Correlates, University of California, San Diego.

Kintsch, W., & van Dijk, T. A. (1978). Toward a model of text comprehension and production. *Psychological Review, 85*, 363–394.

Laird, J. D., Wagenar, J. L., Halal, M., & Szegda, M. (1982). Remembering what you feel: Effects of emotion on memory. *Journal of Personality and Social Psychology, 42*, 646–657.

Lamb, M. E., Thompson, R. A., Gardner, W. P., Charnov, E. L., & Estes, D. (1984). Security of infantile attachment as assessed in the "strange situation": Its study and biological interpretation. *The Behavioral and Brain Sciences, 7*, 127–171.

Liben, L. S. (1977). Memory in the context of cognitive development: The Piagetian approach. In R. V. Kail, Jr. & J. W. Hagen (Eds.), *Perspectives on the development of memory and cognition* (pp. 297–331). Hillsdale, NJ: Erlbaum.

Main, M., Kaplan, N., & Cassidy, J. (1985). Security in infancy, childhood, and adulthood: A move to the level of representation. In I. Bretherton & E. Waters (Eds.), Growing points of attachment theory and research. *Monographs of the Society for Research in Child Development, 50,* 66–104.

Markman, E. M. (1977). Realizing that you don't understand: A preliminary investigation. *Child Development, 48,* 986–992.

Markman, E. M. (1979). Realizing that you don't understand: Elementary school children's awareness of inconsistencies. *Child Development, 50,* 643–655.

Markman, E. M., & Gorin, L. (1981). Children's ability to adjust their standards for evaluating comprehension. *Journal of Educational Psychology, 73,* 320–325.

Miller, N. E. (1983). Behavioral medicine: Symbiosis between laboratory and clinic. In M. R. Rosenzweig & L. W. Porter (Eds.), *Annual Review of Psychology* (pp. 1–31). Palo Alto, CA: Annual Reviews.

Miyake, K., Chen, S., & Campos, J. J. (1985). Infant temperament, mother's mode of interaction and attachment. In I. Bretherton & E. Waters (Eds.), Growing points of attachment theory and research. *Monographs of the Society for Research in Child Development, 50,* 276–297.

Nisbett, R. E., & Wilson, T. D. (1977). Telling more than we can know: Verbal reports on mental processes. *Psychological Review, 84,* 231–259.

Ricks, M. (1985). The social transmission of parental behavior: Attachment across generations. In I. Bretherton & E. Waters (Eds.), Growing points of attachment theory and research. *Monographs of the Society for Research in Child Development, 50,* 211–227.

Rozin, P. (1976). The evolution of intelligence and access to the cognitive unconscious. *Progress in Psychobiology and Physiological Psychology, 6,* 245–280.

Saarni, C. (1979). Children's understanding of display rules for expressive behavior. *Developmental Psychology, 15,* 424–429.

Saarni, C. (1984). Observing children's use of display rules: Age and sex differences. *Child Development, 55,* 1504–1513.

Saarni, C. (1987). Psychometric properties of the Parent Attitude Toward Children's Expressiveness Scale (PACES). Unpublished manuscript, Sonoma State University, Department of Counseling, California.

Sagi, A., Lamb, M. E., Lewkowicz, K. S., Shoham, R., Dvir, R., & Estes, D. (1985). Security of infant–mother, –father, and –metapelet attachments among kibbutz-reared Israeli children. In I. Bretherton & E. Waters (Eds.), Growing points of attachment theory and research. *Monographs of the Society for Research in Child Development, 50,* 257–275.

Schacter, S., & Singer, J. (1962). Cognitive, social and physiological determinants of emotional state. *Psychological Review, 69,* 379–399.

Zabrucky, K., & Ratner, H. H. (1986). Children's comprehension monitoring and recall of inconsistent stories. *Child Development, 57,* 1401–1418.

8   The case of ambivalence:
the interface between emotional
and cognitive development

GRAZIA ATTILI

Introduction

The capacity to coordinate conflicting feelings toward the same person plays a crucial role in human development insofar as it is related to the capacity of forming stable relationships with others. The integration of positive and negative feelings toward the attachment figure in the early years of life in fact leads to integrated internal models of self and of the major caregiver that prevent individuals from suffering from psychological disturbances and permit them to deal appropriately with other human beings. Thus, an individual lacking the capacity for ambivalence may be vulnerable to conditions that lead to pathological development.

The importance of acquiring this capacity has been stressed mainly by psychoanalytic theorists (A. Freud, 1965; S. Freud, 1955/1909; Klein, 1948; Mahler, Pine, & Bergman, 1975) and by attachment theorists (Ainsworth, 1982; Ainsworth, Bell, & Stayton, 1972; Bowlby, 1969; 1973; 1980; Bretherton, 1985; Main, Kaplan, & Cassidy, 1985; Main & Weston, 1982). Recently scholars dealing with linguistic metaprocesses and sociocognition have contributed to this topic of research (Donaldson & Westerman, 1986; Harris, 1983; Harris, this volume; Harter, 1980; Harter & Buddin, 1987; Selman, 1980). The focus of these three perspectives is, of course, different. Emotional development is the concern of the first two traditions, cognitive development that of the sociocognitive approach. Although feelings of ambivalence are clearly based on the interplay between emotional and cognitive factors, the two aspects are unconnected topics of research of these three approaches. Psychoanalysts and attachment theorists are mainly concerned with the nature of the information that leads to feelings of ambivalence; sociocognitive psychologists are mainly interested in the mechanisms responsible for evaluating the information that includes contrasting aspects in order to form an organizing construct. Furthermore, contributions from these perspectives are based on findings related to different issues. The first two research

214

traditions focus on the expression of ambivalence through the organization of behavior, the second on the child's insight into it or on the child's understanding of ambivalence. I believe that findings based on the production of expressive behavior and on the development of concept related to this emotion, once integrated, can help to explain this complex phenomenon and can throw new light on the mechanisms underlying the development of those processes that lead to emotional disturbances.

How early does the capacity for ambivalence appear? How early should individuals be able to integrate contrasting feelings toward one target in order to develop a healthy social and emotional life? Several other related questions arise. Do developmental processes underly the achievement of this capacity? In other words, do age-appropriate constraints to the acquisition of this capacity exist, and if so, are the processes underlying the expression of ambivalence similar to those underlying the understanding of it?

In this chapter I shall review recent research that examines ambivalence as an emotional behavior (mainly attachment research and some psychoanalytic work) and research that examines the development of the concept related to such a complex emotion. Both perspectives seem to move from a consideration of ambivalence as the result of a situational appraisal. Focusing on the nature and function of emotions involved in mixed feelings, I shall consider the definition and specification of the processes involved in the development of the appraisal leading to the expression of ambivalent feelings, and I will compare it with those involved in the understanding of ambivalence.

The word *ambivalence* has often had an ambivalent meaning. In fact, it has been used both for describing the capacity for integrating contrasting feelings toward the same person and/or situation, and for the lack of this capacity. The activation of mechanisms that lead individuals to exclude defensively from conscious processing a kind of information that once accepted lets them suffer more or less severely is based on these individuals' inability to integrate contrasting feelings toward parents – that is, feelings of ambivalence.

I shall try to demonstrate that the sensitive period in which defensive processes may occur is not limited within the first 3 years of life. Vulnerability to conditions initiating defensive exclusion of unacceptable information may be considered high until adolescence. In fact, vulnerability is not, as attachment theorists and psychoanalysts claim, entirely and only dependent upon the nature of information to be excluded. Conversely, it depends upon the interaction between the amount and consistency of information of a certain kind and the appropriate cognitive capacities, which need many years to develop.

Expressing ambivalence: an attachment pattern

Studies by Ainsworth and colleagues (Ainsworth & Bell, 1970; Ainsworth, Bell, & Stayton, 1971; 1972) on infants' behavior during reunion with the mother following a short separation are well known. Ainsworth devised a naturalistic laboratory procedure, consisting of a standard series of episodes in an unfamiliar playroom (the strange situation), in order to assess the quality of mother–infant attachment when infants reach the age of 12 months. Attachment is measured in terms of the effect of maternal absence on the infant's exploration during a brief separation from her. Furthermore, reunion patterns following separation are assessed. On the basis of this procedure, three main types of attachment have been identified: a securely attached relationship characterized by infants approaching the mother at reunion and seeking physical contact with her (Group B, secure babies); an avoidant relationship with infants avoiding mother on her return (Group A, insecure-avoidant babies); and a resistant relationship with infants showing angry and resistant behavior at reunion combined with contact-seeking behavior toward the mother (Group C, insecure-resistant babies).

Even though these three types of attachment qualify the mother–child relationship and not the members of the dyad individually, the A, B, and C patterns concern the organization of the attachment system within the attached person, the infant. The Group C pattern displayed by some infants is labeled by attachment theorists "ambivalent behavior." According to them it reflects (as do the other attachment patterns) the history of the mother–infant relationship of a particular group of babies in the home during the first year of life. In fact, the passage from a dyadic emotional system to an individual one may not be completed at this age. (Unfortunately little is known about how early dyadic attachment patterns become organized into more traitlike styles of interaction; for a more extended discussion on whether and when attachment patterns are interactional and/or individual, see Bretherton, 1985.) However, it could also be that even though the Group C behavior pattern is very well documented by the end of the first year of life it may have appeared earlier albeit in a less structured form.

Stability of each of the three major attachment types has been found during the development of the child: infants who exhibit a Group C reunion pattern at 12 months show a similar pattern when they are 18 months old (Main & Weston, 1982; Waters, 1978). Indeed, in assessments of attachment that consider the different meanings of being secure, insecure/avoidant, or insecure/ambivalent at 1 year of age and at 6 years, stability has been found from 12 months to 6 years of age.

Attachment-related behaviors of 6-year-old children, who had been tested at 12 and 18 months by the strange situation procedure, were measured in a laboratory by means of a multiple technique. Among other measures, the investigators obtained children's behavioral and verbal reactions to reunion with the parent following a brief separation, and assessed their emotional openness in talking about a child's feelings about being away from parents, by presenting pictures of child–parent separations (for details of the procedure, see Main et al., 1985). Children who had been classified as insecure/resistant at 12 and 18 months displayed at reunion with the parent either a punitive behavior or an anxious inappropriate behavior toward the mother or father. Their discourse was disorganized and not fluent, with false starts by child (and by parent too). Their emotional openness according to the separation anxiety test was "ambivalent": They were claiming that the pictured child left alone by the parents would feel well, but at the same time they were giving signs of stress and anger.

However, some changes in the course of development have been reported. For some children, the mother–child interaction pattern changes over time. Although insecure with the mother in infancy, some children became secure when they were 6 years old – that is, by the end of the 5-year period during which Main et al. (1985) carried out their longitudinal study. Moreover, when adults' attachment patterns to their parents were assessed by means of retrospective reports available from a semistructured interview (the Adult Attachment Interview), some revealed a change in the attachment pattern in the course of development: They were classified as secure, despite their recollection of unhappy experiences with the mother when they were young.

The more or less explicit and complete integration of unhappy memories with positive ones was used as a criterion for classifying the adults' attachment toward their parents. In discussing their attachment experiences in fact, these adults were displaying a coherency of positive and negative aspects of feelings and memories. Many adults reported having had a rebellious period during their adolescence (Main et al., 1985).

In summary, attachment theorists claim that the Group C children's insecure attachment pattern is ambivalent. They maintain that the capacity for feeling ambivalence is acquired at least by 12 months. Furthermore, they maintain that this capacity is stable over years. Nevertheless, some changes in attachment status were found. From being insecure in infancy some children became secure at 6 years of age. Some adults seemed to have moved from an insecure attachment pattern in infancy to a secure one when adults.

Indeed, it seems that it is not necessarily the case that unhappy experiences in infancy should lead to insecure attachments to parents once individuals grow older. How can these changes be explained? Are they related to a lack of consistency in individuals' exposure to unhappy experiences or to the development of cognitive capacities in the course of life?

Before answering these questions, we should try to define what does feeling ambivalent exactly mean. When attachment theorists claim that Group C children at 12 months feel ambivalence, what do they assume children to feel? A definition of "feeling ambivalence" might in fact reduce the contrast between attachment theorists' findings and those by scholars working on social cognition who maintain that the capacity for understanding the concept of ambivalence is not acquired as early as the assumed capacity for expressing it.

Insight into emotion: being aware of contrasting feelings

According to research in social cognition (Donaldson & Westerman, 1986; Harris, 1983; Harris, this volume; Harter, 1980; Harter & Buddin, 1987; Selman, 1980), understanding ambivalence is an achievement that appears late in the course of development, after about 12 years. A developmental sequence based on three main stages was identified. Younger children (around 4 to 5 years of age) deny mixed feelings. Older children (around 6 to 8 years of age) do not admit to mixed feelings. If they do, they explain them in terms of two distinct aspects of a situation. Children around 10 to 12 years of age acknowledge ambivalent feelings and explain them as two facets of the same situation. Furthermore, at this stage they recognize that conflicting feelings interact and understand that internal states mediate emotional responses (Donaldson & Westerman, 1986). These findings on the developing ability to acknowledge mixed feelings are based mainly on indirect techniques. Subjects are invited to invent or recall situations or they are told about situations likely to evoke ambivalent feelings. If children are questioned when they are confronted by a situation (e.g., starting at a new boarding school) that actually leads to mixed feelings, the results are somewhat different. Both 8- and 13-year-olds admit to mixed feelings (this is not the case when feelings are recalled). But still the three-stage sequence is maintained. Younger children explain ambivalence in terms of two distinct aspects of their current situation (Harris & Guz, 1986, discussed in Harris, this volume).

These findings raise questions related mainly to the mechanisms underlying the acquisition of the concept of ambivalence. However, answers to these questions may throw light on the mechanisms underlying the development of the expression of ambivalence and may well be integrated into attachment theory. They may provide new arguments for studying the development of internal working models within the theory of defensive processes developed by Bowlby (1980).

Ambivalence: an ambivalent word

Ambivalence has a double meaning for scholars studying emotional development with regard to the expression of patterns. First, by ambivalence they refer to the capacity of integrating contrasting feelings toward the same person. Attachment theorists and psychoanalysts, even though within different frameworks, claim that at least by 3 years of age *normal (secure) children* possess the capacity for contradictory feelings and integrate good and bad inner representations of self and of others (Bowlby, 1980; Klein, 1948; Mahler et al., 1975). Psychoanalysts view ambivalence as the *positive* resolution of the part objects that are formed during infancy. In this view ambivalence is achieved as a result of nonrepression of part objects with consequent integration of the models of the mother into an integrated "mother object" (A. Freud, 1965; S. Freud, 1955/ 1909; Klein, 1948; Korner, 1984; Mahler et al., 1975).

Second, as noted previously, ambivalence is called the behavior of *insecurely attached* children. "Ambivalent" describes the attachment pattern displayed by some children (the Group C children) in the strange situation. These children had been experiencing inconsistent parenting already at an early age. Attachment theorists claim that exposure to a parent who unexpectedly rejects and accepts activates in the course of development defensive mechanisms, leading individuals to exclude from conscious processing information that, if accepted, would cause the person to suffer. Therapy, in fact, can reveal individuals who have a favorable image of the parent at a conscious level, but at an unconscious level a contrasting image according to which the parent is rejecting and neglectful.

Defensive processes and the consequent deactivation of attachment behavior is initiated during the early years, although it increases during later childhood and adolescence. In fact, during the second half of the first year of life and the subsequent two years, attachment is highly activated and the need for being comforted the greatest (Bowlby, 1980). Similarly, although within a different framework, psychoanalysts maintain that some children divide the object world into good and bad, and that by means of this division the good object is defended by an individual's aggressive drives (Klein, 1948; Mahler et al., 1975).

Thus, by 3 years of age, "normal children" feel "ambivalence." Implicitly these scholars say that at least by the age of 3 children have the capacity for ambivalence. This capacity is blocked when the nature of the relationship a child has with the parent is such that the most painful of two contrasting informations available to the child is excluded from awareness. Vulnerability to conditions that result in defensive exclusion is highest as long as a child is in the process of acquiring the capacity for integrating conflicting feelings (i.e., during the first 3 years of life). Still insecure attachment patterns are symptoms of "ambivalence."

According to the sociocognitive theorists' definition, which seems to me very reasonable, ambivalence means to have contrasting feelings simultaneously toward the same person and/or situation. It seems to me that the "ambivalence" displayed by insecure children, the Group C children, is the symptom of *a lack of ambivalence* as already defined. In fact Group C children's experiences, when consistent in time, give rise to defensive processes, or repression. That is, they prevent ambivalence, leading to a lack of ambivalence; which explains the *one-sided* view of mother by clients in therapy (see Korner, 1984).

If we accept this position, we can explain changes in attachment patterns through the findings of sociocognitive psychologists concerning the understanding of ambivalence.

Appraisal

Harris (this volume) suggests that when children are interviewed about their understanding emotions associated with a particular situation they consciously engage in a situational appraisal that leads them to analyze it for components. Children usually face situations characterized by components belonging to one emotional category. When they have to analyze situations containing conflicting emotional components, they have difficulty in making an exhaustive analysis because they encounter components belonging to contrasting categories. The process that characterizes changes during development in the ability to acknowledge ambivalence is slow and gradual insofar as it reflects children's difficulty in carrying out an exhaustive analysis. By contrast, only through an exhaustive analysis can children realize that two or more components may be concurrently associated with one given situation.

This argumentation may be used to explain changes in attachment patterns. The process underlying the appraisal that leads to a display of ambivalence may be very similar to that which underlies its acknowledgment. The two appraisal systems are both slowly developing even though one is conscious and the other is not. The activation of an affect such as ambivalence is based on a cognitive appraisal system that –

similarly to that underlying the insight into it – successfully operates an exhaustive analysis of the contrasting components associated with a given situation or person. The analysis cannot be exhaustive at early ages because individuals lack crucial cognitive capacities. If we use as a framework the skill theory by Fischer (Fischer & Lamborn, this volume), we may say that individuals need to develop the capacity to construct abstract mappings (two abstractions related to each other) in order to coordinate two opposite components in one concept – that is, they must be around 15 years of age. Thus, a three-stage developmental process, similar to that hypothesized by sociocognitive psychologists for the understanding of the concept ambivalence, may underly the development of expressing emotion.

Processes underlying "ambivalent" behavior of very young children and those underlying the understanding of ambivalence cannot be related through a decalage between "réussir et comprendre" (Piaget, 1974), as Harris's successive argumentation (Harris, this volume) seems to imply. Harris, in fact, argues that the capacity of being engaged in a more exhaustive analysis is prompted by children from an early age being able to have mixed feelings, even when they are able to acknowledge only one emotion explicitly. By realizing that their social partners react to the emotion that they cannot acknowledge, children can learn that they themselves are behaving ambivalently. By that they are forced to engage in a mental search for the emotion eliciting the partners' reaction. According to this position, children engage in two types of appraisal systems. One develops rapidly and immediately translates itself into ambivalent behavior. The other is slow in development and is responsible for conscious appraisal. Harris, in accord with attachment theorists, assumes that when 12-month-old children express "ambivalence" upon reunion with their mothers, as do the insecure Group C children tested in the strange situation by attachment scholars, they feel "ambivalence." Furthermore, he assumes that all babies by that age, given an appropriate target, can exhibit ambivalence – as if to say that they are already able, albeit unconsciously, to detect simultaneously the different and contrasting facets associated with the mother's return (components may be either actually present or reminded).

By contrast, I think that findings by sociocognitive psychologists may be used to present a different argument. I think that the "ambivalent" behavior of Group C children is not an "action" and is not ambivalence – that is, it is not based on children detecting simultaneously two contrasting facets associated with the mother's return. By contrast, it is possible to argue that at that age children detect the two contrasting facets of that situation as two distinct aspects.

Processes operating between the domains of sociocognitive and emotional development might be hypothesized in the following terms. Understanding that internal states mediate emotional responses helps children to acquire the ability to understand ambivalence. On the other hand, children may be motivated to understand ambivalence to make sense of their alternating feelings (Donaldson & Westerman, 1986). For fully understanding and feeling ambivalence they need to have acquired the ability, when they appraise a situation, of exhaustively analyzing it for contrasting components (Harris, this volume). According to the skill theory, we may say that they even should have developed the capacity to construct abstract mappings (as happens during adolescence) in order to coordinate two opposite abstractions in one concept (Fischer & Lamborn, this volume). Once they have developed this capacity, children can integrate their contrasting feelings in one emotion and can develop, as we will see later, integrated models of self and others. The domains of sociocognitive and emotional development are interrelated. Changes in attachment patterns might be due to a developmental sequence in acquiring the capacity of integrating contrasting feelings toward the same person similar to that found in the children's capacity of understanding ambivalence. Similar mechanisms may characterize it. An integration of cognitive and emotional factors characterizes both affective and cognitive development.

Affect activation

A controversial issue in emotion theory (Lazarus, 1984; Zajonc, 1984) is the question of whether cognitive appraisal is a necessary antecedent for affect activation (Schacter & Singer, 1962; Zivin, 1986) or whether emotion can be activated without cognitive appraisal (Izard, 1984; Izard & Haynes, 1986). Despite disagreement between these positions, both consider emotion in terms of a cause–effect sequence: The eliciting context or stimulus affects the emotional state that affects the expressive behavior. Recently a third position has been taken: Emotion and cognition are strictly interwoven in a continuing interaction within an individual (Decarie, 1978; Dunn, 1982). Furthermore, emotional behavior is often interpretable in terms of interaction between an interindividual cognitive-affective interactive process and a partner participating in the social exchange (Hinde, 1983). The interconnection between affect and cognition within an individual and the dialectic between this and that of the partner is also crucial for emotions that are much simpler than ambivalence. When we attempt to determine how the appraisal system that leads to the expression of ambivalence works, we are analyzing a system that is affected by multiple factors. This is especially true if ambivalence is displayed within an attachment relationship. In this case, ambivalence cannot be studied as only reflecting the emotional repertoire of children. It also mirrors aspects of the relationship children have with the social environment.

Secure children's ambivalence

Unfortunately, we do not have empirical findings on infants' and very young children's feelings of ambivalence. Attachment theorists and psychoanalysts theorize that normal (secure) children have the capacity for ambivalence at least by 3 years of age on the basis of *negative evidence* related to children's organization of behavior toward the parent: Secure children's behavior is *not* characterized by the contrasting aspects exhibited by the insecure children. It must be stressed that since their early age normal children are exposed to mothers highly consistent, sensitive to their signals, and mostly positive toward them. The possibility of children facing contrasting aspects of their parents is minimal. That these children detect simultaneously bad aspects as well as good aspects in their parents is still to be proved. My argument is that the integration of a good object and a bad object in one representation (Mahler et al., 1975) may make the contrast between the two aspects of the parent irrelevant and not consistent.

Insecure children's ambivalence

The point is different when we analyze the second meaning of ambivalence, which refers to the behavior of insecure/ambivalent infants, the Group C children tested in the strange situation. The forms of behavior that reflect ambivalent feelings (of individuals both within their attachment relationships and in any other type of relationship) imply not only a range of internal states but also a negotiating function between the child and his or her parent. Hinde (1985) suggests that emotional behavior has several functions in *a continuum* that ranges from behavior that is more expressive of internal states to behavior whose function is concerned primarily with negotiation between individuals. Relationships affect both emotional expression and emotional negotiation. The latter can be seen as a way of controlling the partner and/or adapting one's own behavior to that of the partner.

The "ambivalence" expressed by Group C children is an unconscious negotiating strategy, which is the result of a long history of interactions within the particular relationship that children have with their mothers (and/or fathers). These children have experienced conflict over close contact with their parents. In fact, the mothers of these children have been found to be highly inconsistent and insensitive to their children's signals although these mothers enjoy close contact with them (Ainsworth, Blehar, Waters, & Wall, 1978). This type of strategy adopted in the first year of life might be described as follows: The baby wants bodily contact and approaches the mother; the mother reacts inconsistently, often not in accord with the child's actual needs. For example, the mother picks up the baby when he or she does not wish to be held or does not hold the baby for as long as he or she wishes. The child becomes angry and resists that contact.

When the attachment system is activated, as happens within the strange situation, babies need to be comforted. They approach their mother; Group C children get angry if picked up because they have learned to expect to be frustrated by the person they should be comforted by. They lack confidence in their mother's responsiveness (Ainsworth, 1982).

Internal working models

Through the history of early interactions, the child constructs internal working models of the world and the self. By the second half of the first year, these models are going to guide a child in appraising new situations and in letting him behave within them (Bowlby, 1969; 1973; 1980). Internal working models operate outside conscious awareness. They allow individuals to generate interpretations of the present and evaluate a future course of action. The attachment behaviors of "ambivalent" children, as well as all other attachment behaviors, carry implications about not only the affective states of the infant but also the cognitive structures that, in the form of a working model of the attachment figure, guide his or her actions.

What happens when a child's efforts to make contact with the mother are not consistently accepted? What sort of working model does the child develop? What are the cognitive prerequisites that might lead during the development to an alteration of the internal working model of this particular relationship?

According to the theory of defensive processes (Bowlby 1973; 1980), as I have noted, some emotional disturbances might be explained in terms of an individual sometimes operating with two or more incompatible models of the same attachment figure. These models are the product of incompatible interpretations of experience and they become defensively dissociated. The defensive exclusion from awareness of representations that provoke pain provides emotional relief. This exclusion from aware-ness, however, makes it difficult to restructure the model and leads to emotional disturbance. Bowlby (1973) assumes that the model that has greatest influence on the disturbed person's feelings and behavior de-velops during the early years; the second incompatible model is based on an idealized image of the attachment figure and develops much later.

Findings based on studies of insight into ambivalence might lead to a different argument. We might argue that the appraisal system that leads to the display of "ambivalence" is based at an unconscious level on the same underlying mechanism as that which underlies the understanding of ambivalence. Similarly, this system does not develop rapidly. The 12-month-old Group C children (and this is especially true for avoidant children displaying the Group A attachment pattern) detect the con-trasting aspects associated with one given emotional stimulus (the mother) as though they are two situations. The behavior of the mother throughout the first year of the child's life is alternately perceived by her baby as "good" and as "bad," that is, as two situations. On the basis of this argument, we may assume that already at a very early age, children develop two working models of the same attachment figure. When the attachment system is activated, as happens within the strange situation, ambivalence and its conflicting motivations are expressed by postures, gestures, and facial expressions that change according to the aspects detected in and/or cued by the situation. Whereas secure babies develop an internal schema in which the good and the bad images of the mother are affectively combined in one person (cf. Main et al., 1985), ambival-ent children develop two working models that reflect their having been consistently exposed to *two contrasting mothers*. These working models include affective as well as cognitive components.

The mechanisms underlying the situational appraisal may lead to a change in the working models that guide attachment behaviors. Re-lationship-related behaviors are affected both by individuals' internal working models and by the patterns of interactions in which they are involved (Bowlby, 1973; Main et al., 1985). The fact that some children change from being insecure with mother in infancy to being secure at 6 years of age may be explained in terms of positive changes in children's life circumstances *and* in terms of their superior cognitive capacities. The first implies an increase in the mother's sensitivity to her infant's signals, the second that children become aware that mixed feeling can be elicited by a single situation. At this age children become conscious that ambiva-lent feelings are generally possible. However, they are still guided by two working models.

Once a child has reached the stage in which he or she admits positive and negative feelings concurrently associated with one given stimulus, the two working models that guide his ambivalent behavior can be integrated into one. On the basis of this complex working model, older children can see the attachment figure as one person including both good and bad aspects.

The acquired capacity at 11 years of age of engaging in an exhaustive situational analysis may explain alterations in adolescents' attachment patterns. In the study by Main and Kaplan, some adults were considered secure despite having experienced early negative relationships with their parents. They indicated that their adolescence was a time of rebellion. The attainment of the stage of abstract mappings by 14- to 15-year-olds (Fischer & Lamborn, this volume) may well permit the integration of two simple contrasting models into a far more complicated model.

In conclusion, vulnerability to conditions initiating defensive exclusion of information that leads individuals to suffer is not at a maximum only during the first 3 years of life. Vulnerability may be considered high until adolescence. Age-appropriate cognitive capacities constrain the possibility of integrating contrasting information. Defensive exclusion is determined not only by the nature of the information processed but also by the amount of contrast between the aspects that should be included in the internal models. The consistency of exposure to contrasting affective information also affects the capacity for ambivalence. Adolescence may be considered a period in which the formation of one integrated working model is possible.

But in cases where the affective components in the course of development have been consistently in contrast to the extent that they greatly disturb the formation of a child's personality, the integration of the two working models into one might be impossible in spite of the acquired cognitive capacity. The individual remains unaware of the model that causes painful feelings. The second incompatible model becomes more sophisticated. It becomes conscious and is assumed by the person to be dominant.

Individual differences: integrating research efforts

These studies on the development of the concept of ambivalence are mostly concerned with the general development of psychological functioning. By contrast, research on attachment refers to differential development. The integration of work in these two fields could provide interesting results. There are many avenues for future research. The most pressing need is for longitudinal studies. Understanding the transition mechanisms underlying the link between the expression of emotion and insight into it needs to be based on long-term longitudinal studies using multiple techniques in data collection. Observational techniques in real life situations, laboratory procedures, and interviews should be conducted on the same children at different ages. Observational measures of both the child's and the mother's behavior in the natural setting of the home before the end of the first year of life and until adolescence are required to provide an assessment of behaviors antecedent to and concomitant with behaviors of patterns identified in the strange situation. The identification of further dimensions, both cognitive and emotional, that contribute to individual differences in mother–child attachment could be achieved by the use of interviews, such as those used for assessing the development of the understanding of emotion. To help in understanding emotional development, the assessment of individual differences in recognizing mixed feelings is also essential. In fact, individual differences in acknowledging ambivalence need to be related to variation in the appraisal of those aspects that give rise to opposite feelings.

Cross-sectional studies alone do not help us to understand when attachment patterns can change and what the factors are that bring about such changes. Cognitive components offer constraints on the time at which changes in attachment can appear. To what extent do emotional factors affect the development of cognitive capacities? Should transitional mechanisms underlying emotional development be interpreted in terms of emotion preventing, at a given stage, the appearance of already developed cognitive capacities? By contrast, should changes be interpreted in terms of emotion influencing the development of cognition itself? What exactly does it mean to claim that emotion and cognition are strictly interwoven?

A deeper definition and specification of the processes involved in the situation appraisal that underlies both the expression of ambivalence and insight into ambivalence should help us to understand the question of sensitive periods in the formation and transformation of internal working models of attachment. Furthermore, it may contribute to the theory of defensive processes that lead to emotional disturbances.

Individual differences in acknowledging emotion should be linked to individual differences in expressing emotion. The multiple factors affecting emotional development, of course, need to be taken into consideration. An integration of experimental techniques and observational methods within longitudinal studies is a step toward understanding the complexity of a phenomenon that depends on the inseparable intertwining of emotion and cognition.

NOTE

I am deeply grateful to F. Antinucci, P. Harris, and E. Mueller for their comments.

REFERENCES

Ainsworth, M. D. S. (1982). Attachment: Retrospect and prospect. In C. M. Parkes & J. Stevenson-Hinde (Eds.), *The place of attachment in human behavior* (pp. 3–30). New York: Basic Books.

Ainsworth, M. D. S., & Bell, S. M. (1970). Attachment, exploration and separation: Illustrated by the behavior of one-year-olds in a strange situation. *Child Development, 41*, 46–67.

Ainsworth, M. D. S., Bell, S. M., & Stayton, D. J. (1971). Individual differences in strange situation behavior of one-year olds. In H. R. Schaffer (Ed.), *The origins of human social relations* (pp. 17–51). London: Academic Press.

Ainsworth, M. D. S., Bell, S. M., & Stayton, D. J. (1972). Individual differences in the development of some attachment behaviors. *Merrill-Palmer Quarterly, 18*, 123–143.

Ainsworth, M. D. S., Blehar, M. C., Waters, E., & Wall, S. (1978). *Patterns of attachment: A psychological study of the strange situation.* Hillsdale, NJ: Erlbaum.

Bowlby, J. (1969). *Attachment and loss: Vol. 1: Attachment.* New York: Basic Books.

Bowlby, J. (1973). *Attachment and loss: Vol. 2. Separation.* New York: Basic Books.

Bowlby, J. (1980). *Attachment and loss: Vol. 3. Loss, sadness and depression.* New York: Basic Books.

Bretherton, I. (1985). Attachment theory: Retrospect and prospect. In I. Bretherton & E. Waters (Eds.), *Growing points of attachment theory and research, SRCD Monographs, 50* (1–2, Serial No. 209), 3–35.

Decarie, T. G. (1978). Affect development and cognition in a Piagetian context. In M. Lewis & L. A. Rosenblum (Eds.), *The development of affect.* New York: Plenum Press.

Donaldson, S. K., & Westerman, M. A. (1986). Development of children's understanding of ambivalence and causal theories of emotions. *Developmental Psychology, 22*, (5), 655–662.

Dunn, J. (1982). Comment: Problems and promises in the study of affect and intention. In E. Z. Tronick (Ed.), *Social interchange in infancy* (pp. 197–206). Baltimore: University Park Press.

Freud, A. (1965). *Normality and pathology in childhood: Assessments of development.* New York: International Universities Press.

Freud, S. (1955). Notes upon a case of obsessional neurosis. In J. Strachey (Ed.), *Standard edition* (Vol. 10, pp. 153–249). London: Hogarth Press. (Original work published 1909)

Harris, P. L. (1983). Children's understanding of the link between situation and emotion. *Journal of Experimental Child Psychology, 36*, 490–509.

Harris, P. L., & Guz, G. R. (1986). *Models of emotion: How boys report their emotional reactions upon entering an English boarding school.* Unpublished manuscript, University of Oxford. Department of Experimental Psychology, Oxford.

Harter, S. (1980). A cognitive-developmental approach to children's use of affect and trait labels. In F. Serafica (Ed.), *Social cognition and social relations in context* (pp. 27–61). New York: Guilford Press.

Harter, S., & Buddin, B. (1987). Children's understanding of the simultaneity of two emotions: A five-stage developmental acquisition sequence. *Developmental Psychology, 23,* 388–399.

Hinde, R. A. (1983). *What is emotion?* Paper presented at the Seventh Biennial Meetings of the IISBD, Munich, W. Germany.

Hinde, R. A. (1985). Expression and negotiation. In G. Zivin (Ed.), *The development of expressive behavior* (pp. 103–116). New York: Academic Press.

Izard, C. E. (1984). Emotion-cognition relationships and human development. In C. E. Izard, J. Kagan, & R. Zajonc (Eds.), *Emotions, cognition and behavior* (pp. 17–37). Cambridge: Cambridge University Press.

Izard, C. E., & Haynes, M. O. (1986). A commentary on emotion expression in early development: An alternative to Zivin's framework. *Merril-Palmer Quarterly, 32* (3), 313–319.

Klein, M. (1948). On the theory of anxiety and guilt. *International Journal of Psychoanalysis, 29.*

Korner, A. (1984). *Object relations and developing ego in therapy.* Aronson.

Lazarus, R. S. (1984). On the primacy of cognition. *American Psychologist, 39* (2), 124–139.

Mahler, M. S., Pine, F., & Bergman, A. (1975). *The psychological birth of the infant.* New York: Basic Books.

Main, M., Kaplan, N., & Cassidy, J. (1985). Security in infancy, childhood and adulthood: A move to the level of representation. In I. Bretherton & E. Waters (Eds.), *Growing points of attachment theory and research, SRCD Monographs, 50* (1–2, Serial N. 209), 66–104.

Main, M., & Weston, D. R. (1982). Avoidance of the attachment figure in infancy: Descriptions and interpretations. In C. M. Parkes & J. Stevenson-Hinde (Eds.), *The place of attachment in human behavior* (pp. 31–59). New York: Basic Books.

Piaget, J. (1974). *Réussir et comprendre.* Paris: Presses Universitaires de France.

Schachter, S., & Singer, J. E. (1962). Cognitive, social and psychological determinants of emotional state. *Psychological Review, 69,* 379–399.

Selman, R. L. (1980). *The growth of interpersonal understanding: Developmental and clinical analyses.* New York: Academic Press.

Waters, E. (1978). The reliability and stability of individual differences in infant–mother attachment. *Child Development, 49,* 483–494.

Zajonc, R. B. (1984). On the primacy of affect. *American Psychologist, 39* (2), 117–123.

Zivin, G. (1986). Processes of expressive behavior development. *Merrill-Palmer Quarterly, 32,* 103–140.

IV Motor development

9 Transition mechanisms in sensorimotor development

CLAES VON HOFSTEN

Introduction

During growth, the sensorimotor system of the child is substantially changed. The sophisticated and skilled movements of the adult seem to have very little in common with the rudimentary movements of the neonate. How is the sensorimotor system of the neonate transformed into the sensorimotor system of the adult?

The development of coordinated movements is in no way a smooth and linear function of age. On the contrary, it is characterized by several apparent regressions. A theory of sensorimotor development has to take such phenomena into account, as well as the increase in skill during other periods.

The development of sensorimotor control has traditionally been considered to be genetically determined (Gesell & Amatruda, 1964; McGraw, 1945). Gesell considered the construction of the action system to be governed by lawful growth forces.

Behavioral patterns are not whimsical or accidental by-products. They are the authentic *end*-products of a total developmental process which works with orderly sequence. They take shape in the same manner that the underlying structures take shape. They begin to assume characteristic forms even in the fetal period, for the same reason that the bodily organs themselves assume characteristic forms. (Gesell & Amatruda, 1964, p. 4)

The maturational hypothesis was supported by systematic observations of the developmental sequence and by a number of empirical studies on infants where training was manipulated. McGraw's (1940) failure to find any effects of training on toilet behavior and Gesell and Thompson's (1929) failure to find any significant effects of training on one member of a twin pair in stair climbing are classical examples. The main conclusion was that even if environmental factors might support

233

and under certain conditions specify development, they do not engender the basic forms and sequence of it.

What is the effect of experience on the development of sensorimotor control? First, experience seems to be necessary for calibrating the sensorimotor systems. In a series of experiments, Held and Hein (see, e.g., Hein, 1974; Hein & Held, 1967; Held & Hein, 1963) demonstrated the importance of self-produced movements for the establishment of coordinated movements in kittens. In another series of experiments Bauer and Held (1975) showed that visual feedback from the upper limbs were necessary for the establishment of eye–hand coordination in the rhesus monkey. However, both these lines of research also demonstrated that very little experience was needed for the establishment of coordination at the time when animals raised in a normal environment already had it. Already after a few days of normal experience, Held and Hein's (1963) kittens and Bauer and Held's (1975) rhesus monkeys moved normally, even if this occurred after as much as 6 months of deprivation. Bauer and Held (1975) therefore concluded that it was more appropriate to describe their kind of learning as a form of calibration of the metrical relation between space of vision and the motor space than to characterize it as motor learning in an ordinary sense.

Another effect of experience is to affect the rate of development. Studies on the establishment of walking in infants (André-Thomas & Saint-Anne-Dargassies, 1952; Zelazo, Zelazo, & Kolb, 1972) have demonstrated the importance of experience for sensorimotor development. Zelazo et al. (1972) showed that brief daily exercise of primary walking in the young infant leads to a significantly earlier onset of walking alone.

These experiments do stress the importance of environmental factors for supporting development and for the specification of coordinated movements, but they do not really upset the hypothesis that maturation provides the basic forms and sequence of ontogenesis. More serious for the strong maturational hypothesis are observations of inconsistencies in the development sequence of normal children. Touwen (1976) studied the development of 51 low-risk infants each fourth week during their first 21 months of life. He found many inconsistencies in the developmental sequence. Some infants developed an ability to stand up before they could sit independently and some infants did not crawl at all before walking free. It is clear from these results that the developmental sequence as described by Gesell should not be taken too literally. It is a description of a probable course of development and evidence for a strong maturational component in development, but development is never the result of a single cause. It is always an interaction between the genotype, the phenotype, and the environment.

Biomechanical constraints

Sensorimotor development not only includes the emergence of neuro-structures for motor control but also the growth of the body through which movements are implemented. As the body grows, the biomechanical constraints on movement production will change too. An understanding of this change constitutes an important prerequisite to understanding of the problems that sensorimotor systems are set to solve at different ages.

Recently, there has been an increasing interest in the importance of biomechanical constraints on sensorimotor development (Kugler, Kelso, & Turvey, 1982; Newell, 1986). It is obvious that the biomechanical constraints are different for a large and a small organism and that these differences will affect the problem of movement production. In standing erect, for instance, it is necessary to control body sway. A short body sways with a higher frequency than a tall one and to keep balance, a small child will therefore require a control mechanism that responds much quicker than the one required by the adult. The biomechanical constraints will also be a function of environmental factors. They will, for instance, be different for a body immersed in water because of the reduced effect of gravity. Thelen, Fisher, and Ridley-Johnson (1984) studied the stepping of young infants whose legs were submerged in water. They found that the stepping of 3-month-old infants, who normally step very little, would be about equal to newborn rates in a comparable group. They could show that the disappearance of newborn stepping is a function of a specific biomechanical constraint – namely the dramatic postnatal increase in weight of the infant's legs.

As the body grows, at least two kinds of problems will be encountered. First, there are tuning problems. As the body is scaled up, there has to be continuous readjustment of the sensorimotor systems to keep them calibrated to each other and to the external world. However, if the calibration process in general is as efficient as found by Bauer and Held (1975), this should not be a great problem for the growing child. There is also the possibility that at least some sensorimotor systems are based on body-scaled information, insensitive to growth. A sensorimotor system based on such body-scaled information obviously has great advantage during a period when growth is very rapid. In the manual domain, vergence-controlled arm movements seem to represent such a case. The growth of the arm is almost completely compensated for by the increase over age in the interocular distance and the decrease over age in the angular displacement of the foveas relative to the visual axes (Hofsten, 1977). Convergence at arm's length is approximately the same throughout the first year of life.

The second problem has to do with qualitative changes with growth. Whenever we are dealing with a system whose determinants are changing in a continuous way but where the system itself only will assume a limited number of stable states, we will observe phase shifts as we scale up the determining variables. A good example of a phase shift is the change from walking to running as the speed of propelling increases. Kelso (1984) has performed an elegant example of this kind of reorganization in an experiment in which he asked subjects to flex one index finger simultaneously while extending the other and do that while increasing the speed of the action. This resulted in a rather abrupt change in the organization of movements. The fingers continued to move synchronously but now they extended and flexed together. Within a range of values the system was stable but as the system approached these boundaries instability resulted.

Are the nonlinearities observed in sensorimotor development phase shifts? They have at least some properties in common with phase shifts (Kugler et al., 1982). As the child grows, the sensorimotor system will approach its boundaries of stability. For a period its output will become variable and less efficient until it enters a new phase of stability. This description of sensorimotor development fits with the one given by Gesell (1954) and the one given by Piaget (1970). However, Gesell preferred to discuss such periodicity in terms of maturation of neurostructures and Piaget in terms of development of cognitive structures. The weakness with a pure biomechanical approach is that it does not explain very much. Specifically, it does not explain a crucial aspect – why sensorimotor control becomes more refined and sophisticated with age.

The fact that biomechanical constraints do not explain everything about motor development does not, of course, mean that we should disregard the effects of biomechanical constraints on development. On the contrary, it is necessary to take them into account, as shown by the research by Thelen and associates (Thelen & Fisher, 1982; 1983; Thelen et al., 1984) on neonate stepping. Another good example of dramatic changes in the biomechanical constraints on the sensorimotor system is birth. If there is any truth to the notion of phase shifts, the newborn period should truly be characterized by variability and change in the production of movements. However, this does not fit at all with the traditional description of newborn behavior. It is supposed to consist of a number of reflexes that are described as stereotyped, triggered, and automatic. Although such reflexes are found in the newborn – for instance, the knee tendon reflex – is that typical newborn behavior? I would say no. In a number of studies that I performed on newborn infants (Hofsten, 1982; 1984), I have been struck by the variability of my subjects' movements. Touwen (1978) has also described newborn behavior as variable. He points out that the fallacy of describing newborn behavior as stereotyped originates from the fact that the early neurological models of the newborn infant came from adult models of pathological behavior. Reappearing reflexes in brain-damaged older children or adults are typically stereotyped.

Differentiation and integration of perception–action systems as a framework for sensorimotor development

It is not possible to conceive of a motor action isolated from perception. Perception is such an essential part of any action system that the description of the perceptual mechanisms that drive the system is as important as the description of the motor mechanisms that execute the movement. This is true for the newborn as well as the adult. At no time during development is perception separated from the motor system. On the contrary, the basic machinery for biological movements is always based on perception–action.

It is reasonable to assume that perception and action evolved together. Evolution seems to work essentially by solving specific action problems for the animal demanding specific perceptual skills rather than by designing general capacities. The evolution of an adaptive skill would include the construction of a perceptual mechanism especially designed for obtaining the information needed to solve the action problem in question. In lower animals this is rather obvious. According to Arbib (1981) the frog may be said to possess a number of specific visual systems working in parallel – for example, one for threat avoidance, or one for barrier negotiation. In humans, the tie between perception and action is undoubtedly less rigid than that. According to Rozin (1976), this is a general evolutionary trend. Capacities first appear in narrow contexts and may later become extended into other domains. However, there is still reason to believe that sensorimotor systems will function optimally in the tasks for which they originally evolved. Therefore, problems of motor skills and perception in humans may be better understood in this perspective.

The view that motor skills are made up of more or less specific, biologically given, perception–action systems has important implications for the study of sensorimotor development. The problem is not any more how the motor mechanisms make contact with perception. Rather, it is a question of how sensorimotor systems differentiate and integrate into the sophisticated and synchronized perceptuomotor system of the adult. These processes would occur in the motor domain as well as in the perceptual domain. They are complementary in the sense that any part of a system that undergoes differentiation and refinement will necessitate a new synthesis (Fentress, 1986). Integration and synchronization of previously independent systems will make new differentiations and refinements possible.

An important kind of integration in development is the one between action and posture (Reed, 1982). Most skilled actions require not only an elaborate control of posture but also an intimate integration between movement control and postural control. A major achievement during the first year of life is to be able to support trunk, limbs, and head and to integrate that support with various other kinds of perception–action systems.

The perception–action systems of the neonate

If the origin of coordinated action is in itself a set of coordinated actions, they should appear early in development. There is, in fact, an increasing awareness of the rich variety of sensorimotor coordinations present in the newborn. Early knowledge about the sensorimotor systems of the newborn was mainly gained in connection with the standardized neurological testing procedures (see, e.g., Brazelton, 1973; or Prechtl, 1977). The stimuli used were mostly tactile, vestibular, and kinesthetic. Knowledge about visually controlled movements, which are of such importance later in life, has only recently been gained. Recent research shows that many of the visually based sensorimotor systems are functioning at birth, however imperfectly.

The newborn infant will follow an attractive moving target with eye and head movements (Aslin, 1981; Bullinger, 1977; Hofsten, 1982). Pursuit eye movements are not smooth, however. They consist of a jerky series of saccadic refixations on the moving target. Pursuit eye movements that are smooth do not appear consistently until around 2 months of age (Aslin, 1981). Further, vergence eye movements (Slater & Finlay, 1975) and accommodation (Banks, 1980) are present in the neonate. Aslin (1977) also showed some convergence and divergence in 1-month-olds to approaching and receding targets. Vergence eye movements are further coordinated with accommodation from an early age. Aslin and Jackson (1979) measured binocular alignment under both binocular and monocular viewing conditions. In the monocular conditions there was only an accommodative stimulus present. Infants at 8 weeks of age showed reliable convergence under these conditions. The function of eye movement is not only to direct the eye to interesting events in the environment, but also to enable the eye to maintain fixation irrespective of head and body movements. Such eye movements depend on vestibular function. They are present at birth even in blind infants (Peiper, 1963).

Eye and head movements of the neonate may also be controlled by the auditory and haptic systems. A reasonably complex sound presented to the side of the infant's head will evoke an appropriate movement of the head and eyes toward the source of the sound (Alegria & Noirot, 1978; Mendelson & Haith, 1976). The sound does not need to be a human voice. A bottle of popcorn shaken will also evoke the same response (Field, Muir, Pilon, Sinclair, & Dodwell, 1980). A slight touch on the infant's arm will also evoke a head turning toward the source of stimulation (Humphrey, Muir, & Dodwell, 1981).

Contrary to traditional belief (e.g., Piaget, 1953) the neonate has an ability to control visually his or her arm movements (Hofsten, 1982). I monitored infants' arm movements quantitatively with a technique that took the three-dimensional properties of the movements into account. The analysis demonstrated that movements performed while the neonate fixated a target were aimed much closer to it than movements performed while the neonate looked somewhere else or closed his or her eyes. The effect could not be explained in terms of head–arm coordination or any explanation based on head position or object position.

The ability of the neonate to control visually the movements of the arms also demonstrates that visual space and proprioceptive space are connected at this age. As the arm is not placed in a stereotyped position before the initiation of the movement, both the position of the target and the position of the arm need to be defined for the production of an aimed movement. The infant fixates the target, which means that the starting position of the aim needs to be defined by some other means – that is, proprioceptively.

The neonate also has the ability to direct his or her arm movements toward the mouth through purely kinesthetic means (Butterworth, 1986; Rochat, Blass, & Hoffmeyer, 1987). Butterworth reported that the mouth was significantly more likely to be open throughout the arm movement when the hand went directly to the mouth than when the hand first contacted other parts of the face. Butterworth also found that the hand could be guided to the mouth after first having contacted other parts of the face. He found no evidence of rooting after contact; the head was held still and the hand moved "immediately in the direction of the mouth" (p. 28).

The most specialized kind of sensorimotor system found in the neonate up to now is the ability to imitate facial gestures (Dunkeld, 1978; Maratsos, 1973; Meltzoff & Moore, 1977; Vinter, 1985). Certain specific actions, like the protrusion of the tongue and opening of the mouth, will evoke corresponding actions in the neonate. Such an ability presupposes very specific perceptual mechanisms for extracting information from the visual array and a very specific mapping of perception and action. Neonatal imitation is an excellent example of a phylogenetically determined, specific, and intelligent perception–action system.

Sources of incoordination

The various sensorimotor coordinations just described are seldom distinct and clear. One reason for this is that the different perception–action systems need to be calibrated and stabilized in their new environment, which imposes very different biomechanical constraints on the system. The question of calibration is especially crucial for visually linked perception–action systems, which for obvious reasons have not been functioning before birth.

A specific coordination may require a certain amount of postural control that the neonate does not have and will therefore only be demonstrable if the neonate is supported in certain ways. Again, neonate walking is a good example. To be able to walk freely, the infant needs to master the balancing of upright posture and integrate that with the production of walking movements. Fentress (1984) has given us another example. When supporting neonatal mice in an upright position, already from Day 1, rich but poorly coordinated grooming-like movements were seen.

An important reason for a sensorimotor system not to function appropriately at birth is that the neurostructures involved are not differentiated enough. This is apparently the case with neonatal reaching. An appropriately coordinated reach and grasp requires the arm to extend and the hand to flex around the object. The neonate will not do that. Instead, the arm and hand will extend and flex in a synergy (Hofsten, 1982). The synergistic properties of neonatal reaching do not seem to be influenced by vision. In a majority of cases the reaching hand was found to open before or during the extension of the arm, whether the infant looked at the target or not. In the extended phase of the arm, the subjects were never observed to flex the hand to grasp the target, not even when the hand ended up with the object on its palm. The earliest reaching attempts of the rhesus monkeys studies by Lawrence and Hopkins (1972; 1976) also showed some of these characteristics.

Neonate reaching is undifferentiated in yet another way. The motor mechanisms controlling the arm are in certain ways coupled to the motor mechanisms controlling the neck. The asymmetric tonic neck response, which can be most clearly seen during the second and third month postnatally, is a classical example of this coupling (Touwen, 1976). Grenier (1980; 1981) suggested that the neck impotence of the neonate would also hamper the other part of the synergy, the movements of the arm. Grenier held the neonate's neck in position for a certain time and found much more coordinated reaching than otherwise.

Differentiation and integration of sensorimotor systems as exemplified in the development of manual coordination

The emergence of manual coordination takes place mainly during the first year of life. It is a dramatic development. In a matter of months, the crude aiming of arm movements in the newborn will change into the delicate pincer grasp of the 1-year-old.

Hofsten (1984) studied the early part of this development longitudinally in infants from 1 week of age to 19 weeks of age. The infants were seen every third week. He found that the first transformation occurred already around 2 months of age. Then the extension synergy of the newborn broke up. Instead of extending the fingers when the arm extended, the fingers would instead flex as the arm extended. The occurrence of this latter kind of behavior increased from less than 10% in the neonates to around 70% in the 2-month-olds. Visual fixation of the target did not affect this tendency. Apparently, the hand is gaining independent status at this age. When a few weeks older, the infants started to open the hand again when extending the arm but this time only when fixating the target. At the same time, the amount of reaching attempts increased greatly.

Parallel to this development, better means of obtaining precise visual information about spatial relations in reaching space emerge. The sensitivity to binocular disparity develops very rapidly between 3 and 5 months of age. Fox, Aslin, Shea, and Dumais (1980) found that 3.5-month-olds but not 2.5-month-olds would track a moving virtual object specified by binocular disparity in a dynamic random-dot stereogram. Held and colleagues (Birch, Gwiazda, & Held, 1982; Held, Birch, & Gwiazda, 1980) showed the same developmental trend using a modified preferential looking technique. They showed a rapid rise in detection of fine disparities from 3 months of age to an adultlike level between 5 and 7 months of age.

Two other factors contribute to the development of successful reaching. The first is the uncoupling of head and arm movements. This coupling seems to be strongest around 2 months of age when the infant has gained control over the neck muscles. The asymmetric tonic neck reflex is easily demonstrated at this age (Touwen, 1976). In the next 2 months, however, arm movements will be increasingly independent of neck movements and the neck reflex becomes more and more difficult to elicit. This uncoupling will allow for more flexible integration between eye–head movements and manual coordination. The other factor that contributes to the emergence of successful reaching is the appearance of postural stability of the upper trunk at around 4 months of age (Gallahue, 1982). This will enable the infant to sit with support and will constitute an appropriate base for the construction of reaching movements.

The differentiation of the sensorimotor systems for approaching and grasping, the sensitivity for binocular disparity, the decoupling of arm and neck movements, and the postural stabilization of the upper trunk all appear around the same age. They are essential for the emergence of successful reaching. Therefore, in a way, the emergence of successful reaching could be described as an emergent property of several converging developments. Thelen (1985) has discussed the development of coordinated leg movements from this perspective. She proposed the existence of an early coordinative structure for leg movements leading to a highly patterned output. This coordinative structure would undergo elaboration and differentiation during development allowing for more flexible movements. At any point in development, however, movements are not specified by this pattern generator alone, but by the systems outcome of a number of interacting components, each with its own developmental course and acting within definite constraints and opportunities defined by the context. In the case of locomotion, she mentions seven such components apart from pattern generation itself: tonus control, articulator differentiation, extensor strength, postural control, visual flow sensitivity, body constraints, and motivation.

Differentiation requires integration. The differentiation of the sensorimotor systems for approaching and grasping an object necessitates a new integration of these two systems for smooth and efficient action. Ideally, the approach system should carry the hand close to the target where the grasp system should be prepared to take over with a final adjustment as the target is grasped (Jeannerod & Biguer, 1982). This development was studied longitudinally by Hofsten (1980) in infants from 15 to 36 weeks of age. He observed that when infants started to reach for and grasp objects successfully at around 4 months of age, the reaches typically consisted of several steps or phases and the approach was awkward and crooked. However, during the months to follow this picture changed dramatically. Figure 9.1 shows, for individual subjects, how the approach path straightened up: Individual differences in performance were stable during the period studied but the developmental

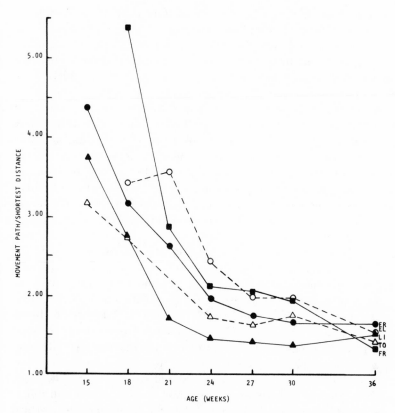

MOVEMENT PATH/SHORTEST DISTANCE

AGE (WEEKS)

Figure 9.1. Relative length of movement path as a function of age for five different subjects. The relative movement path was defined as the length of the movement path divided by the shortest distance from the beginning to the end of the reach.

function was similar for all five infants depicted. Further analysis showed that the steps or phases of the reaches observed diminished in number. The first step grew in importance. More and more of the approach and the power of the reach became concentrated to this step. Subsequent steps became more and more subordinate to the first one, having less to do with the approach and more with increasing the precision of the reach. At around 6 months of age the adultlike reaching pattern started to dominate.

Although vision of the hand is not needed for controlling the approach of the target, it is a prominent factor in the guidance of precise grasping (Hofsten & Lee, 1982). As infants approach 6 months of age they are becoming increasingly dependent on seeing the reaching hand, indicating a focusing on the grasping phase. Lasky (1977) had infants reach for an object seen through a horizontally placed mirror. At the proper place underneath the mirror, an object identical to the reflected one was placed. In the control condition a panel of clear plastic replaced the mirror. Lasky found that in the control condition, 6-month-olds contacted the target nine times more often and retrieved the object three times more often than in the mirror condition.

When infants are still older they seem to become less dependent on seeing the reaching hand. Reaching has become more precise and more automatized. The subject might even look away while reaching and does not seem to be as bothered as the 6-month-olds when sight of the reaching hand is disrupted (Bushnell, 1985). However, in reaching for small targets, where control of individual finger movements is essential, visual guidance is always a prominent factor in controlling the movements. The fine pincer grasp appearing around 9 months of age presupposes delicate visual guidance.

How is the infant adjusting the hand in preparation of grasping the object? There are at least two basic adjustments that can be observed from the age when reaching starts to become successful. First, the orientation of the hand is adjusted to the orientation of object to be grasped (Hofsten & Fazel-Zandy, 1984; Lockman, Ashmead, & Bushnell, 1984). In a longitudinal study, Hofsten and Fazel-Zandy presented infants, 18 to 34 weeks old, with a vertical or a horizontal rod. At group level, we found preparatory adjustments to the orientation of the rod at all ages including the youngest one. Individual results are shown in Figure 9.2. The dependent variable in these graphs is the mean difference in hand orientation between reaches for horizontal and vertical objects at a certain time during the approach of the object. A positive score denotes a difference in the direction predicted by object orientation. A score increasing over time means that the hand rotates toward the orientation of the object during the approach. Figure 9.2 shows that at the end of the approach, 11 of the 15 subjects in the study oriented the hand in the direction of the object at 18 to 22 weeks of age and that this was true for all infants at 30 to 34 weeks of age. However, apart from that, Figure 9.2 also shows that individuals differed much in the way that this end-point correspondence was achieved. Some adjusted the hand during the measured part of the approach and some at an earlier stage. The result proves that the preparatory adjustment is not achieved through some rigid mechanism but rather through a very flexible perception–action system that is functioning at the time when infants start reaching for objects.

The second kind of preparatory adjustment observed in early successful reaching is the timing of the grasp to the encountering of the object.

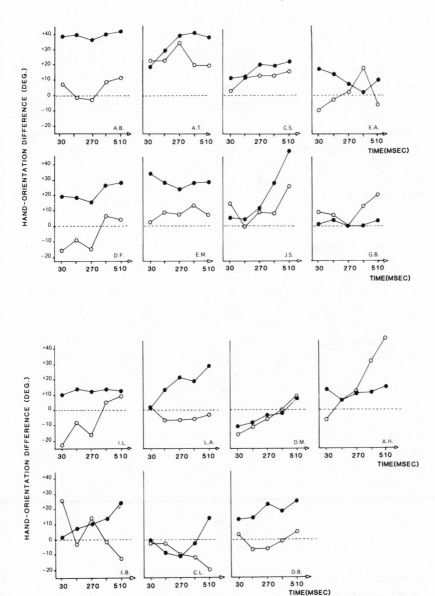

Figure 9.2. Mean difference in hand orientation (degrees) between reaches for horizontal and vertical objects at different times during the last 540 msec. of the approach. A positive score denotes a difference in the direction predicted by object orientation. Curves with unfilled circles are the pooled results from 18- and 22-week sessions and curves with filled circles are the pooled results from the 30- to 34-week sessions. Each diagram depicts the results from one subject (from Hofsten & Fazel-Zandy, 1984).

This is important for efficient grasping of the object. If the hand is closed too early, the object will bounce on the knuckles of the hand. If the hand is closed too late, the object will bounce on the palm of the hand and eventually be lost. Traditional belief has been that infants initially only close the hand as a reaction to the tactile encounter with the object in the same way as the hand closes in a grasp reflex. Hofsten and Rönnquist (1988) studied infants from 5 months of age as they reached for different-sized objects. The distance between the thumb and the index finger was monitored during the approach with an optoelectronic technique. We found that all infants including the youngest would typically time the grasping of the object rather precisely to the encounter of it. Figure 9.3 shows the distribution of timing of grasps for the 5 and 9 months age groups.

The development of basic reaching skill is a prerequisite for the functioning of a number of more specialized perception–action systems. Catching is a good example of such a skill. Developmental psychologists who have been studying the ontogenesis of catching skills have mostly been struck by the complexity of the task. Kay (1970), for instance, suggested that catching ability appears at the earliest around 5 years of age. However, in a series of studies I have found that young infants already possess a remarkable capacity to catch objects (Hofsten, 1980; 1983; Hofsten & Lindhagen, 1979). Hofsten and Lindhagen (1979) studied this problem longitudinally in a group of 11 infants. They were 12 to 24 weeks old at the first session, were seen at 3-week intervals until 30 weeks old, and were finally seen at 36 weeks of age. The subjects were presented with objects moving in front of them at 3.4, 15, or 30 cm/sec. We found that from the very age when infants start to master reaching for stationary objects, they will also reach successfully for fast-moving ones. Eighteen-week-old infants caught the object as it moved 30 cm/sec. To be able to catch such an object, at least some predictive ability is necessary. As the length of the infant's arm at that age is less than 20 cm, the infant needs to start reaching for the target before it is actually within reach.

Major transitions in the sensorimotor functioning of the young child

Differentiation of proprioception

When studying the development of postural stability in children, Shumway-Cook and Woollacott (1985) found that 4- to 6-year-olds

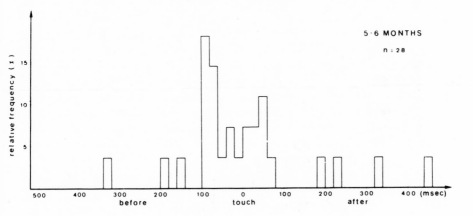

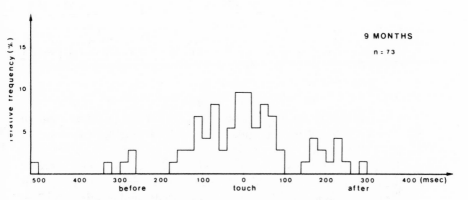

Figure 9.3. Relative distributions of timing of grasping movements relative to the moment of touch for individual reaches performed by 5- to 6-month-old and 9-month-old infants (from Hofsten & Rönnquist, 1988).

appeared to regress in their postural response organization. Their leg postural response synergies were more variable and more delayed as compared with those in a group of children aged 15 to 31 months, a group of 7- to 10-year-olds, or adults (Figure 9.4).

When comparing the different age groups in other respects, they noted that children in the youngest age group (15 to 31 months) were much more visually dependent than children in the older age groups. Dorso-flexing ankle rotation in the absence of visual change did not produce a postural response in gastrocnemius/hamstrings, as is true in older chil-

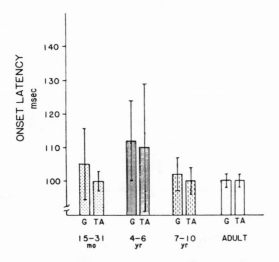

Figure 9.4. Average onset latency (± SD) in the appropriate distal muscle in response to a forward sway translation (G) or backward sway translation (TA) as a function of age. Response latencies are slower and more variable in children 4 to 6 (from Shumway-Cook & Woollacott, 1985).

dren and adults. Heavy reliance on vision for balance in young children has also been found by Lee and Aronson (1974) and Butterworth and Hicks (1977).

Children 4 to 6 years old did produce a postural response to dorso-flexing ankle rotation, but in the absence of congruent visual change this response was much delayed, sway increased significantly, and "in several instances children fell" (Shumway-Cook & Woollacott, 1985, p. 146). These results suggest that in the period between 4 and 6 years of age, there is an increasing sensitivity to proprioceptive inputs mediating postural responses. This will result in a shift away from an established and predominantly visual control of posture. This will evidently lead to an integrated visual-proprioceptive control of balance, but during the transition the efficiency of the system will regress.

In the manual domain, a parallel transition seems to occur at the same age. Hofsten and Rösblad (1987) studied visual and proprioceptive control of pointing movements in children 4 to 12 years of age. The task of the subject was to place drawing pins underneath a table top at the locations of four dots placed on the upper side of the table top. In the visual condition the subject could see the dots but not the hand placing

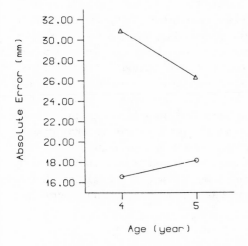

Figure 9.5. Mean absolute error for visually directed pointing (*circles*) and proprioceptively directed pointing (*triangles*) for the 4- and 5-year-old children studied by Hofsten and Rösblad (1988).

the drawing pins. The mode of control in this condition is "visual–proprioceptive" – the location of the target is visually determined, and the movement of the hand is proprioceptively determined. To be able to use this strategy, the visual space and the proprioceptive space have to be congruent.

In the proprioceptive condition, the subject placed the index finger of the other hand on the dot to be pointed to, closed the eyes, and placed the drawing pin underneath the dot. This was done for each of the four dots. In this condition, both the location of the target and the movement of the hand were proprioceptively determined. The mode of control was thus purely proprioceptive. To be able to use this strategy, the proprioceptive space of the left hand has to be congruent to the proprioceptive space of the right hand.

Thirty subjects were tested at each age level. The results show that the purely proprioceptive control of pointing movements – that is, pointing at a felt target – increases in accuracy during the whole age period studied and especially between 4 and 5 years of age. At the same ages, the visual–proprioceptive control of these movements – pointing at a seen target – does not improve at all. This is depicted in Figure 9.5.

These experiments suggest that proprioception undergoes substantial

differentiation and integration during the preschool age. The proprio-
ceptors from the different parts of the body become better integrated into
one unified body space and the subject becomes better able to use
proprioceptive signals in an appropriate way. Posture as well as manual
behavior are mainly visually controlled in younger children. Vision,
however, has a number of functions apart from controlling posture and
movement. It would therefore be of great advantage if at least some
aspects of motor tasks could be controlled by a purely proprioceptive
mode. This is what seems to happen around 5 years of age. Proprioception is starting to play a more prominent role in movement control. The
apparent regression in postural organization and in the visual control of
pointing that occur between 4 and 6 years of age seems to be associated
with the acquisition of an integrated and versatile visual and proprio. cep-
tive sensorimotor system.

Changes in the continuity of arm movements

Another apparent regression in the sensorimotor development of the
child concerns the accuracy and continuity of arm movements and was
first observed by Hay (1978; 1979) in studies of children, 4 to 11 years of
age. In her first study, Hay (1978) measured the accuracy of horizontal
pointing movements with the outstretched arm resting on a cradle. The
pointing was made in the dark and only the target to be pointed at was
visible. She found that younger children of 4, 5, and 6 years of age
performed very accurate movements. In the 7-year-olds, accuracy suddenly decreased, after which it progressively increased until the age of 11
when levels close to those of adults were obtained.

In a second study, Hay (1979) found that the decrease in accuracy at
7 years of age was accompanied by an increased reliance on visual
guidance in reaching. The subjects were required to wear displacing
prisms that allowed Hay to determine the visually guided part of a
reaching movement. The hand will move in the wrong direction determined by the prism spectacles until the subject sees the hand and
corrects the movement. Seven-year-olds started to correct their reaches
earlier than the 5-year-olds and the 9- and 11-year-olds.

How should these findings be interpreted? Is it possible to assume a
similar origin for these phenomena and those studied by Hofsten and
Rösblad (1988) and Shumway-Cook and Woollacott (1985)? The major
difficulty for such an interpretation is, of course, that the regressions
occur at different ages in the different studies reported. However, the

tasks were also different. For instance, Hofsten and Rösblad used a pointing task with fine final adjustments involving proximal as well as distal movements of the arm and the hand, while Hay (1978) used a pointing task mainly consisting of adjusting the direction of the arm at the shoulder. The amount of error, especially at 6 and 7 years of age, is also much greater in Hay's pointing task than in Hofsten and Rösblad's.

Woollacott and Bressan (1986) discuss the possibility that changes in body size – that is, purely biomechanical factors – cause the disruption of visual–proprioceptive control of reaching. I have great difficulty with such an interpretation. There is no reason that the mode of control of reaching movements should suddenly change from a visual–proprioceptive mode to a purely visual mode as body size increases, after which the visual–proprioceptive mode again regains importance as body size increases still more.

Another type of interpretation of Hay's observation is a cognitive one. Mounoud and associates have elaborated this point of view in a number of papers (see e.g., Mounoud, 1976; 1983; Mounoud and Vinter, 1981). The general idea is that action is governed by representations and that sensorimotor development is characterized by a number of representational reorganizations that will result in more and more sophisticated movement control. One such reorganization should occur around 7 years of age. In the late preschool age, substantial changes occur in the cognitive system of the child, which among other things make him or her able to analyze the spoken word into phonemes and letters. Mounoud argues that similar reorganizations should take place in the sensorimotor system. Many activities deteriorate on some measures and do not completely recover until the age of 9 years. This is true for weight lifting (Gachoud, Mounoud, Hauert, & Viviani, 1983) as well as for circle drawing (Mounoud, 1986). Hay's reaching movements are also supposed to be a part of this reorganization of procedures for action. The problem with this kind of explanation, however, is that it is rather vague. It may give us a rationale for thinking about apparent regressions in sensorimotor development in a general way but it does not predict the character of the regressions. Not only did Hay's subjects become more visually dominated at 7 but so did Mounoud's circle drawers (Mounoud, 1986). No cognitive theory can predict that.

The way to solve these problems in a satisfactory way is to study the development of various sensorimotor tasks in a longitudinal fashion during the preschool and early school age. Only by doing that will we be able to see what changes in sensorimotor skills occur together in a single subject.

How is sensorimotor development related to cognition?

Every perception–action system from the simplest to the most sophisticated has some adaptive function that requires knowledge about the world and about the organism of which it is a part. In that sense they are also cognitive systems. However, the cognition involved is rarely of a general nature – that is, it is not accessible to other domains than the one it has been designed for. As stated earlier, there is reason to believe that evolution works by solving specific action problems for the animal demanding specific perceptual skills rather than designing general capacities. In another domain, Fodor (1983) has extensively discussed this kind of knowledge and its domain specificity. He also finds that input processes are best described as modularized or encapsulated.

A major reason for perceptual processes to be modularized or encapsulated is that it allows speed (Hofsten, 1985). Speed is needed in the context of action, because actions are geared to the environment and the events therein. As the environment exists independent of ourselves, adaptive coordination is only possible if we can time our actions relative to the properties of the environment. That requires fast and efficient predictive processing. What is optimal for one task may not be optimal for another. Specialization makes for more efficient functioning but also for less accessible processes.

Take catching, for example. To catch a ball with one hand you not only need to get your hand into the right place but you also have to close your fingers at the right time. The ball will hit the palm of your hand and bounce out if you close too late, or it will bang you on the knuckles if you close too early. Alderson, Sully, and Sully (1974) found that the timing accuracy in the catching of a ball had to be around 14 msec. Just getting the hand to the right place at the right time seems complicated. The catch must be aimed for some point ahead of the object where the hand and the target would meet. How does the subject do that? Does he calculate future positions of the object together with the time it would take him to get there? It seems improbable. An infant does not seem to be able to perform this predictive calculation, but an infant of 5 months will be able to catch a fast object. Instead of being accomplished by a general cognitive calculation, the prediction involved in catching could be accomplished by a much simpler but specialized sensorimotor mechanism. Hofsten (1983; 1987) has discussed the catching of a fast target in terms of a combination of an approach and a tracking action. If the tracking component correctly matches the velocity and direction of the target, the hand is bound to get to the meeting point with it.

The problem with a cognitive approach to sensorimotor development is that the specialized intelligence that evolved through a long biological history may have little in common with prediction and decision making derived through general, accessible cognitive processing. The development of the specialized modules for sensorimotor control and the differentiation and integration of them seem to require their own rules rather than just being a part of a general cognitive development.

The longitudinal approach

The aim of the present chapter has been to give an overview of the problems and transitions encountered in sensorimotor development and to exemplify them with research in the manual domain. However, only a small fraction of the research reviewed has been achieved through the longitudinal method. The cross-sectional method is dominating. It has its advantages in the early stages of the research process. It is much less complicated and resource demanding than the longitudinal method and it is still able to give us a rough idea of how development proceeds and where transitions might occur. However, it will never be able to answer the more specific questions about the transitions and how they fit into the developmental function of each individual. Only the longitudinal approach will be able to do that.

As the rate of development differs between individuals, group values handled by the cross-sectional method will tend to distort and occlude important transitions. In the longitudinal study of prereaching infants by Hofsten (1984), it was found that reaching frequency decreased up to 2 months of age and then increased. Individual data proved that this increase was dramatic and occurred between two visits (i.e., within 3 weeks) for all infants, but at different ages for different infants. For eight infants it occurred at 10 weeks of age, for six infants at 13 weeks of age, for five infants at 16 weeks of age, and for one infant at 19 weeks of age. With the aid of the longitudinal method we can ask what other developmental changes – neurological, bodily, or behavioral – might accompany this dramatic transition and why some individuals are early and some late. Such questions are crucial for our understanding of this phenomenon, as it is of developmental phenomena in general.

The confounding between developmental function and rate of development in the age norms provided by the cross-sectional method has serious consequences for our ability to understand individual differences in development. For instance, it makes it impossible to distinguish pathology and late development. Today, children with functional disturbances are often mistaken for being late developers with the consequences that they are not properly treated for their problems. A functionally

254   HOFSTEN

disturbed child may be a late developer, but the important thing is that the developmental function is abnormal. Only the longitudinal method can help us disentangle such phenomena.

REFERENCES

Alderson, G. J. K., Sully, D. J., & Sully, H. G. (1974). An operational analysis of a one-handed catching task using high speed photography. *Journal of Motor Behavior, 6,* 217–226.

Alegria, J., & Noirot, E. (1978). Neonate orientation behavior towards human voice. *International Journal of Behavioral Development, 1,* 291–312.

André-Thomas, X., & Saint-Anne-Dargassies, S. (1952). *Etudes neurologiques sur le nouveau-né et le jeune nourrisson.* Paris: Masson.

Arbib, M. A. (1981). Perceptual structures and distributed motor control. In V. B. Brooks (Ed.), *Handbook of physiology, The Nervous System II: Motor Control* (pp. 1449–1480). Bethesda, MD: American Physiological Society.

Aslin, R. N. (1977). Development of binocular fixation in human infants. *Journal of Experimental Child Psychology, 23,* 133–150.

Aslin, R. N. (1981). Development of smooth pursuit in human infants. In D. F. Fisher, R. A. Monty, & J. W. Senders (Eds.), *Eye movements: Cognition and visual perception.* Hillsdale, NJ: Erlbaum.

Aslin, R. N., & Jackson, R. W. (1979). Accommodative-convergence in young infants: Development of a synergistic sensory-motor system. *Canadian Journal of Psychology, 33,* 222–231.

Banks, M. S. (1980). The development of visual accommodation during early infancy. *Child Development, 51,* 646–666.

Bauer, J., & Held, R. (1975). Comparison of visually guided reaching in normal and deprived infant monkeys. *Journal of Experimental Psychology: Animal Behavior Processes, 1,* 298–308.

Birch, E. E., Gwiazda, J., & Held, R. (1982). Stereoacuity development for crossed and uncrossed disparities in human infants. *Vision Research, 22,* 507–513.

Brazelton, T. B. (1973). *Neonatal behavioral assessment scale* (Clinics in Developmental Medicine No. 50). Philadelphia: Heinemann Medical Books.

Bullinger, A. (1977). Orientation de la tête du nouveau-né en présence d'un stimulus visuel. *L'Année Psychologique, 2,* 357–364.

Bushnell, E. (1985). The decline of visually guided reaching during infancy. *Infant Behavior and Development,* 139–156.

Butterworth, G. (1986). Some problems in explaining the origins of movement control. In M. G. Wade and H. T. A. Whiting (Eds.), *Motor development in children: Problems of coordination and control* (pp. 23–32). Dordrecht: Martinus Nijhoff.

Butterworth, G. E., & Hicks, L. (1977). Visual proprioception and postural stability in infancy: A developmental study. *Perception, 6,* 255–262.

Dunkeld, J. (1978). *The function of imitation in infancy.* Unpublished doctoral dissertation, University of Edinburgh, Edinburgh.

Fentress, J. C. (1984). The development of coordination. *Journal of Motor Behavior, 16,* 99–134.

Fentress, J. C. (1986). Development of coordinated movement: Dynamic, relational and multileveled perspectives. In M. G. Wade & H. T. A. Whiting (Eds.), *Motor development in children: Problems of coordination and control* (pp. 77–106). Dordrecht: Martinus Nijhoff.

Field, J., Muir, D., Pilon, R., Sinclair, M., & Dodwell, P. (1980). Infants' orientation to lateral sounds from birth to three months. *Child Development, 51*, 295–298.

Fodor, J. A. (1983). *The modularity of mind*. Cambridge: MIT Press.

Fox, R., Aslin, R. N., Shea, S. L., & Dumais, S. T. (1980). Stereopsis in human infants. *Science, 207*, 323–324.

Gachoud, J. P., Mounoud, P., Hauert, C. A., & Viviani, P. (1983). Motor strategies in lifting movements: A comparison of adult and child performances. *Journal of Motor Behavior, 15*, 202–216.

Gallahue, D. L. (1982). *Understanding motor development in children*. New York: Wiley.

Gesell, A. (1954). The ontogenesis of infant behavior. In L. Carmichael (Ed.), *Manual of child psychology* (pp. 335–373). New York: Wiley.

Gesell, A., & Amatruda, C. S. (1964). *Developmental diagnosis: Normal and abnormal development*. New York: Paul B. Hoeber Medical Division.

Gesell, A., & Thompson, H. (1929). Learning and growth in identical infant twins: An experimental study by the method of co-twin control. *Genetic Psychology Monographs, 6*, 1–124.

Grenier, A. (1980). Révélation d'une expression motrice différente par fixation manuelle de la nuque. In A. Grenier & C. Amiel-Tison (Eds.), *Evaluation neurologique du nouveau-né et du nourrisson*. Paris: Masson.

Grenier, A. (1981). "Motricité libérée" par fixation manuelle de la nuque au cours des premières semaines de la vie. *Archives Françaises de Pediatrie, 38*, 557–561.

Hay, L. (1978). Accuracy of children on an open-loop pointing task. *Perceptual and Motor Skills, 47*, 1079–1082.

Hay, L. (1979), Spatial–temporal analysis of movements in children: Motor programs versus feedback in the development of reaching. *Journal of Motor Behavior, 11*, 189–200.

Hein, A. (1974). Prerequisite for development of visually guided reaching in the kitten. *Brain Research, 71*, 259–263.

Hein, A., & Held, R. (1967). Dissociation of the visual placing response into elicited and guided components. *Science, 158*, 390–391.

Held, R., Birch, E. E., Gwiazda, J. (1980). Stereoacuity of human infants. *Proceedings of the National Academy of Sciences U.S.A., 77*, 5572–5574.

Held, R., & Hein, A. (1963). Movement-produced stimulation in the development of visually guided behavior. *Journal of Comparative and Psyiological Psychology, 56*, 872–876.

Hofsten, C. von (1977). Binocular convergence as a determinant of reaching behavior in infancy. *Perception, 6*, 139–144.

Hofsten, C. von (1980). Predictive reaching for moving objects by human infants. *Journal of Experimental Child Psychology, 30*, 369–382.

Hofsten, C. von (1982). Eye–hand coordination in newborns. *Developmental Psychology, 18*, 450–461.

Hofsten, C. von (1983). Catching skills in infancy. *Journal of Experimental Psychology: Human Perception and Performance, 9*, 75–85.

Hofsten, C. von (1984). Developmental changes in the organization of pre-reaching movements. *Developmental Psychology, 20,* 378–388.

Hofsten, C. von (1985). Perception and action. In M. Frese & J. Sabini (Eds.), *Goal directed behavior: The concept of action in psychology* (pp. 80–96). Hillsdale, NJ: Erlbaum.

Hofsten, C. von (1987). Catching. In H. Heuer & A. F. Sanders (Eds.), *Tutorials on perception and action* (pp. 33–46). Hillsdale, NJ: Erlbaum.

Hofsten, C. von, & Fazel-Zandy, S. (1984). Development of visually guided hand orientation in reaching. *Journal of Experimental Child Psychology, 38,* 208–219.

Hofsten, C. von, & Lee, D. N. (1982). Dialogue on perception and action. *Human Movement Science, 1,* 125–138.

Hofsten, C. von, & Lindhagen, K. (1979). Observations on the development of reaching for moving objects. *Journal of Experimental Child Psychology, 28,* 158–173.

Hofsten, C. von, & Rönnquist, L. (1988). Preparation for grasping an object: A developmental study. *Journal of Experimental Psychology: Human Perception and Performance.*

Hofsten, C. von, & Rösblad, B. (1988) *Development of visual and proprioceptive control of manual spatial ability. Neuropsychologia.*

Humphrey, D., Muir, D., & Dodwell, P. (1981). *Touch localization in newborns.* Unpublished manuscript.

Jeannerod, M., & Biquer, B. (1982). Visuomotor mechanisms in reaching within extrapersonal space. In D. J. Ingle, M. A. Goodale, & R. J. W. Mansfield (Eds.), *Analysis of visual behavior.* Cambridge: MIT Press.

Kay, H. (1970). Analyzing motor skill performance. In K. Connolly (Ed.), *Mechanisms of motor skill development.* London: Academic Press.

Kelso, J. A. S. (1984). Phase transitions and critical behavior in human bi-manual coordination. *American Journal of Physiology, 246,* 1000–1004.

Kugler, P. N., Kelso, J. A. S., & Turvey, M. T. (1982). On the control and coordination of naturally developing systems. In J. A. S. Kelso & J. E. Clark (Eds.), *The development of movement control and coordination.* New York: Wiley.

Lasky, R. E. (1977). The effect of visual feedback of the hand on reaching and retrieval behavior of young infants. *Child Development, 48,* 112–117.

Lawrence, D. G., & Hopkins, D. A. (1972). Developmental aspects of pyramidal motor control in the rhesus monkey. *Brain Research, 40,* 117–118.

Lawrence, D. G., & Hopkins, D. A. (1976). The development of motor control in the rhesus monkey: Evidence concerning the role of corticomotorneuronal connections. *Brain, 99,* 235–254.

Lee, D. N., & Aronson, E. (1974). Visual proprioceptive control of standing in human infants. *Perception & Psychophysics, 15,* 529–532.

Lockman, J. J., Ashmead, D. H., & Bushnell, E. W. (1984). The development of anticipatory hand orientation during infancy. *Journal of Experimental Child Psychology, 37,* 176–186.

Maratsos, O. (1973). *The origin and development of imitation in the first six months of life.* Unpublished doctoral dissertation, University of Geneva, Geneva.

McGraw, M. B. (1940). Neural maturation as exemplified in achievement of bladder control. *Journal of Pediatrics, 16,* 580–590.

McGraw, M. B. (1945). *The neuromuscular maturation of the human infant.* New York: Columbia University Press.

Meltzoff, A. N., & Moore, M. K. (1977). Imitation of facial and manual gestures by human neonates. *Science, 8,* 75–78.

Mendelson, M. J., & Haith, M. H. (1976). The relation between audition and vision in the human newborn. *Monographs of the Society for Research in Child Development, 41* (Serial No. 167).

Mounoud, P. (1976). Les revolutions psychologiques de l'enfant. *Archives de Psychologie, 171,* 103–114.

Mounoud, P. (1983). L'évolution des conduites de préhension comme illustration d'un modèle du développement. In S. de Schoenen (Ed.), *Les débuts du développement.* Paris: P.U.F.

Mounoud, P. (1986). Action and cognition: Cognitive and motor skills in a developmental perspective. In M. G. Wade & H. T. A. Whiting (Eds.), *Motor development in children: Problems of coordination and control* (pp. 373–390). Dordrecht: Martinus Nijhoff.

Mounoud, P., & Vinter, A. (1981). Representation and sensorimotor development. In G. Butterworth (Ed.), *Infancy and epistemology: An evaluation of Piaget's theory.* Brighton: The Harvester Press.

Newell, K. M. (1986). Constraints on the development of coordination. In M. G. Wade & H. T. A. Whiting (Eds.), *Motor development in children: Problems of coordination and control* (pp. 341–360). Dordrecht: Martinus Nijhoff.

Peiper, A. (1963). *Cerebral function in infancy and childhood.* New York: Consultants Bureau.

Piaget, J. (1953). *The origins of intelligence in the child.* New York: Routledge.

Piaget, J. (1970). Piaget's theory. In P. H. Mussen (Ed.), *Carmichael's manual of child psychology* (Vol. 1, pp. 703–732). New York: Wiley.

Prechtl, H. (1977). *The neurological examination of the full-term newborn infant* (2nd ed.) (Clinics in Developmental Medicine No. 63). London: Heinemann Medical Books.

Reed, E. S. (1982). An outline of a theory of action systems. *Journal of Motor Behavior, 14,* 98–134.

Rochat, P., Blass, E. M., & Hoffmeyer, L. B. (1987). Oropharyngeal control of hand–mouth coordination in newborn infants. Unpublished manuscript.

Rozin, P. (1976). The evolution of intelligence and access to the cognitive unconscious. *Progress in Psychobiology and Physiological Psychology, 6,* 245–279.

Shumway-Cook, A., & Woollacott, M. (1985). The growth of stability: Postural control from a developmental perspective. *Journal of Motor Behavior, 17,* 131–147.

Slater, A. M., & Finlay, J. M. (1975). Binocular fixation in the newborn baby. *Journal of Experimental Child Psychology, 20,* 248–273.

Thelen, E. (1985). Developmental origins of motor coordination: Leg movements in human infants. *Developmental Psychobiology, 18,* 1–18.

Thelen, E., & Fisher, D. M. (1982). Newborn stepping: An explanation for a "Disappearing" reflex. *Developmental Psychobiology, 18,* 760–775.

Thelen, E., & Fisher, D. M. (1983). From spontaneous to instrumental behavior: Kinematic analysis of movement changes during very early learning. *Child Development, 54,* 129–140.

Thelen, E., Fisher, D. M., & Ridley-Johnson, R. (1984). The relationship between physical growth and a newborn reflex. *Infant Behavior and Development, 7,* 479–493.

Touwen, B. C. L. (1976). *Neurological development in infancy* (Clinics in Developmental Medicine No. 58). London: Heinemann Medical Books.

Touwen, B. C. L. (1978). Variability and stereotypy in normal and deviant development. *Clinics in Developmental Medicine, 67*, 99–110.

Vinter, A. (1985). *L'imitation chez le nouveau né*. Paris et Neuchatel: Delachaux et Niestlé.

Woollacott, M., & Bressan, E. S. (1986). The development of sensory-motor integration: Some implications from eye–hand coordination and balance control. In J. Clark (Ed.), *Current selected research in motor development II*. Washington, DC: AAHPERD.

Zelazo, P. R., Zelazo, N. A., & Kolb, S. (1972). Newborn walking. *Science, 177*, 1058–1059.

10 On early coordinations and their future

HENRIETTE BLOCH

Introduction

The picture provided by behavioral studies on sensorimotor coordinations at the beginning of life – their strength, their stability, and their possible evolution – is far from clear. Perceptual development is commonly stated to be linked, at least in its initial phases, to the development of local and general motor abilities. However, when viewed from the perspective of what motor development owes to sensory information gathering, the ties appear to be less well related and less clearly determinant. The weight of the motor machinery, the complexity and the diversity of its components (muscle, bone, tendon, joint, nerve), and the relays implicated in the organization of movement may give the impression that motor development is relatively autonomous. In humans, the role of sensory activity in the development of kinematic mechanisms and displacement activities is generally written off in terms of feedback corrections, and reported to occur fairly late.

The growing evidence that sensorimotor coordinations occur during the first days of life in the human newborn points to the need for considerable theoretical reconsideration. Data of this type challenge the notion of a purely reflex origin of movement, a point of view adopted among others by Wyke in 1975 and Vurpillot and Bullinger in 1983. This position has been seriously weakened by both neurological and behavioral arguments (see Bloch, 1983; Touwen, 1985). Second, the existence of early coordinations refutes classical sensorimotor development schemata, which view coordination as organizations arising progressively from the previously autonomous activities of each system involved. In classical theories, sensory and motor systems are gradually paired and combined until general and unified coordination is achieved by the end of the second year of life. Data indicative of early sensorimotor coordination and those demonstrating intermodal transfers cannot be accommodated by such models.

The crucial issue is to specify whether the emergence of early coordinations has an effect on later behaviors, and whether they are in fact their prerequisites. Current data are far from conclusive when it comes to identifying what becomes of early coordinations during the first months of life, thus making the task of charting a coherent overall description even more arduous.

One study lends itself well to illustrating these difficulties. Bower, Broughton, and Moore (1970) reported that 7-day-olds exhibited anticipatory hand shaping when an object was placed near them in their visual field. However, these same subjects never looked at objects placed directly in their hand. Other authors' attempts at replicating the shaping results, which clearly suggest coordination between vision and reaching, have failed, as Hofsten (1982) points out. On the other hand numerous studies have corroborated the second finding, although there is a lack of agreement as to the age at which a change takes place – for example, at 13 weeks for Bower (1974), but not before 8 months for Lockman, Ashmead, and Bushnell (1984).

The persistence of stereotypic, rhythmic motor activities, which were traditionally considered to be "archaic" reactions and as such destined to fade rapidly, complicate the issue even further. The frequency of rhythmical stereotypies as a function of infant state or arousal and context (see Thelen, 1981) as well as the fact that they do not appear to respond adaptively to external stimulation has led researchers to consider that they interfere with the emergence of possible expressions of sensorimotor coordinations. This demonstrates the value of examining the status of early coordinations, their role in the behavioral repertoire, and their functions, as well as conducting fine analyses of the course of these coordinations to shed light on their persistence, or to identify the factors that transform or cause them to disunite.

The major questions can be summarized as follows:

> Are early coordinations the precursors of unified sensorimotor development, or do they form the common substrate for autonomous development of their perceptual and motor components?
> Are they indicative of indifferentiation or do they constitute the first manifestation of adaptive organization?
> Can it be shown that they orient and lay the groundwork for behaviors that appear later in life?

Dealing with early sensorimotor coordinations requires an appropriate methodology. Cross-sectional studies often provide a sound basis because they can capture major trends at each age and trace developmental vectors. The drawback to cross-sectional studies is that they only identify a sequence of states. Processes of change are not directly observable, and can only be deduced from the fact that they are consecutive. This is why they should be complemented by longitudinal studies, particularly in the first years of life when numerous and rapid changes take place. The advantage of longitudinal methods, even short-term ones, is that they furnish a means of dating these changes more accurately, and yield information on the way(s) in which these changes take place.

The aim of this chapter is to focus on the earliest forms of sensorimotor coordinations, to identify the factors presiding over change and the outcomes of these changes, and to discuss the methods that are the most likely to reveal them.

Status and function of early coordinations

It is no easy matter to demonstrate convincingly that sensorimotor coordination really exists in the newborn. Methodological difficulties are augmented by conceptual problems. Hofsten (1982) has cataloged these difficulties and has clearly shown that they can be overcome. One of the major methodological difficulties is measurement of the motor component, which must be distinguished from background noise formed by mass agitation and rhythmic stereotypies. In addition, it must be measured at a distance from the source, to avoid interfering with spontaneous behavior. Assessment of neonate perceptual activity is scarcely easier. The duration of sensorial focus on a stimulus is not informative as to the type of exploration or stimulus analysis the infant is performing.

The problems of conceptualizing sensorimotor activity stem from the fact that coordination in infants is not an ipso facto indication of level of performance. How should an infant's actions be characterized or defined? It is often difficult to avoid assigning a priori meaning to action, as can be seen in discussion sections in the literature. Manual extension toward an object is often described as attempted prehension. When the infant fails, there is a danger of attributing this failure to a lack of coordination. This is what Di Franco, Muir, and Dodwell (1978) in fact do: They conclude that there is no real eye–hand coordination at the beginning of life because this form of coordination does not accomplish the goal it succeeds in doing later on. More sensitive to the direction of hand movement than to its "success," Amiel-Tison and Grenier (1985) introduce the notion of intentionality. Aside from the fact that this is a loaded term, it may also erroneously imply that coordination is the epiphenomenon of a covert representation.[1]

The persistence of these difficulties underscores the fact that sensorimotor coordinations in the newborn are not easily captured. The specific conditions in which coordinations can be observed, and their main

features, must be measured by an approach that is free from precon-
ceived ideas as to their functions.

The first forms of sensorimotor coordination emerge in contexts that
elicit a quiet state of alertness (behavioral state no. 3 according to
Prechtl's classification). They also require specific postural conditions:
semivertical position, with the head held in an upright position. The fact
that posture – and in particular the upright position of the head, which
is the support for most teleonomic sensory captors – plays an important
role suggests that posture may be the framework necessary for the
organization of coordination. I will return to this point and its related
hypotheses later on in the chapter.

The most clear-cut features of early forms of coordination appear to be
negative ones: Joint head and eye movements do not prevent visual
pursuit from being discontinuous; hand–eye coalitions do not enable the
infant to touch or take a fixated object; hand–mouth movements are
ill-directed, hesitant, and often miss.

When sensory pointing is apparently precise, as assessed by accurate
measures of visual fixation, this does not ensure that coordinated action
will be carried out. Hofsten (1982) has shown that the hand comes closer
to a fixated than to a nonfixated object, but that the absolute frequency
of contact in both cases does not differ. This seems to indicate that
arm–hand movement is more immature than gaze, and raises the issue of
differences in maturation of associated systems. One important and
perhaps specific feature of early coordinations is that in most cases they
associate two systems that are not on the same maturational level, a
characteristic Goldman-Rakic (1985) rightly draws to our attention.
This is a crucial point for the understanding of the status of early
coordinations, and for the investigation of their functional relationships.

Two examples – eye–head and eye–hand coordination – provide an
overview of the different hypotheses that can be generated from a given
set of data.

Eye–head coordination

Neuromuscular maturation of the head is relatively incomplete at birth.
Although the visual system is not entirely mature, ultrasound study has
shown that eye movement is present from the 16th gestational week.
Associated movement of both eyes is common in newborns and is used to
detect events in the periphery of the visual field and to track moving
objects or targets.

In recent years a series of experiments has been carried out in the
laboratory (Bloch, 1983; Bloch, Mellier, & Fuenmajor, 1984; Fuenmajor,
1985) on visual pursuit in full- and preterm infants in order to detect

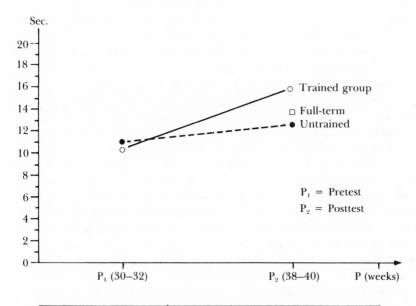

Figure 10.1. Comparison of trained and untrained neonates for visual pursuit (mean duration). Unfilled circles represent a trained group of premature infants; filled circles, an untrained group of premature infants; and squares, a full-term reference group.

Gestational age		Stimulation		F	p
		Trained	Untrained		
30–32	pretest	10.5 $t = 5.33$	10.92 significant at p .001	12.26	> .01
38–40	posttest	15.48 $t = 2.86$	12.48 significant at p .02		

maturational differences of the visual system, and to investigate whether early visual experience results in a gain in premature infants. The sample was composed of low-risk, healthy premature infants born 30 to 32 weeks gestational age, with good Apgar scores (seven or higher at 5 minutes after delivery). Subjects were randomly assigned to the experimental or the control groups.

Both groups were given a pretest during the first week of life (mean age, 5 days) and a posttest upon hospital discharge when they had reached the normal full-term age. The experimental group was given daily pursuit training using mobiles that were changed between tests. Full-term newborns served as a reference group. This group was only tested once during the first week of life (mean age, 4 days).

No differences were observed on the pretest between the two groups of premature subjects. However, the groups of premature infants differed on the posttest and from the reference group in both span and duration of tracking (see Fig. 10.1).

A qualitative difference was also observed. In full-term infants pursuit was generally shaped by a sequence of eye displacements and head rotations, whereas in untrained premature infants it was only ocular. Training sessions in the experimental group were videotaped and performance scored. Videotape analysis showed a gain due to a transition from ocular to oculocephalic activity: In a supine position, the infants were initially only able to follow the moving target with their eyes, until reaching maximal orbital eccentricity. This excentric position triggered a lateral fall of the head, which induced a vestibular-ocular reflex. The eyes then moved rapidly in the opposite direction. This deviation was followed by a slower orbital recentration. Experience was responsible for the change in organization. After 6 to 10 days of training, a regulation of vestibular-ocular reflex was observed; the infants became able to stop the rapid deviation, thus facilitating recentration. The head straightened up in the median plane and began to rotate toward the stimulus. Although pursuit remained discontinuous, the stimulus was lost for shorter periods of time and less frequently. This improvement demonstrates the role played by eye–head coordination, which appears to be triggered and governed by visual practice. Visual goal directedness aids perceptual processing. When the head drops, randomization of gaze ensues. Head rotations that occur in the horizontal plane thus may serve to establish a system of spatial coordinates, which become the basis for perceptual information processing (see Fig. 10.2).

This view is supported by other findings. Some years ago, Barten, Birns, and Ronch (1971) reported individual differences in the amount of eye–head pursuit in full-term 48-hour-old newborns. Their subjects were presented with two different stimuli in identical conditions and were observed for pursuit. The major implication in the authors' words is that "head-and-eye pursuit is a more flegged form of pursuit," which is affected by the attractiveness value of the stimulus.

Eye–hand coordination

The second example is provided by early eye–hand coordination in open situations. Grenier (1981) reports that 1- to 2-week-old infants, when brought to a quiet state of alertness and held in a sitting position with the head upright and the arms free, exhibit obvious signs of interest in a nearby object located on a small table immediately in front of them but

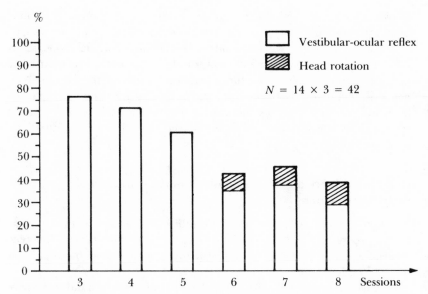

Figure 10.2. Progressive vestibular-ocular-reflex regulation as a function of practice and emergence of first head rotations in the experimental group of premature infants.

slightly to the left or the right, so as to be easily accessible to reach. Subjects focus on the object for relatively long periods of time and while doing so, initiate a slow and nonballistic reaching movement. At times, the arm describes a curve in space before orienting toward the object. No anticipatory hand shaping is observed. When the hand reaches the vicinity of the object, the movement stops and the hand lands on the table, or pushes the object toward the center of the table with small sweeping movements. Grasping, handling, or tactual exploration are absent or rare and fleeting. These observations suggest that the infant's goal in reaching is not manipulation, but rather a contribution to visual activity. Stopping or pushing with the hand may serve to bound off the useful visual field or localize the object better.

Hofsten (1982) has obtained congruent findings in his studies on newborns and argues that "the function of neonate reaching seems to be attentional rather than manipulative," an opinion shared here. This hypothesis can be extended by studying what favors perceptual and, more particularly, visual attention. The point of view I put forward here is that attentional processes in the baby are subsumed to a spatial framework, which orders the environment. Posture and line of gaze are the sources of a horizontovertical coordinate system that enables coding of object locations. It is likely that the earliest sensorimotor coordinations serve this purpose and help reinforce the efficiency of the system.

To sum up, what we know about early coordinations appears to indicate that they do not involve reciprocal or symmetrical relationships, because of differences in maturational level between the two components. Rather, early coordinations seem to be driven by the more mature form and serve initially to structure or reinforce the activity of the leader system. This suggests that, from the outset, sensorimotor coordinations have specific features.

Current evidence on factors involved in the evolution of early coordinations

The first set of issues surrounding primitive asymmetries is their persistence, progressive fading, or sudden extinction. The second involves determining the relationships between these features and the organization of development.

It is easier to pinpoint the latter than the former. In hand–eye coordination, authors situate the earliest changes at about 4 to 5 months of age. As of this age, the role of coordination is object prehension. The groundwork for this change is apparently laid from the third month and is accompanied by changes in prior organization. Gaze, which had formerly triggered manual approach movement but did not control it, now provides true guidance, at least in the final phases of movement. Coordination thus gains in accuracy and synchrony.

This does not imply that asymmetry has been overcome; Hofsten (this volume) points out that vision still predominates even beyond the first year of life. Recent work by Bushnell and Weinberger (1987) corroborates these findings: In a study of intermodal transfer, the authors show that at age 11 months, visual information gathering sets the parameters for manual exploration. More important, object qualities (such as texture), which seemingly appeal directly to the tactual mode, do not give rise to tactual control when apprehended visually.

There are numerous indications that beyond the first year of life sensorial information gathering still governs sensorimotor coordinations. However, coordination clearly becomes more harmonious and fluid. This may be due to the fact that motor development takes place at a different pace than perceptual development, motor development apparently accelerating later. The infant appears to be a mosaic of biological ages, and behavioral development is based on heterochronies.

The importance of stable postural organization in all displacement activities has often been stressed. Results indicate that the development of directed motor performance is tightly linked to postural stability. This leads to two implications: The first is related to constraints and limitations that apparently govern the slow emergence of what is termed postural maturation; the second involves the organizational role of the postural frame as a spatial system of reference.

Biomechanical constraints

In general, research over the past few years has stressed the importance of biomechanical constraints over motility at the beginning of life and their impact on early sensorimotor coordination. These constraints play a role in the development of oculomotor coordination, even before the head can be maintained in an upright position: over the course of the first 2 months, the ratio of head weight to the weight of the trunk and the limbs is modified, which is thought to facilitate mobility and favor synchronization with eye movements. With respect to development of hand movement in hand–eye coordination, Hofsten, as we have seen, puts forward an alternative explanation based on "body-scaled" information. Another example is found in motor reactions observed at birth that disappear and then reappear after a relatively long interval in an integrated sensorimotor structure. The most striking example is walking, which is automatic in the newborn and part of what are termed the "archaic reflexes" that fade during the course of the second month. The rhythmic alternation of leg extension and flexion reappear in autonomous walking at about 11 to 12 months, when they are part of a sensorimotor coordination because the step is visually guided. A biomechanical explanation for this pattern of development has been put forward (Thelen, Fischer, & Ridley-Johnson, 1984; Thelen, 1986), but a certain number of findings do not support this contention.

Biomechanical constraints are clearly related to allometrics during the growth process. They change as a function of size and weight relationships between parts of the body, and have an effect on local and global tonicity. They are thought to control the appearance and disappearance of certain spontaneous reactions, in particular those that are assumed to be under low-level central nervous system control. It is plausible for instance that biomechanical constraints are responsible for both the onset of automatic walking in the neonate – because of the disproportionality of head weight – and for its extinction at around the end of the second month because of the rapid increase in the size of the limbs. However, this explanation is not entirely satisfactory, because the strength of the response, variation in weight, hyper- or hypotonicity (as André-Thomas & Autgaerden, 1952, have shown) do not appear to have a decisive influence on its extinction. Our own observations on automatic walking confirm that pronounced individual differences persist even when all subjects are tested at the same time of day, and behavior state is controlled for.

Evidence with respect to the relationship between automatic walking and autonomous walking is also problematical. When compared with a control group of infants untrained in automatic walking after the response had faded, the test group that had received practice tended to walk independently earlier than the untrained babies (André-Thomas & Autgaerden, 1952; Bower, 1974; Zelazo, 1976; 1983). This slight but systematic precocity suggests that practice helped the test group overcome the constraints countering the persistence of this response, and thus prepared the groundwork for autonomous walking in a way that still remains unclear.

Thelen, Kelso, and Fogel (1987) argue that identical dynamic properties govern automatic walking and autonomous walking and that locomotion responds to a metric that changes continuously with growth – that is, with the lengthening of the legs. Is it sufficient to argue that autonomous walking is simply a question of changes in biomechanical constraints?

To examine the evolution in behavior from automatic to autonomous walking, and to track what can change during the course of regular practice in autonomous walking, we set up the following experiment: Newborns selected on the basis of good stepping reflex (André-Thomas's evaluation criteria) during the postnatal neurological examination were randomly assigned to either the test or the control group. For each group, subjects were matched for size and weight. The experimental group was given daily practice in walking between the ages of 2 weeks and 3 months. Sessions were filmed every 3 weeks. The control group was only given practice once every 3 weeks (for a total of four sessions) between the second week and the third month of life. The training procedure and the testing sessions were as follows: The infant, in an upright position, was held under the armpits by the experimenter situated behind him or her, such that the infant's feet rested on a uniform surface. In this position, the neonate immediately began to walk automatically. A rigid plexiglass plate with a uniform, nonskid surface was placed on a table and used as a route surface. The infants were filmed from above by a camera located facing them, at the far end of the plate. The training as well as the control session lasted approximately 2 to 2.30 minutes.

To obtain within-group measures, the subjects in both groups were retested in identical conditions when they began to be able to stand erect unaided. Age of onset of autonomous walking was recorded. Over-

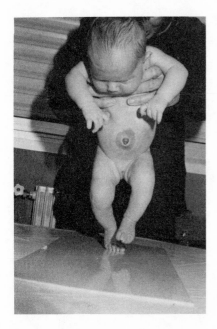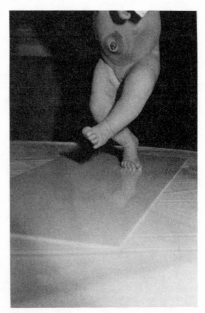

Figures 10.3*a* and *b*. Automatic walking: characteristic positions of a 3-week-old control-group infant.

all posture, positions, and limb movements were scored from videotapes using a double-blind procedure, and processed on computer. Within- and cross-group comparisons were performed for each test.

The changes observed in the test group that can be attributed to practice effects are the following:

> Between the ages of 3 and 12 weeks, posture became upright, the head was held erect, and the trunk was stabilized. The shoulders became perpendicular to the orientation of the feet when walking. Gaze was oriented in the same direction as steps and clearly focused beyond the feet, in most cases on a line with the head.
>
> Position and movement of the limbs composing the dynamics of overall movement also changed. The legs remained parallel, the knees and ankles no longer crossed, the foot was lifted without torsion, and the heel was placed down first. Stepping was well defined.

At the age of 12 weeks, the overall range of within-group responses was smaller for the experimental group than for the control group, for all measures tested (see Figs. 10.3 and 10.4).

When we tested infants from the same groups at the age of 8 to 13

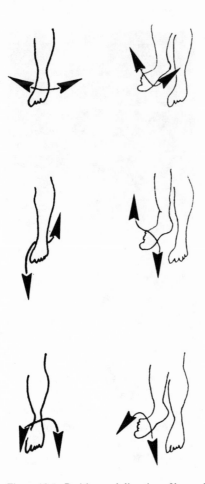

Figure 10.4. Position and direction of leg and foot movement in 12-week-old untrained infant.

months using the same technique used to train newborns to walk, we were surprised to observe that all subjects behaved like those in the control group. They bent forward and exhibited frequent leg crossing and torsion. The benefits of practice in infants who had received training in automatic walking had apparently disappeared, and the same handicaps that prevent neonates from walking were apparently operating in these toddlers. The effects of early training in automatic walking and the high degree of similarity at very different ages (growth differences are enormous) raise doubts as to whether motor activity is under the sole,

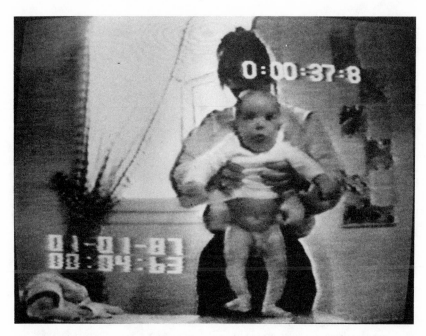

Figure 10.5. Characteristic position of 12-week-old infant trained daily in autonomic walking.

rigidly determined agency of biomechanical constraints. The data suggest that the precocity of trained 10-month-olds, which is clear-cut in terms of posture and perception at 4 to 5 months (see Maciaszczyk & Bloch, 1986), may be due to faster reactivation than to conservation of an acquired organization. Nevertheless, although within-group comparisons are not yet available, the only differences between infants with prior training and those who were trained appears to be the greater erectness of the trained group (see Figs. 10.5 and 10.6).

Thus, it is far from clear that overcoming biomechanical constraints at a given point in time will have long-term effects. Other data tend to undermine the contention of a decisive role of biomechanical constraints on the course of sensorimotor development. These data concern, first, the persistence of rhythmic movements. Prechtl (1984) bases his arguments for a continuity between fetal and postnatal motility on the persistence of rhythmic movements. A purported continuity of this type is contradictory with the notion of determinism exerted by constraints

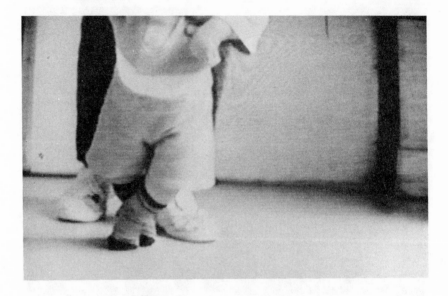

Figure 10.6. Characteristic position of 9-month-old infant immediately prior to autonomous walking. No differences in leg–foot position were observed between trained and untrained subjects.

that change dramatically from the fetal (aquatic) environment to the postnatal (aerial) environment.

Second, the prevailing assumption that the four major stages of postural maturation – head upright, sitting, standing, and autonomous walking – are an invariant sequence, if Touwen (1978) is right, may not be ordered universally. A number of studies have shown that crawling and creeping are not prerequisites for standing or walking. These behaviors are not considered to endanger the foundations of the developmental edifice because they are seen as epiphenomena of previously formed organizations. The cases described by Touwen of children who display the reverse order – who stand up before they sit – are more disturbing. The implications of this type of evidence are difficult to assess. When a so-called normal behavior does not appear spontaneously, should it be concluded that the functional capacity to perform this behavior is absent, or should the conditions favoring the emergence of this behavior be incriminated first? This question also applies to heterodox cases, reported by Touwen, involving infants who, because of prematurity or perinatal dysfunction, were kept in one body position and may have had more limited early postural experience.

The third and perhaps most sensitive issue concerns the implicit or explicit relationships between the strength of biomechanical constraints and the level of control they exert over certain movements. It is significant that considerations on the role of these constraints have focused almost exclusively on behaviors qualified as "reflexes" or on behaviors in which control is assumed to be purely subcortical, with limited degrees of freedom.

In this theoretical framework, early sensorimotor coordination is viewed as being prewired, and dependent upon a common motor program controlled by the superior colliculus (Roucoux, Crommelinck, Guerit, & Meulders, 1981). These coordinations can only become flexible and be transformed through higher-level control structures (see Tyschen & Lisberger, 1986). Globally the data do not disconfirm this thesis. However, various indexes – the presence of sections of smooth pursuit in a pursuit activity in the newborn (Kremenitzer, Vaughan, Kurtzberg, & Dowling, 1979), the fact that the neonate can adapt the number of saccades as a function of the trajectory of the mobile he or she is tracking (Bloch & Jouen, 1986), and perhaps the rich repertoire of arm–hand movements described by Grenier and Hofsten – cast a number of doubts on this assumption. Some data suggest that prior to the third month, visuomotor activity is under cortical control (Atkinson, 1984).

Postural maturation and coordinations

The postural framework in which early coordinations develop and function is critical. Disagreement lies in the nature of the relations between posture and sensorimotor coordination during the first 2 years of life. When a new posture and a new form of coordination emerge simultaneously, this coincidence is occasionally interpreted causally. Only a few authors have credited the emergence of an early coordination with a new posture.

Spontaneous maintenance of the head in the geovertical position, which intervenes at 3 months, is thought to cause a change in the pattern of visual scanning (Hainline & Lemerise, 1982) and a considerable widening of the useful visual field (MacFarlane, Harris, & Barnes, 1976; Barnes, 1983).

Eye–hand coordination has been explored in our laboratory in a series of experiments on prehension in 4- to 8-month-olds (Pieraut-le Bonniec,

Hombessa, & Jacquet, 1987). The findings show that both the ability to sit alone and the stability of the sitting position play a crucial role in the organization of movement: Arm displacement and reach of the arm and the hand toward the fixated object vary as a function of the acquisition of the sitting posture; bilateral equilibrium of arm extension is more fluid when the infant can sit cross-legged with the trunk erect than when he or she is only capable of sitting with the legs spread far apart and the trunk bent slightly forward. Arm bilateral balance in turn affects manual capture in the surrounding space. These findings clearly indicate that posture plays a role in determining the organization of movement spaces. Similarly, it can be postulated that a vertical position of the head, oriented to the geographical vertical and not to the body axis, is primordial in the structuration of visual space. Thus, the infant's ability to keep the trunk upright is essential to the structuration of visual–kinesthetic space.

For a sensorimotor coordination to emerge and for it to be efficient, regardless of its function, an identical framework must govern its sensory and motor components. The verticality of the head constitutes one of the axes of the reference system for visual perception in the newborn. This has been shown for tracking, anticipating places (Bloch, 1977; Jouen, Lepecq, & Bloch, 1984), computing distances (Lepecq, 1986), and perhaps analyzing forms (Hainlin & Lemerise, 1982).

The diversity of arm–hand movements in the newborn, which Grenier (1981) interprets as being a precursor of the future organization of reaching, may thus be related to postural immaturity, and diversity may be an indicator of randomness in the directionality of movement; randomness in this case would fade when the trunk could be maintained upright. Hence, control of movement must take spatial coordinates into account and thus requires a spatial frame of reference. Paillard and Beaubaton (1978) attribute the organization of prehension at the age of 4 to 5 months precisely to the emergence of a "geocentric frame of reference." This is congruent with the regularities of positioning observed by White (1970) at this same age. More testing and validation are necessary to confirm this hypothesis. It is likely, however, that relationships between posture and sensorimotor coordination take on a significance through the elaboration of spatial frames of reference.

Spatial frameworks were traditionally considered to be indicative of stable or achieved states. In Piagetian theory, spatial egocentrism characterizes a form of perceptual activity whose ultimate stage of development is exocentrism. It is not my intention to dwell on the ambiguities of the notion of egocentrism. The real issue is the status of these referents:

Should they be seen as the outcomes of developmental process, or are they themselves part of this process? My position is that they are factors in the organization of sensorimotor coordination and, as such, play a role in sensorimotor development.

Orientation and mechanisms of sensorimotor development

Existing studies, for the most part cross-sectional, indicate that there is increasing accuracy and convergence of sensorial activity and the movements performed under sensory guidance. This is a very global perspective. Little is known about the mechanisms underlying functional and structural changes.

The data give rise to contradictory interpretations and hypotheses (see Butterworth, this volume), and raise the issue of whether changes in sensorimotor coordination take on one or several forms although following the same general trend.

Focus on one sensorimotor coordination rather than another gives a different picture of type of change and even type of initial development. Eye–head coordination, once established, appears stable. During the first 2 months, it gains in precision through a tighter temporal organization of eye movement and head rotation and becomes more flexible: During pursuit, eye–head coordination can be coupled or uncoupled. It is doubtless a prerequisite for the extension of saccadic pursuit and the transition to smooth pursuit. During the first months, its apparent stability in fact conceals a change in control mechanisms: Eye–head coupling, governed first by a common, collicular program, may be transferred to hierarchically higher and more diversified control. This hierarchization is responsible for both the synchronization and the flexibility reported at about age 3 months (Roucoux & Crommelinck, 1984).

The earliest eye–hand coordinations do not seem to follow the same pattern. Between the first and fourth months, reaching movements change but do not appear to progress. The arm–hand movement becomes ballistic and of a piece. At 3 to 4 months, the hand often contacts the object but lands on it heavily, which either produces grasping, pushing the object away, bumping – in short, misses. The features of this movement, clearly far removed from what is observed in the neonate, have prompted certain authors to interpret this behavior as a manifestation of a primitive reflex (White, Castle, & Held, 1964). Does this imply that the behavior observed at the age of 3 to 4 months is a regression, with respect to neonate performance? Is this apparent regression a change in function?

Can this type of assumed change in function only take place through remodelization? Could this change be related to the onset of cortical control, whose most visible effect would be a reduction in the number of degrees of freedom of reaching movements? This idea is not unrelated to Bernstein's (1967) position. Nevertheless, the fact that prehension only develops gradually, over a period of months, leaves doubts as to the total determinism of a hierarchization of this type.

It should be recalled, however, that cortical control has been used as an explanation for locomotor development (André-Thomas & Autgaerden 1952). This does not seem to be incompatible with reorganizations, and is in fact considered to be responsible for them. It is reasonable to assume that the effects of cortical control can be measured by qualitative changes. Traditional theories of sensorimotor development drew heavily on this hypothesis when situating the hierarchization process within the more general framework of maturation. An indication can be found in the pattern attributed to sensorimotor development, which overlaps that of postural maturation.

Although agreement on this point is fairly general, this is not the case for the concept of maturation, or for the relationships between maturation and experience, to which it is traditionally opposed. Clearly, maturation is no longer considered to be a purely endogenous program (Gesell & Amatruda, 1945) and is seen as a set of constitutive properties whose actualization is regulated by experience (Piaget, 1976; Weiss, 1939). The widespread adoption of the notion of epigenesis is illustrative of this change in interpretation. In addition, experience is no longer seen as a source of accommodation, but rather in terms of active practice.

Nevertheless, researchers continue to find it difficult to adhere to the idea that sensorimotor development is a process that integrates maturation and experience. The major problem is the way maturation and experience are related over time. Piagetian theory provides one example. Piaget (1936; 1952) stressed the role of "assimilatory activity," which is thought to "broaden the range of application of reflexes" during the first months of life (1952, pp. 120, 127). But is this wider range of application sufficient to produce eye–hand coordination at a specific date (at 4.5 months, according to Piaget)? Piaget provides a detailed account of the benefits of this new form of coordination. However, he does not account for what triggers its onset. This leads inevitably to recourse to maturation, and the assumption that it sets the turning points for sensorimotor development.

After the second year, practice is assumed to transform coordination, and govern the steady gains in performance. References are made to skill acquisition rather than to development. The general hypothesis is not that there is development of performance, but that experience (i.e., practice) only acts on stable organizations.

The data, however, do not fit with a sequential picture of this type. Hofsten has shown that performance gains between the ages of 2 and 9 years in pointing tasks involving eye–hand coordination form a jagged rather than a smooth continuous curve. On the other hand, the role of experience as a building block appears to be corroborated by a certain number of accelerations in development produced by practice for the first 2 years of life.

Nevertheless, neither of these arguments totally disconfirms the necessity of a stable organizational basis on which practice can operate. The acceleration of the establishment of eye–head coordination in premature infants may only be possible because eye movement is already well organized (at 34 to 35 gestational weeks, as shown by consistency of within-subject responses). The ages at which regressions have been observed (much later, at 5 and 7 years) and ensuing changes suggest that they affect stable organizations, and that they are indicative of internal modifications in these structures (Hay, 1979). The argument for a continuity that gives way to a period marked by discontinuities no longer seems tenable.

Which methodologies for further research?

Areas of uncertainty and gaps in our knowledge prevent us from forming a detailed description of sensorimotor development and from gaining an understanding of the process(es) that presides over successive organizations. This suggests that methods of investigation should be reappraised and a better choice made of those that are the most appropriate to extending our knowledge in this field. There is clearly a relationship between methods and hypotheses, and it is simply worth drawing attention here to the impact that the notion of "stage of development" has had on the use of cross-sectional studies in developmental psychology. However, cross-sectional studies are responsible to a great extent for current uncertainties, not only with respect to discontinuities or continuity of change, but also with respect to control mechanisms.

Paradoxically, the success of cross-sectional studies is an argument against their exclusive use. By establishing "key" ages below and above which behavior differs, they encourage researchers to determine patterns of change, and to test whether a given behavior corresponds to a pronounced discontinuity or has a bearing on future behavior. This points to the necessity of complementing cross-sectional studies with longitudinal studies. During the first 2 years of life, when the rhythm of change of all types is extremely rapid, discrete variations do not always provide enough coherency to point clearly to "development," to a program of temporal successions. The difference in dates for the onset of sensorimotor development testifies amply to this: at the age of 2 months for some authors, at birth for others.

This lack of agreement is based on the assumption of a relationship or lack of relationship between these two ages. Vurpillot and Bullinger (1983) define the neonate as a collection of "innate sensorimotor reflex loops" and argue that the onset of development is dependent upon a control of exchanges with the environment that has its onset at the age of 2 months. According to these authors, this agency has no effect on innate sensorimotor loops that persist over the entire lifetime and are nearly independent of the other modes of functioning. Only a longitudinal study from 0 to 2 months can confirm or refute such a total discontinuity of this type.

The value of longitudinal studies also comes to the fore when attempting to account for the processes involved in development, in particular the relationships assumed to exist between maturation and practice. We have seen an example of this with regard to walking. At this point, two methodological precautions should be pointed out:

> Subjects should be matched according to other criteria than age, regardless of the definition used.
> The design should include within-group comparisons for responses tested at different points in time.

The reticence in using longitudinal methods in developmental studies often derives more from cost considerations due to their length than to design issues. This justifies examining the advantages of short-term longitudinal studies. The overall rhythm of development during the first 2 years lends itself well to short-term studies designed either to test for the onset of a behavior, or factors involved in the onset, or alternatively to define a period of establishment or stabilization of a form of behavior, or its possible association. This widens the scope of longitudinal methodology.

The use of longitudinal methods cannot be justified purely by the desire to adhere closely to duration, as Zazzo has pointed out (1956), nor is duration a sole explanation for behavior. This suggests that systematic and sole recourse to longitudinal studies and even their prolonged use over the entire course of a type of development should be avoided. On the other hand, short longitudinal studies that are clearly focused on well-defined behaviors can be fruitful. This word of warning leads to a second, which is to restrict the use of longitudinal studies to hypothesis testing. In this area, caution is the byword. Naturally there are no logical arguments against the use of longitudinal studies in exploratory research. But it is likely that they are less suited to reducing the range of possibilities than cross-sectional studies.

These arguments presented in favor of longitudinal studies are general ones, which apply more to a period of life than to a specific area of development. However, there is no reason to restrict them to the first 2 years of life. On the contrary it would be of great interest to use longitudinal studies to investigate other key periods more systematically than has been done. Furthermore, sensorimotor coordinations are ideally suited to this type of investigation because they are revealed through action. The unfolding of action in space and time can thus be indicative of changes in modes of organization.

The findings reported by Hay (1979) and Hofsten and Rösblad (1987) confirm the interest of this type of approach. Both authors observed regressions in eye–hand pointing tasks in highly comparable conditions. However, in one case the regression is situated between the ages of 7 and 9 and in the other between 5 and 7. The two authors come to the conclusion that regression is indicative of a transition in coordination mechanisms. According to Hay, this is due to a temporal displacement of visual control of corrections in hand movement, which intervenes in the final phase of reaching in subjects below age 7 but at the start of the movement in subjects aged 7. Hofsten and Rösblad (1987) center their explanation on the convergence between the haptic and visual spaces. Longitudinal studies focused on the ages of 5 to 7 should provide a means of gaining crucial information on the modalities of change involved.

Longitudinal studies of this type nevertheless run a certain number of risks. Task repetition may induce skill acquisition. If the learning process only alters the rhythm of expected changes, comparisons obtained through cross-sectional methods are applicable. However, if the learning process cancels out changes, no conclusions can be drawn. Thus, it is illusory to believe that only one method can increase our knowledge of developmental mechanisms.

NOTE

1 Bower et al. (1970) were the first to use the term *intention*, but their definition referred to a specific criterion: anticipatory hand shaping.

REFERENCES

Amiel-Tison, C., & Grenier, A. (1985). *La surveillance neurologique au cours de la première année de la vie*. Paris: Masson.

André-Thomas, X., & Autgaerden, S. (1952). Les deux marches. *La Presse Medicale, 61*, 582–584.

Atkinson, J. V. (1984). How does infant vision change in the first three months of life? In H. F. R. Prechtl (Ed.), *Continuity of neural functions from prenatal to postnatal life* (pp. 159–178). Oxford and Philadelphia: S.I.M.P.

Barnes, G. R. (1983). The effects of retinal target location on suppression of the vestibulo-ocular reflex. *Experimental Brain Research, 15*, 364–385.

Barten, S., Birns, B., & Ronch, J. (1971). Individual differences in the visual pursuit behavior of neonates. *Child Development, 42*, 313–319.

Bernstein, N. (1967). *The coordination and regulation of movement*. London: Pergamon.

Bloch, H. (1977). Quelques données sur les possibilités de structuration spatiale chez le bébé. In *Psychologie experimentale et comparée* (pp. 353–362). Paris: P.U.F.

Bloch, H. (1983). Les relations entre les paliers de maturation biologique et les organisations comportementales. In S. de Schonen (Ed.), *Le développement dans la première année* (pp. 208–224). Paris: P.U.F.

Bloch, H. (1987). There is more in our movements than in your theory. *Cahiers de Psychologie Cognitive, 2*, 136–142.

Bloch, H., & Jouen, F. (1986). *Direction du stimulus et poursuite visuelle chez le nouveau-né*. Paper presented at the Colloque National des Neurosciences, Bordeaux.

Bloch, H., Mellier, D., & Fuenmajor, G. (1984). Organization of visual pursuit in pre-term infants and regulation of the V.O.R. *Infant Behavior and Development, 7*, 38.

Bower, T. G. R. (1974). *Development in infancy*. San Francisco: W. H. Freeman Co.

Bower, T. G. R., Broughton, J. M., & Moore, M. K. (1970). Demonstration of intention in the reaching behavior of neonate humans. *Nature, 228*, 679–681.

Bushnell, E. W., & Weinberger, N. (1987). Infants' detection of visual–tactual discrepancies: Asymmetries that indicate a directive role of visual information. *Journal of Experimental Psychology: Human Perception and Performance, 13*, 601–608.

Di Franco, D., Muir, D., & Dodwell, P. (1978). Reaching in very young infants. *Perception, 7*, 385–392.

Fuenmajor, G. (1985). *La poursuite visuelle chez le prématuré*. Thèse de doctorat de l'Université René Descartes, Paris.

Gesell, A., & Amatruda, C. S. (1945). *The embryology of behavior: The beginnings of human mind*. New York: Harper.

Goldman-Rakic, P. S. (1985). Towards a neurobiology of cognitive development. In J. Mehler & R. Fox (Eds.), *Neonate cognition* (pp. 285–325). Hillsdale, NJ: L.E.A.

Grenier, A. (1981). Motricité libérée par fixation manuelle de la nuque au cours des premières semaines de la vie. *Archives Françaises de Pédiatrie, 38*, 557–562.

Hainline, L., & Lemerise, E. (1982). Infants' scanning of geometric forms varying in size. *Journal of Experimental Child Psychology, 33*, 235–256.

Hay, L. (1979). Spatial–temporal analysis of movements in children: Motor programs vs. feedback in the development of reaching. *Journal of Motor Behavior, 11*, 189–200.

Hofsten, C. von (1982). Eye–hand coordination in the newborn. *Developmental Psychology, 18*, 450–461.

Hofsten, C. von, & Rösblad, B. (1987). The synchronization of sensory information in the development of precise manual pointing. Unpublished manuscript.

Jouen, F., Lepecq, J. C., & Bloch, H. (1984). Place learning in five-month-old infants. In *Future trends in developmental psychology* (Part II, pp. 49–55). Lancaster: British Society of Psychology.

Kremenitzer, J., Vaughan, H., Kurtzberg, D., & Dowling, K. (1979). Smooth-pursuit eye movements in the newborn infant. *Child Development, 50*, 442–448.

Lepecq, J. C. (1986). Localisation et estimation de distance chez le nourrisson en déplacement passif. *Psychologie Française: Espace et cognition chez l'enfant, 31*, 35–42.

Lockman, J. J., Ashmead, D. H., & Bushnell, E. W. (1984). The development of anticipatory hand orientation during infancy. *Journal of Experimental Child Psychology, 37*, 403–404.

MacFarlane, A., Harris, P., & Barnes, I. (1976). Central and peripheral vision in early infancy. *Journal of Experimental Child Psychology, 21*, 532–538.

Maciaszczyk, S., & Bloch, H. (1986). *Les effets sensori-moteurs et cognitifs de l'expérience posturale.* Paper presented at the Communication au Colloque National des Neurosciences, Bordeaux.

Paillard, J., & Beaubaton, D. (1978). De la coordination visuo-motrice à l'organisation de la saisie manuelle. In H. Hecaen & M. Jeannerod (Eds.), *Du contrôle moteur à l'organisation du geste* (pp. 225–260). Paris: Masson.

Piaget, J. (1936). *La naissance de l'intelligence.* Geneva: Delachaux et Niestlé.

Piaget, J. (1952). *La psychologie de l'intelligence.* Paris: Armand Colin.

Piaget, J. (1976). *Le comportement, moteur de l'évolution.* Paris: Gallimard.

Pieraut-le Bonniec, G., Hombessa, E., & Jacquet, A. Y. (1987). *Le comportement de prise d'objet chez le bébé: Rôle de la maîtrise de la posture et effet de l'entraînement à la manipulation.* Communication à XXIè Symposium A.P.S.L.F., Toulouse.

Prechtl, H. F. R. (1984). Continuity and change in early neural development. In H. F. R. Prechtl (Ed.), *Continuity of neural functions from prenatal to postnatal life* (pp. 1–15). Oxford and Philadelphia: S.I.M.P.

Roucoux, A., & Crommelinck, M. (1984). La coordination oeil-tête. In J. Paillard (Ed.), *La lecture sensori-motrice et cognitive de l'expérience spatiale* (pp. 45–62). Paris: Ed. du C.N.R.S.

Roucoux, A., Crommelinck, M., Guerit, J. M., & Meulders, M. (1981). Two modes of eye–head coordination and the role of the V.O.R. in these two strategies. In A. Fuchs & W. Becker (Eds.), *Progress in oculo-motor research: Development in neuroscience* (Vol. 12, pp. 309–315). Amsterdam: Elsevier.

Thelen, E. (1981). Kicking, rocking and waving: Contextual analysis of rhythmical stereotypies in normal human infants. *Animal Behavior, 29*, 3–11.

Thelen, E. (1986). Treadmill-elicited stepping in seven-month-old infants. *Child Development, 57*, 1498–1506.

Thelen, E., Fisher, D. M., & Ridley-Johnson, R. (1984). The relationship between physical growth and a newborn reflex. *Infant Behavior and Development*, 7, 479–493.

Thelen, E., Kelso, J. A. S., & Fogel, A. (1987). Self-organizing systems and infant motor development. *Developmental Review*, 7, 39–65.

Touwen, B. C. L. (1978). Variability and stereotypy in normal and deviant development. In J. Appley (Ed.), *Care of the handicapped child* (pp. 99–110). London: Heinemann Medical Books.

Touwen, B. C. L. (1984). Primitive reflexes: Conceptional or semantic problem In H. F. R. Prechtl (Ed.), *Continuity of neural function from prenatal to postnatal life* (pp. 115–125). Oxford and Philadelphia: S.I.M.P.

Tyschen, L., & Lisberger, S. G. (1986). Maldevelopment of visual notion processing humans who had strabismus with onset in infancy. *Journal of Neurosciences*, 6, 2495–2508.

Vurpillot, E., & Bullinger, A. (1983). Y-a-t-il des âges-clefs dans la première année? In S. de Schonen (Ed.), *Le développement dans la première année*. Paris: P.U.F.

Weiss, P. (1939). *Principles of development*. New York: Holt and Rinehart.

White, B. L. (1970). Experience and the development of motor mechanisms in infancy. In K. Conolly (Ed.), *Mechanisms of motor skill development* (pp. 95–134). New York and London: Academic Press.

White, B. L., Castle, P., & Held, R. (1964). Observations on the development of visually-directed reaching. *Child Development*, 35, 349–364.

Wyke, B. (1975). The neurological basis of movement. In K. S. Holt (Ed.), *Movement and child development* (pp. 19–34). London: S.I.M.P.

Zazzo, R. (1956). Diversité, réalité et fiction de la méthode longitudinale. Rapport introduit au Symposium *Etudes longitudinales en Psychologie de l'Enfant*, XVIIIè Congrès International de Psychologie, Moscow.

Zelazo, P. R. (1976). From reflexive to instrumental behavior. In L. Lipsitt (Ed.), *Developmental psychobiology: The significance of infancy*. Hillsdale, NJ: L.E.A.

Zelazo, P. R. (1983). The development of walking: New findings and old assumptions. *Journal of Motor Behavior*, 15, 99–137.

11   On U-shaped and other transitions in sensorimotor development

GEORGE BUTTERWORTH

Introduction

In reviewing recent evidence on transition mechanisms in early sensori-motor development, this chapter begins with an attempt to characterize the origins of sensorimotor control and then offers some hypotheses on alternative ways of considering transitions. It will end with an attempt to show that a cognitive approach is compatible with biological or matur-ationally based explanations for some of the transitions that can be observed in human infancy. Studies concerned with the early origins of behavior are relatively few and the longitudinal method has been applied to only a small proportion of them. Nevertheless, the evidence reveals important continuities and discontinuities in development from the ear-liest age. Another aim of this chapter will be to offer a comprehensive framework, based on Changeux's (1986) model of neuronal growth, within which the variety of transitions in early behavioral development may be understood.

On how to describe the origins of development

Perhaps the first problem is to characterize the starting point for de-velopment. The skilled movements of an adult may seem to have little in common with the rudimentary movements of the neonate. However, the lack of obvious skill in most newborn behavior may actually give a misleading picture of the origins of motor competence because the neonatal period is itself a time of transition from the intrauterine en-vironment. The characteristically unskilled movements of the newborn may at least in part reflect the need to adapt to a new environment. The developmental transition brought about by birth creates new possibilities for action in which the extent of movement, the additional weight of one's own body, and the use of vision to control activity are all factors that did not exist before. Hence, it is not surprising that we may characterize the activity of the neonate as limited, because behavior is in transition to a new form of independent movement in the world.

Prechtl's description of fetal movement patterns

Information about the extent and importance of movement in the intrauterine environment is becoming available from real-time studies using ultrasonic scanning. De Vries, Visser, and Prechtl (1984) have evidence for 15 distinctly different movement patterns in the fetus by the 15th gestational week. Their descriptions of complex, well-coordinated fetal movement patterns illustrate the point that sensorimotor activity observed at its origins may lead to a better understanding of the nature of subsequent transitions in development.

Among the movements observed are isolated arm or leg movements that can be seen as early as the 9th gestational week, hand-to-face contacts by the 10th week, head retroflexion by the 10th week and antiflexion by the 12th week, and an integrated yawn and stretch pattern of the arms by the 10th week. The stretch pattern is described as follows:

A complex motor pattern, always at a slow speed, consists of forceful extension of the back, retroflexion of the head, external rotation and elevation of the arms.

The yawn pattern is described as follows:

Similar to yawn observed after birth; prolonged wide opening of the jaws followed by quick closure, often with retroflexion of the head and sometimes elevation of the arms. Non-repetitive.

The rotation of the fetus at 10 weeks from one position to another is described as follows:

Rotation occurs around sagittal or transverse axis, complete change of position around transverse axis is achieved by complex general movement, including alternating leg movements which resemble neonatal stepping. Rotation around longitudinal axis can result from leg movements with hip rotations, or from rotations of head followed by trunk. Total change in position can be achieved in as little as two seconds but may take longer. (De Vries et al., 1984, pp. 50–53)

Conjugate lateral eye movements and downward eye movements are observed at around 18 weeks of age. These are a separate category from those observed in rapid eye movement (REM) sleep, where the eyelids are closed.

The new technology of ultrasonic scanning makes visible the spontaneous movements of the fetus in the natural environment for the first time. The character of these movements is surprisingly different from what we have been led to expect by the classical description of a limited number of reflexive movements elicited in the exteriorized fetus. Even the principle of cephalocaudal development is breached by observing the fetus in the natural environment. Spontaneous activity is observed in the whole fetus with no privileged direction of development from head to tail. Furthermore, movement is differentiated from an early age into a variety of postures, movement synergies, and programmed sequences. The hypothesis that the neonatal period marks a behavioral transition becomes quite plausible.

Starting from this perspective, the first few weeks after birth may be considered a period that bridges two states of adaptation, an earlier one that encompasses behaviors most suited to the intrauterine environment and a later one involving adaptation to the extrauterine environment.

The neonatal period as a time of transition

Given the hypothesis that the neonatal period is itself a time of transition between states of adaptation, it becomes possible to classify various behavioral capacities and incapacities of the newborn in a new way. Recent advances in developmental neurology give an insight into the selective processes that occur as the nervous system develops in the embryo. This can be one source of useful hypotheses to explain observed behavioral transitions. Changeux (1986) describes development of the nervous system as an epigenetic process involving selective stabilization of synapses. He suggests that synaptic connections in the developing nervous system can exist in three states: labile, stabile, and degenerate. Neural activity can occur only in labile or stabile states; it may initially be spontaneous but is eventually evoked by the interaction of the newborn with the environment. In the development of the nervous system, a number of transitions are possible:

> from labile to stabile states, which result in stabilization of the developing system;
>
> from stabile to labile states of the system, which involve labilization of the system;
>
> from labile to degenerative states, and these involve regression.

This neurological model can support a large variety of possible behavioral transitions. Although some transitions may occur for purely maturational reasons, it is also possible to argue that others will occur because a radical change in environment requires new adaptation to occur, while earlier, ontogenetic adaptations may actually become redundant. Prechtl (1981) has suggested five possible mechanisms of de-

Table 11.1 *Changeux's transition model*

	Labile	Stabile	Degeneration
Labile		Stabilization	Regression
Stabile	Labilization		

Note: Prechtl's (1981) five possible mechanisms of developmental transition in sensorimotor behaviors:

1. Sensorimotor machinery may disappear totally (regression in the diagram above).
2. It remains intact but comes under permanent inhibition from higher centers (perhaps a process of stabilization).
3. Sensory channels become ineffective and are replaced by other sensory channels eliciting the same response (labilization of sensory systems).
4. The same sensory mechanisms become connected with different motor systems (labilization of motor systems).
5. Two neural machineries may develop rivalry with each other and eventually become separated.

A number of motor patterns remain unchanged, e.g. sneezing, yawning, hiccuping, breathing, stretching movements.

velopmental regression and transformation of intrauterine sensorimotor behaviors. These are summarized in relation to Changeux's model in Table 11.1.

The table shows that intrauterine machinery may disappear totally (regression in the diagram); it remains intact but comes under permanent inhibition from higher centers (perhaps a process of stabilization); sensory channels become ineffective and are replaced by other sensory channels that elicit the same response (labilization of sensory systems); the same sensory mechanisms become connected with different motor systems (labilization of motor systems); two neural machineries may develop rivalry with each other and eventually become separated and recoordinated (perhaps this corresponds to a process of differentiation and hierarchical integration?). Of course, a number of motor patterns remain unchanged such as sneezing, yawning, hiccuping, breathing, and stretching movements.

The point is that newborn behaviors may be characterized according to any of these classifications. Some newborn behavior may exist as the temporary continuation of an intrauterine activity soon to drop out, with no further implications for development. Such behavior will prove to be an ontogenetic adaptation to the intrauterine environment (Oppenheim, 1981). Other behavior develops from birth and is not present in the intrauterine environment. An example is the Moro reflex, which, it has been suggested, appears as a result of the onset of vestibular functioning (Prechtl, 1984). On the other hand, some newborn behavior may exist as a continuation of intrauterine activity and may anticipate in some degree the needs of later development. This class of behavior may undergo a transition with an accompanying dip, drop, or U-shaped function as the neural, sensorimotor, or other reorganizations involved in making the transition occur. The behavior will reappear, perhaps in modified form, in later development, and this is the class of phenomena that has been of particular interest to the developmental psychology of human infancy.

These possibilities may be elaborated by extending the discussion of three examples already offered by Hofsten (this volume). These concern the development of walking, hand–mouth coordination, and neonatal imitation of mouth and hand movements.

Illustration of transitions involved in walking, hand–mouth coordination, and imitation

There is now good evidence for each of these examples of newborn behavior: Neonatal stepping is well established (Thelen, 1984), neonatal imitation has been shown by a number of authors (Maratos, 1982; Meltzoff & Moore, 1976; Vinter, 1986), and hand–mouth coordination has recently been extensively studied (Butterworth & Hopkins, 1988). Each of these behaviors "disappears" during the first 3 months of life, to reappear on a variable timetable later in the first year. The aim here is to analyze the nature of the transition that each may undergo.

Neonatal stepping

Hofsten (this volume) has extensively discussed neonatal stepping and its possible relation to later walking. It has been traditional to consider the innate stepping movements of the newborn baby as reflexive movements that will become inhibited by higher cortical centers as the infant matures. Typically, this motor pattern cannot be elicited after the first 2 months of life. Zelaso, Zelaso, and Kolb (1972) in a longitudinal study extending from birth over several months showed that practicing the innate stepping reflex in one of a pair of identical twins led to a significant acceleration in onset of walking compared with the unpracticed control twin. This study showed that practicing the behavior may help to maintain it when it would otherwise "disappear." It has also been taken as evidence for a continuity between neonatal stepping movements and walking. Thelen's (1984) major contribution has been to demonstrate that this "disappearing" reflex does not disappear at all. Rather, the baby's legs grow so rapidly after birth and they become so heavy that, when supported in the upright posture, the baby simply lacks the strength to lift them. This is demonstrated by the reappearance of the stepping movement when the baby is tested with the legs suspended in a tank of water, which helps support their weight. Furthermore, Thelen (1981) has shown that rhythmical kicking movements are isomorphic in their patterning to the stepping movements but kicking (which occurs when the baby is supine) does not disappear from the repertoire. She suggests that more force is required to move the legs when the baby is held upright than when supine, and it is the biomechanical demands that differ between the two postures. There is no need to postulate that a developmental transition occurs within the motor control system. She argues that the pattern generator for walking is innate and that the apparent regression in development is illusory: Infants walk when they do because only then do the biomechanical constraints on the system allow it.

Now this is an extremely parsimonious view because the question why humans walk when they do is answered mainly by reference to mechanical constraints, such as body proportion and weight, that prevent it. The account definitely lacks any "cognitive component" as an explanation of the apparent transition between earlier and later walking. However, when the locomotor pattern involved in the stepping reflex is examined closely, it becomes apparent that other factors are involved. The posture of the feet for instance in the innate stepping reflex, in which the toes touch the ground first, is consistent with quadrupedal movement. In skilled walking, the heel touches the ground first in the typical bipedal posture. Furthermore, mature walking must overcome the fetal tendency for the feet to cross as they touch the ground. There are other important differences between neonatal stepping and mature walking in the dynamic properties of movement concerning the hip and knee joints (Thelen, 1984). The important point is that before the U-shaped transition from neonatal stepping to walking can be understood, it is necessary to consider the adaptive function of neonatal stepping itself.

In fact, it seems very likely that the innate stepping movement pattern plays an important role in allowing the fetus to change position easily in utero, hence preventing adhesion and allowing normal development of limbs and joints. Biomechanical constraints arising from rapid growth after birth may indeed explain the apparent disappearance of the behavior, but the fact that it can be reelicited when the constraints change argues against a regression model or cortical inhibition model for the transition. Furthermore, before the pattern generation for reflexive stepping can be related to walking, it may be necessary to consider whether it may be more directly related to crawling. The quadrupedal posture of crawling, especially in the orientation of the toes, is actually more similar to the intrauterine movement pattern than the bipedal posture of walking, which may require a further transition between locomotor control systems involved in crawling and walking.

How can walking be linked to cognitive growth? Zelaso (1984) has suggested that cognitive growth may enter the timetable for walking, not because cognition is involved in the detailed control of the behavior but because it provides a motive for it. He notes the tight coupling in humans between the onset of bipedal locomotion, tool use, and the beginnings of language and suggests that humans walk when they do because a general cognitive change allows each of the constituent motor systems to be used instrumentally. That is, walking occurs as a means to an end and, in that sense, cognitive growth is ordinarily but not necessarily implicated in the control of bipedal locomotion. Cognitive and motor systems, in this case, are loosely coupled. One only has to note that decapitated chickens engage in running movements to make the same point that the pattern generating mechanism for locomotion may easily be dissociated from other systems that are necessarily but more generally involved in motor control.

Hand–mouth coordination

About 15% of the spontaneous arm movements of the awake, newborn infant result in the hand contacting the mouth, an interesting coordination that has been known for some time (Preyer, 1896) but which has received little study until recently (Butterworth & Hopkins, 1988).

Several functional explanations have been offered for hand–mouth movements in the newborn. Piaget (1953) suggested that contacts of hand with mouth arise from impulsive movements that serve to exercise the innate grasping reflex, which, after constant repetition, differentiates into the primary circular reactions involved in tactile exploration of the face in the second month of life. Kravitz, Goldenberg, and Neyhus (1978) have also suggested that hand-to-head movements may serve the function of tactile self-exploration, although, unlike Piaget, they consider facial exploration to be innate. They describe a consistent order of emergence of movements of the hand to the face in the hours after birth, starting with movements to the ears, eyes, and nose. It has also been suggested that hand–mouth contact may serve a self-calming function through sucking the fingers and that mouth touching may be related to prandial condition (Feldman & Brody, 1978). Korner and Beason (1972) performed a frame-by-frame analysis of 1,000 feet of film of spontaneous movement in 2- and 3-day-olds and noted concurrence of visual alerting before and after hand–mouth contact, which led them to suggest that mouth contact may occur under visual guidance. None of these explanations has sought to locate the behavior in prenatal activities, even though the fetus of 24 weeks is known to be able to bring hand to mouth and has been shown to engage in thumb sucking (Hofer, 1982).

Butterworth and Hopkins (1988) observed that the baby, lying with the head to one side, opens the mouth and then moves the arm and hand ipsilaterally to the orientation of the head so that the hand enters the mouth. The eyes are equally likely to be shut as open; hence it seems that visual guidance is not necessary. Hand–mouth coordination may be described as "orally elicited reaching," analogous to the "visually elicited" reaching described by Hofsten (this volume).

It would be interesting to establish in a longitudinal study what the course of development of hand–mouth coordination may be. In an unpublished observation, Hopkins (personal communication) has suggested that the movement seems to become less accurately targeted on the mouth toward the end of the second month of life. Of course, detailed observations would be needed to establish what the cause of such an inaccuracy may be, but it does suggest that a developmental transition may be occurring, as is so often found with other neonatal coordinations.

What of the developmental antecedents of newborn hand–mouth coordination? The previous analysis of neonatal stepping would suggest that a precursor may be found in the behavioral repertoire of the fetus and, indeed, this is the case. De Vries et al. (1984), in a study of fetal movement patterns, found that between 50 and 100 hand-to-face contacts per hour occur in fetuses aged between 12 and 15 weeks. They observed at 12.5 weeks gestational age contact of hand with mouth in association with ipsilateral head movement, a description remarkably similar to the behavior observed in neonates by Butterworth and Hopkins (1988). It seems possible therefore that hand–mouth coordination in newborns may be an innate, centrally organized movement synergy that has its origins in prenatal activity and is controlled proprioceptively. Prenatal practice may be responsible for the highly organized behavior observed soon after birth; detailed longitudinal studies would reveal more of the time course of development of this coordination.

A possible function that has not been considered is that hand–mouth coordination may be an early form of orally targeted reaching that might be a precursor of self-feeding activity. Feldman and Brody (1978) compared hand–mouth contacting before and after feeding and found it to be more frequent preprandially. Thus, the innate behavior pattern may be a developmental precursor of self-feeding just as it has been argued the stepping movements in the newborn may be developmentally embedded in later voluntary walking (Zelaso, 1983). Hypotheses of this kind asserting developmental continuity are notoriously difficult to test but, nevertheless, Rochat (1986, n. 1) has reported some preliminary data suggesting that application of sucrose to the tongue of the newborn significantly increases the incidence of hand–mouth contact. We may speculate that the movement synergy may be a component of an alimentary control system, which, with practice and when skilled, will eventually be used in self-feeding. In any event, self-feeding develops toward the end of the first year of life (Connolly, 1970) and is soon socialized by the instrumental use of spoons as intermediaries, which again illustrates how action systems that are innate may eventually become embedded within instrumental control processes that appear later in development.

The methodological difficulties associated with proving the link between neonatal and later behavior are great. One hypothesis, of course, is that hand–mouth coordination does not "disappear" but is simply prevented by the weight constraints of the rapidly growing arms. However, this biomechanical explanation seems unlikely to explain the whole phenomenon because there is a differentiated timetable involved in the appearance, disappearance, and reappearance of various aspects of arm movement. Kravitz et al. (1978) noted an emerging order of tactual self-exploration in the first few hours after birth, beginning with the mouth (at 167 minutes), then the face (192 minutes), the head (380 minutes), the ear (469 minutes), the nose (593 minutes), and the eyes (1,491 minutes). There have been no systematic studies of the order of self-exploration of the face in the second 6 months of life. If such ordered exploration should emerge, then this may be taken as evidence against a purely biomechanical explanation of the U-shaped function, because the weight of the arm is constant yet the target for self-exploration is differentiated.

Certainly, self-exploration of the body is differentiated, with finger-to-finger exploration at 12 weeks, finger-to-body at 15 weeks, finger-to-knee at 18 weeks, finger-to-foot at 19 weeks, and Freudian forms of self-exploration at about 23 weeks. The evidence seems more consistent with the hypothesis that self-exploration allows cognitive elaboration of the body image on the basis of sensory input. That is, the differentiated form of self-exploration, despite the constant biomechanical constraint on the arm, suggests that a transition to a new level of representation of the body as a result of self-exploration may be in progress (Kravitz et al., 1978).

This example does not solve the question of whether there is replacement of one system by another in development or integration of an early control system with later behavior. The idea that later appearing control systems may simply modulate, rather than replace, earlier mechanisms is certainly consistent with research on visual control of posture. In the case of visual control of posture, for example, the 12-month-old infant who has recently learned to stand will fall over on every trial in a "moving room" that generates misleading visual feedback consistent with postural instability (Butterworth & Cicchetti, 1980). By 15 months, however, the infant has a concept of self as an independent causal agent and having fallen over once or twice, he will no longer fall but will turn to see who has made the room move. However, even adults are very dependent on congruent visual feedback when in an unfamiliar posture, such as balancing on a beam (Lee & Lishman, 1975). In these examples, "higher-order," cognitive control mechanisms modulate the effect of visual proprioception, without replacing it entirely.

Neonatal imitation

That motor activity cannot be understood in isolation from perception is particularly true in the case of innate imitation of "invisible" gestures, such as tongue protrusion and mouth opening. Furthermore, although there is evidence that tonguing and mouth opening are frequently practiced behaviors in utero, the infant obviously has not seen a tongue in utero and the phenomena therefore raise particular problems in explaining how sensory input relates to motor output without specific visual experience. Vinter (1984; 1986) has carried out one of the most recent investigations of neonatal imitation. She has replicated the findings on imitation of mouth opening and tongue protrusion in neonates, and she has also shown imitation of sequential finger movements. In a longitudinal study, she showed that imitation of finger movements disappears at about 7 weeks to reappear at about 7 months, whereas imitation of tongue protrusion disappears at about 3 months to reappear toward the end of the first year of life. She has also shown that dynamic (not static) models elicit imitation in the neonate and that responses are immediate rather than deferred. There has been no explicit comparison of static versus dynamic models with 1 year-old babies. Piaget's own observations (1951, p. 53) always seem to involve presentation of a dynamic model to the 1-year-old who is capable of deferred imitation. Nevertheless, it seems possible that along with the capacity for deferred imitation at the end of the first year of life will arise the ability to imitate a dynamic gesture given only a static model (a process analogous to going from a part of the object to the whole). In other words, early and later imitation, for example, of tongue protrusion may recruit the same final common path of movement, but there is good reason to suppose that the later form requires long-term memory and other cognitive processes not implicated in the neonatal behavior.

Two further issues are slowly being unraveled concerning transitions in neonatal imitation. More evidence for an overall coordinating mechanism involved in relating perception to action in the neonate comes from demonstrations that very young babies are capable of perceiving information common to several modalities. Meltzoff and Borton (1979) showed that infants less than 1 month of age will prefer to look at an object of the same shape as they have previously sucked than at a dummy of a different shape. Kuhl and Meltzoff (1982) have shown that very young infants also perceive the equivalence between certain auditory stimuli and the mouth posture involved in producing those sounds. Mounoud and Vinter (1981) have suggested that what authorizes such equivalence classes in the neonate is the body schema in its most basic and cognitively unelaborated form.

Bairstow (1986) captures the essential characteristics of such a mechanism admirably as "a superordinate representation at the interface between sensory and motor processes that both externally and internally specify a posture." Such a definition provides the necessary link between sensory and motor domains that would enable us to explain how the newborn infant can reproduce a movement that has never been seen.

As far as sensorimotor transition is concerned, an implication of this analysis is that transitions may occur as the body schema is elaborated. This elaboration may give rise to two types of transition. On the one hand, there is the U-shaped appearance, disappearance, and reappearance of particular responses such as tongue protrusion and hand movement where the similarity between early and later behavior may best be explained in terms of the final common pathway. On the other hand, the differentiated timetable whereby neonatal behaviors apparently disappear and reappear may involve a sequence of sensory replacement. Papousek (1986, personal communication), for example, has suggested that imitation does not disappear at 3 months when tongue protrusion responses become difficult to elicit. Rather, he maintains that the locus of imitative activity shifts to the auditory modality. Thus, considering isomorphic behaviors at different times in development leads to the hypothesis of a U-shaped transition. On the other hand, focusing on different sensory domains suggests sensory substitution. In the case of the decline in imitation of tongue protrusion, biomechanical constraints seem extremely unlikely to apply, because there is no evidence for rapid growth of the tongue leading to an inability to make the appropriate movements.

Conclusion

This essay has illustrated that very many kinds of transitions are possible in sensorimotor development. It has been suggested that the key to the problem of understanding transitions between the neonatal period and later development will be a description of the organization of behavior in the fetus. This repertoire of well-formed, adaptive behaviors may correspond to what Hofsten (this volume) describes as evolved perception–action systems. At least four mechanisms may prove necessary to encompass the variety of transitions that can occur:

First, innate pattern generators may be implicated in the control of locomotion by crawling or walking. Biomechanical constraints arising from rapidly growing limbs (and perhaps other parts of the body) may lead to apparent suppression or regression of these pattern generators, but the same control systems will reappear once the constraints are overcome.

Second, for some sensorimotor processes, isomorphic early and later forms of behavior may prove actually to be unrelated, with similar action merely the final common pathway. Prechtl (1981) gives the example of reflexive and voluntary grasping that he has observed to occur simultaneously in the 3-month infant. Because both are present at the same time, he suggests that there must be separate control systems. If this is the case, then one behavior simply replaces another in development. There need be no underlying continuity in the transition between them and hence no developmental pathway from reflexive to voluntary control of the hand.

A third hypothesis concerns the role of cognitive processes as put forward by Mounoud and the Genevan school. Their argument is that early and later forms of a behavior (e.g., imitation) are related insofar as the early form constitutes a "programming language" for the later form. Mounoud's model of the transitions involved is of a series of "revolutions" in development (Mounoud & Vinter, 1981). This is a model that stresses replacement of representational systems by progressively more elaborate control codes. Verbal regulation of behavior is an example of a radical transition that may be explained within this framework.

Fourth, another version of the cognitive hypothesis does not require replacement of control systems in development. This involves progressive embedding of innate systems in higher-order control processes that modulate them. On this view, core programs given innately are progressively modulated as further control systems are added.

Human infancy is a period of particularly rapid developmental change and hence it offers an ideal opportunity for the study of developmental transitions. It is not yet possible to explain all transitions during the sensorimotor period by a single model. However, there is no doubt that application of the longitudinal method continues to promise rapid progress in our understanding of transitions in human development.

REFERENCES

Bairstow, P. (1986). Postural control. In H. T. A. Whiting & M. G. Wade (Eds.), *Motor skill development in children: Aspects of coordination and control.* Dordrecht: Martinus Nijhof.

Butterworth, G. E., & Cicchetti, D. (1980). Visual calibration of posture in normal and motor retarded Down's syndrome infants. *Perception, 7*, 513–525.

Butterworth, G. E., & Hopkins, B. (1988). Hand to mouth activity in the newborn baby: Evidence for innate sensory-motor coordination. *British Journal of Developmental Psychology, 6* (4).

Changeux, J. P. (1986). *Neuronal man.* Oxford: Oxford University Press.

Connolly, K. J. (1970). Skill development: Problems and plans. In K. J. Connolly (Ed.), *Mechanisms of motor skill development.* London: Academic Press.

De Vries, J. I. P., Visser, G. H. A., & Prechtl, H. F. R. (1984). Fetal motility in the first half of pregnancy. In H. F. R. Prechtl (Ed.), *Continuity of neural function from prenatal to postnatal life* (pp. 46–64). London: Spastics International Medical Publications.

Feldman, J. F., & Brody, N. (1978). Non-elicited newborn behaviors in relation to state and prandial condition. *Merrill-Palmer Quarterly, 24* (2), 79–84.

Hofer, M. (1982). *The roots of human behavior.* San Francisco: William Freeman Co.

Korner, A. F., & Beason, L. M. (1972). Association of two congenitally organized behavior patterns in the new-born: Hand–mouth coordination and looking? *Perceptual and Motor Skills, 35*, 115–118.

Kravitz, H., Goldenberg, D., & Neyhus, A. (1978). Tactual exploration by normal infants. *Developmental Medicine and Child Neurology, 20*, 720–726.

Kuhl, P. K., & Meltzoff, A. N. (1982). The bimodal perception of speech in infancy. *Science, 218*, 1138–1141.

Lee, D. N., & Lishman, J. R. (1975). Visual proprioceptive control of stance. *Journal of Human Movement Studies, 1*, 87–95.

Maratos, O. (1982).Trends in the development of imitation in early infancy. In T. G. Bever (Ed.), *Regressions in mental development* (pp. 81–102). Hillsdale, NJ: Erlbaum.

Meltzoff, A. N., & Borton, R. W. (1979). Inter-modal matching by human neonates. *Nature, 282*, 403–404.

Meltzoff, A. N., & Moore M. K. (1976). Imitation of facial and manual gestures by human neonates. *Science, 198*, 75–78.

Mounoud, P., & Vinter, A. (1981). Representation and sensori-motor development. In G. E. Butterworth (Ed.), *Infancy and epistemology: An evaluation of Piaget's theory* (pp. 201–235). Brighton: Harvester.

Oppenheim, R. W. (1981). Ontogenetic adaptations and retrogressive processes in the development of the nervous system and behavior: neuroembryological perspective. In K. J. Connolly & H. F. R. Prechtl (Eds.), *Maturation and development: Biological and psychological perspectives* (pp. 16–30). London: Spastics International Medical Publications.

Piaget, J. (1951). *Play, dreams and imitation in the child*. London: Routledge and Kegan Paul.

Piaget, J. (1953). *The origins of intelligence in the child*. New York: Basic Books.

Prechtl, H. F. R. (1981). The study of neural development as a perspective on clinical problems. In K. J. Connolly & H. F. R. Prechtl (Eds.), *Maturation and development: Biological and psychological perspectives* (pp. 198–215). London: Spastics International Medical Publications.

Prechtl, H. F. R. (1984). Continuity and change in early neural development. In H. F. R. Prechtl (Ed.), *Continuity of neural function from prenatal to postnatal life* (pp. 1–15). London: Spastics International Medical Publications.

Preyer, W. (1896). *The senses and the will*. New York: Appleton.

Rochat, P. (1986). *Unity of the senses and early development of action*. Paper presented at the 2nd European Conference on Developmental Psychology, Rome.

Thelen, E. (1981). Rhythmical behavior in infancy: An ethological perspective. *Developmental Psychology, 17*, 237–257.

Thelen, E. (1984). Learning to walk: Ecological demands and phylogenic constraints. In L. Lipsitt & C. Rovee-Collier (Eds.), *Advances in infancy, research vol. 3* (pp. 213–250). Norwood, NJ: Ablex.

Vinter, A. (1984). *L'imitation chez le nouveau-né*. Lausanne: Delachaux & Niestlé.

Vinter, A. (1986). The role of movement in eliciting early imitation. *Child Development, 57*, 66–71.

Zelaso, P. R. (1983). The development of walking: New findings and old assumptions. *Journal of Motor Behavior, 15*, 99–137.

Zelaso, P. R. (1984). Learning to walk: Recognition of higher order influences. In L. Lipsitt & C. Rovee-Collier (Eds.), *Advances in infancy, research vol. 3* (pp. 251–256). Norwood, NJ: Ablex.

Zelaso, P. R., Zelaso, N. A., & Kolb, S. (1972). Walking in the newborn. *Science, 177*, 1058–1059.

Epilogue: On the use of longitudinal research in developmental psychology

ANIK DE RIBAUPIERRE

In this epilogue chapter, I will focus on the key points of the book: the issues of developmental transitions (that is, changes as defined by the different authors), of the change or transition mechanisms that have been hypothesized, and of the relevance of a longitudinal perspective. Because the general criterion of a longitudinal-developmental design is repeated individual observation (Baltes & Nesselroade, 1979; Hoppe-Graff, this volume), allowing a study of inter- and intraindividual differences over time, the review will also devote special attention to the role assigned by the authors to individual differences in development.

The chapter begins by calling for a clearer definition and distinction of concepts such as developmental changes, transition principles, and transition mechanisms; then the different content chapters of the book will be briefly reviewed, according to the authors' explicit or implicit definition of transitions and of underlying mechanisms, the role of individual differences, and the specificity of a longitudinal approach. Finally, the scarcity of longitudinal research will be discussed; I will argue, in particular, that its main cause does not lie in practical difficulties as is often mentioned, although they are real, but rather in conceptual problems and in the clear lack of interest for individual differences manifest in developmental psychology at large.

About transitions and transition mechanisms

A transition in its most general meaning implies the passage or change from one state to another. Hoppe-Graff in his introductory chapter specifies that a transition is a change in a well-defined developing system. It therefore requires that one clearly define the states or endpoints under study and describe the intervening changes or transitions; only then can inferences be drawn as to the factors or mechanisms of transition. I see three levels of analysis and inference on the basis of observed performances, from the more descriptive to the more inferential.

First, an important descriptive enterprise has to be conducted at a

297

"surface level," consisting of a clear definition of what the end states of the transition are, by relying on changes in performances with age or/and time. Implicit in the idea of a transition is the hypothesis that some changes in development are more important than others; if the development was simply seen as a slow and continuous increment, it would not be useful to speak of transition (to do so would suggest that the subject was continuously in a transitional state). For Sugarman (1987), for instance, the main agenda of developmental psychology consists in specifying the actual course of development (and not necessarily its cause) and in particular in identifying end states; although this perspective is certainly too restricted, because the agenda of developmental psychology is much larger, it stresses nevertheless the importance of this first step. According to Sugarman, the investigator must treat development as a starting assumption (that is, postulate that older subjects' behaviors are by definition more elaborate) and determine, by comparing younger and older children, what should be considered a significant change. An important facet of this first step would also be to describe the path followed from one end state to the next, that is, the developmental form: For instance, does development consist in a progression in performances (regular or according to a step function), or are regressions such as those seen in U-shaped curves also observed (e.g., Strauss & Stavy, 1982)? Does development only consist in gains or in a mixture of gains and losses (e.g., Baltes, 1987)? It is quite important, even in this first step which actually consists of inferring the meaning of changes in performances, to dissociate clearly between observed performances and underlying processes; one should ask whether changes are quantitative or qualitative (reflecting not so much an improvement as a change in how the task is tackled) and whether a same performance can result from different underlying processes. This is crucial with respect to the form of developmental transitions: A U-shaped curve for instance can reflect a real regression or, on the contrary, a progression in the sense that more elaborate underlying processes are used with age while first resulting in poorer levels of performances.

A second level of inference, not always clearly distinguished from the first one, consists in hypothesizing a "deep structure" for the end states that were defined at the performance level and for their differences, usually by comparing end states in different domains. Typically, the concept of developmental stage corresponds to this second step. Stages are qualitatively distinct levels, presenting an invariable sequence and characterized by a general structure; different stages are also meaningfully related to one another, through integration for instance (e.g., Piaget, 1956). Structural invariants such as stages remain, however, essentially descriptive constructs of task accomplishments; they represent intrinsic constraints on development and account for the range of performances possible at a given level (Campbell & Bickhard, 1986) and for developmental sequences of abilities across domains. This step corresponds to what Flavell and Wohlwill (1969; Flavell, 1984) labeled the formal or morphological aspect of any account of development. Indeed, a basic "structuralist error" (e.g., Campbell & Bickhard, 1986; de Ribaupierre & Pascual-Leone, 1984) has often consisted in considering task descriptions as accounts of internal processes and representations.

The third level consists in defining underlying processes as well as mechanisms of transition – that is, in trying to understand how and possibly why one proceeds from one state to the other. This step requires still greater inferences because mechanisms as such are just never observable. A whole range of mechanisms has been defined in the literature, more or less finely differentiated. For instance, Flavell (1977; 1984) distinguishes between those processes operating within cognitive entities such as differentiation and those processes relating different cognitive entities, such as integration, subordination, coordination, regulation, and equilibration. A further obstacle to a clear consensus in the literature with respect to the term *mechanism*, already alluded to with respect to the status of the stage concept, resides in a frequent confounding between external and internal variables. I suggest reserving the terms *transition processes* and/or *mechanisms* to psychological or organismic variables; as an example, the Piagetian concepts of assimilation, accommodation and equilibration (whatever their operationalization may be) can be seen as true organismic processes. These should be clearly differentiated from external or environmental variables that, even though they may have a causal influence, need to be mediated through some psychological variable. The psychological variables could be referred to as *transition factors*. For instance, accounts of the influence of socioeconomic variables on cognitive development remain purely descriptive as long as one does not try to understand through which psychological processes such external variables are necessarily mediated (e.g., Lautrey, 1980). Another example is the interesting distinction introduced by Rutter (in press) between risk indicator and risk mechanism, the latter being considered as more remote and exerting a causal influence; however, such mechanisms still seem to correspond to external variables, and there remains the need to understand with which internal mechanism they may interact.

This is not to say that only internal or subjective mechanisms should be focused upon; on the contrary, I am arguing for a better differentiation between internal and external variables, which in turn should lead to a better understanding of interactional or transactional phenomena. Keeping with Hoppe-Graff's (this volume) useful distinction, I would consider *transition principles* (defined by Hoppe-Graff as laws of change) as referring essentially to the observer's descriptive account of the developmental changes, whereas the term *transition mechanisms* (defined as those principles explaining the transition) could be reserved to describe organismic variables and changes. A good example of a transition principle from the observer's point of view is provided by Fischer's transformational rules (Fischer & Lamborn, this volume), whereas an example of an organismic variable accounting for developmental change could be found in Pascual-Leone's M-Power (e.g., Pascual-Leone, 1970; 1983; 1987) or Case's Short Term Storage Space (e.g., Case, 1985).

I would like to argue that the issue of psychological internal processes versus external variables is even more problematic when it comes to individual differences in cognitive development, which are crucial when a longitudinal perspective is adopted. Indeed, developmental psychologists increasingly acknowledge the importance of individual differences (e.g., Case, Marini, McKeough, Dennis, & Goldberg, 1986; Fischer & Silvern, 1985; Neimark, 1985); however, the source of individual differences is most often located outside the subjects, such as in tasks, environments, or at best in the subjects' past experience. In turn, these nonorganismic variables are considered to modulate a developmental process that remains essentially conceptualized as unidimensional (for a discussion, see Dasen & de Ribaupierre, 1987; Lautrey, 1985; Pascual-Leone, 1987; de Ribaupierre, Rieben, & Lautrey, 1988; Rieben, de Ribaupierre, & Lautrey, 1986; 1988).

Because the necessity and the specificity of longitudinal studies have been well analyzed by Hoppe-Graff, in the introduction, they do not need to be discussed in detail again. The objectives of a longitudinal design, relative to a cross-sectional design, may be seen as threefold; the very simplistic and not exhaustive classification that follows will be used to review the chapters.

First, one can hope to obtain finer descriptions of change by following the same subjects over time. The conservation paradigm described by Piaget in terms of regulations can be taken as a sketchy example: Piaget claimed, on the basis of cross-sectional studies, that subjects start by centering on one dimension, then on the other, and finally on the two together. One could hope that such shifts could be observed longitudinally. However, such a hope remains in most cases idealistic, because not only does it raise the issue of observability of changes (e.g., Hoppe-Graff, this volume), but the study would require microlongitudinal studies, which for many reasons are unfeasible on a long period and with such paradigms. Further, the specificity of a longitudinal design is not optimalized in such an approach; the same results could probably be obtained via cross-sectional studies, provided a very small age interval is used. In the same vein, and somewhat paradoxically given the reasons usually given for not resorting to a longitudinal design, longitudinal studies may be used for practical purposes, particularly in infancy research: The same babies are seen several times because it is more convenient for a variety of reasons. Once more, the specificity of a longitudinal design (i.e., of intraindividual repeated measurement) is not well exploited. A second objective of longitudinal studies, mainly used in personality and in clinical research and more often in studies covering the life-span than in developmental child psychology (although there is no reason for that but for a different focus of interest), lies in their predictive power. The interest here is to understand which may be the best predictors of a number of behavioral outcomes; in terms of psychopathology for instance, retrospective studies are certainly not sufficient for understanding the causal chain leading to a maladaptive outcome (see Rutter, in press).

A third objective of a longitudinal design is model testing. Usually, hypotheses are first derived from cross-sectional studies and the longitudinal design serves to test them, in terms of the developmental function or/and in terms of individuals, in particular by evaluating whether changes defined in terms of groups (age differences) also apply to individual subjects (intraindividual developmental changes). This is the approach that Schneider and Weinert (this volume) refer to as deductive. Note that, as will be later discussed, this approach requires that the researcher be convinced of the necessity to study individual differences; as long as one postulates universal developmental trends, the cost of longitudinal research may appear too great. It is, however, the only means to assess whether development takes the same form for all subjects.

Review of papers

As mentioned previously, this section will overview the different chapters dealing with content areas, focusing on the developmental end states and forms that are implicitly or explicitly defined by each author, the transition principles, mechanisms or factors that are hypothesized, the meaning assigned to individual differences, and the relevance of a longitudinal perspective. Because few authors explicitly spell out these different aspects, this review will necessarily be very sketchy and may reflect gross misinterpretations on my part with respect to which I ask for the authors' indulgence. A summary of these points is presented in Epilogue Table 1.

Epilogue Table 1. *Comparison of the different approaches*

	Developmental end state	Transition principles	Transition mechanisms	Role of longitudinal studies	Role of individual differences
Fischer and Lamborn	Tiers Levels Steps	Transformation rules: shift of focus, compounding, substitution, differentiation, intercoordination	Optimal level Emotions Task Environmental support	For model testing (implicit)	Inter- and intraindividual differences
Schneider and Weinert	Increment in memory performance	Continuous increment (?)	Basic capacities Strategies Content knowledge Metamemory	For model testing: focus on individual curves and on relative contribution of each source	Inter- and intraindividual differences
Camaioni	Prelinguistic–linguistic One-word utterance and use of syntax	Continuity from sociointeractive to linguistic patterns	Interactions Imitation exchanges	For model testing and to determine precursors	Interindividual differences (in rhythm)
Bryant and Alegria	Nonreading–reading	Rhyming, reading, phonological awareness	Activity —	To establish temporal connections (precursors?)	Intergroup comparisons
Stattin and Magnusson	Nonproblem–problem social behavior	—	Biological factors as mediated through self-perception and interpersonal relationships	For long-term predictions	Interindividual differences

Harris	Three levels from behavioral expression, acknowledgment of ambivalence, and display	Development of two systems of appraisal	Environmental amplification of behavior's variations	To test stability of relative speed of development and to establish precursors	Interindividual differences (in speed)
Attili	Development of expression and acknowledgment of ambivalence	Progressive integration of internal working models	Cognitive capacities as imposing constraints on development of emotions	For model testing	Interindividual differences (in vulnerability)
Hofsten	Development of perception–action systems such as reaching and manual coordination	Breaking up of the extension synergy / Sensitivity to binocular disparity / Uncoupling head–arms / Stability of upper trunk	Maturation / Biomechanical constraints / Environment and practice	To disentangle developmental function and developmental change	Interindividual differences (in speed)
Bloch	Development of early coordinations	Stability / Increasing accuracy / Regressions	Difference in the maturational level of the different components / Biomechanical constraints / Postural development / Experience	For model testing (form of development and continuity–discontinuity)	—
Butterworth	Prenatal–postnatal coordinations	Stabilization / Labilization / Regression / Disappearance / Substitution / Integration	Biomechanical constraints / Cognitive changes	For model testing (continuity)	—

Fischer and Lamborn's essay will be discussed in somewhat greater length than the other papers because it proposes a general model of cognitive and emotional development or a "big picture" of development to use Flavell's term (1984), applied in the present case on the development of social interactions (honesty and kindness). The model focuses on the development of skills throughout childhood and adolescence, and defines three types of levels, from the more general to the more specific: tiers (i.e., main stages), recurrent levels within each tier, and steps within levels. Thus, the model provides for clearly defined and illustrated developmental products or end states, throughout a large developmental range, starting at birth and ending at adulthood (although the present chapter deals mainly with late childhood and adolescence). The distinction between surface and deep structures or mechanisms (i.e., between actual performances and underlying mechanisms) is, however, not always clearly stated in Fischer's model (see also Dasen & de Ribaupierre, 1987). As a consequence, the term *level* seems to refer interchangeably to the observable performance and to the underlying "competence": For instance, optimal level is seen as a "process affecting the complexity of skills" (deep level) and as an observable level of performance reached under high environmental support. Likewise, functional level refers to the highest observable behavior in spontaneous contexts where no environmental support is provided, and it reflects the child's underlying competence in that context (Fischer, personal communication).

Transition principles or laws accounting for the sequence of skill acquisition are described in terms of transformation rules, two of which are analyzed in greater detail in the present chapter, namely, shift of focus and compounding. In other papers (e.g., Fischer & Pipp, 1984), three additional rules are hypothesized: substitution, differentiation, and intercoordination. The first four rules deal with within-level sequence of skill acquisition whereas intercoordination is assumed to account for the transition to a higher level as well as to a higher tier. Although they are sometimes described as processes, these rules merely seem to be good descriptions of changes in the observer's language, particularly as they are described as algebraical rewritings. In this sense, they correspond to the second step suggested previously, and not to transition processes.

Fischer and Lamborn consider four factors, qualified as "mechanisms that produce change": optimal level, emotions, task, and environmental support, construed as both organismic and environmental. These factors certainly play an important role as sources of variation in performances (and as such are undoubtedly both environmental and organismic); however, to refer to them as psychological processes or mechanisms seems disputable. First, to consider optimal level for instance as a mechanism eradicates the distinction between structures and processes: Structures, as already mentioned at the beginning of this chapter, might constrain a theory of processes but should not be considered psychological realities (see Campbell & Bickhard, 1986). Thus, optimal level may well correspond to a processing limit but is not a process or mechanism in itself. Second, considering these four factors as mechanisms attests, in my opinion, to a confounding between subjective and environmental variables and not necessarily to an interactionist perspective as Fischer would defend. Although entirely subscribing to a perspective stated in terms of interactions – and Fischer systematically and rightly emphasizes, throughout the various presentations of his model, the need to conceptualize development in terms of interaction or collaboration between person and environment – I would like to argue (probably on different epistemological grounds) that a truly interactional approach necessarily rests on a clear distinction between internal and external variables; there are some truly organismic processes responsible not only for developmental changes within the individual but also for individual differences, just as there are some truly external variables, both types of variables being in constant interactions. Environmental support just cannot be seen as a psychological mechanism per se, although it can of course influence development of the structures (informational units) that subjects can elaborate; organismic variables need to be posited, such as an increase in processing resources or limits that in turn will interact with environmental or situational variables to produce developmental changes (or/and individual differences). This is of course not to claim that there are solely organismic influences or purely organismic "types of subjects."

Fischer's model, in contrast to several other neo-Piagetian models, assigns an important role to individual differences; repeatedly in the present essay and elsewhere, the authors say that no across-task invariances can be observed unless performance is assessed under high environmental support. This is indeed a merit of Fischer's position to point to a large individual variability as well as to a large situational variability. "Development does not automatically produce broadly applicable schemes, but involves the construction of skills specific to task domains." I would like to argue again, however, that the distinction between individual differences as psychological or organismic variables on the one hand and environmental variables on the other is not clear enough, due to Fischer's immediate emphasis on a "collaborative" approach.

Fischer and Lamborn discuss methods for testing developmental sequences; although they point to the usefulness of longitudinal research for providing assessments of different developmental steps in the same individuals, they seem more convinced by the use of a "strong scalogram analysis." They are correct is suggesting that strong scalogram analysis is not used enough in developmental psychology; they should, however, also note that it is no substitute for a longitudinal approach. As demonstrated by Campbell and Richie (1983; see also Lautrey et al., 1986), within-individuals sequence analysis could yield excellent results (i.e., an excellent Guttman scale could be observed) without there being any common underlying process between the items analyzed. Scale analyses are appropriate for testing the order of items in terms of complexity but are not sufficient for testing developmental sequences. The fact that Fischer and Lamborn have been able to build such well-ordered tasks should not be neglected, however. Longitudinal research would nevertheless still prove necessary to determine whether developmental sequences conform to this order at the individual level – that is, whether subjects follow the ordered tiers, levels, and steps postulated by the authors; furthermore, it would allow analysis of interindividual differences in intraindividual changes.

Finally, I would like to emphasize that Fischer and Lamborn's chapter has the merit of integrating cognitive and emotional development. Not only are emotions seen as susceptible to interfere with or to facilitate the cognitive performances, but they are given a cognitive explanation, too: At the beginning of each tier, subjects are seen as more vulnerable, because they are incapable of coping with all the elements at once.

The Schneider and Weinert essay provides an interesting review of work on memory development, and shows that present-day research does not innovate when it attempts to combine the study of general laws and universal developmental functions with that of individual differences. The essay focuses on identification of factors that may cause variations in memory performances but does not define any precise "developmental product"; it addresses the issue of memory increment in general (which, I assume they would probably consider as continuous). This development is not spelled out in detail, probably because until now no invariances have been found across situations; however, the authors mention models such as Case's that claim to have found such invariances. As a consequence, no transition principle or law describing the changes between end states can be described. However, the Schneider and Weinert essay stresses the three other points that should constitute the focus of the present book – namely, factors causing developmental changes, the importance of individual differences, and the necessity of longitudinal research. Referring to Siegler (1983; 1986; see also Flavell,

1977), they enumerate four sources of change in memory development: basic capacities, strategies, content knowledge, and metamemory. This underlines the need for development to be considered as multidetermined (e.g., Pascual-Leone, 1987; de Ribaupierre, Rieben, & Lautrey, 1988; Rieben, et al., 1986). Not only do they stress this need, but also they argue, on both theoretical and empirical grounds, for the need to assess the relative contribution of each of these sources. Individual differences are also given an important role; it is not always clear, particularly given the role assigned to schooling (i.e., to environmental factors), whether the authors would go as far as considering psychological organismic factors responsible for individual variability. They also stress the magnitude of variability and, like Fischer and Lamborn, seem to postulate that there is no stability across tasks. Finally, the Schneider and Weinert essay is probably the best advocate of the use of longitudinal studies in developmental research, particularly with respect to its model-testing role; they stress the importance of taking into consideration individual curves, especially when the change in performance is not linear.

Camaioni's chapter examines the transition from prelinguistic to linguistic behavior, and from early to more elaborate language. The development end states examined are of a behavioral nature and are not described in terms of stages: nonverbal early interactive patterns versus behaviors on linguistic measures on the one hand, and one-word utterances versus emerging use of syntax on the other hand. The transition is described as a progressive shift from person-focused interchanges toward increasingly object-focused and "standard action" formats, and a continuity is hypothesized from sociointeractive to linguistic patterns. One of the sources of linguistic development would be interactions and imitation exchanges that allow for shared meanings to be constructed; in turn shared meanings form the referents for more advanced and conventional communications signals, that is, for language. On the basis of her research, Camaioni stresses the importance of activity in conventional games for later linguistic development that would thus be interactively shaped. Action – defined not only as activity on physical objects (aspect stressed by Piaget), but also in a social context – thus plays a major role in the transition. Camaioni also emphasizes the importance of interindividual differences (defined in terms of rhythm of development and rate of activity) while asserting that only a longitudinal design can help to test the form of developmental transitions.

The objective of Bryant and Alegria's paper is methodological in that they want to demonstrate the need to combine a longitudinal with an intervention design in order to study developmental transitions and test any hypothesis of causality. Longitudinal studies are considered to help determine a temporal ordering and a "real life" definite relationship between variables; in contrast, training studies, although they may often be artificial, are considered to allow a hypothesis of causality to be tested However, the term *longitudinal*, in Bryant and Alegria's essay, is used too narrowly, because it is equated with correlational designs. If it is true that correlations cannot get at causes, results of longitudinal studies can nevertheless be scrutinized in a more stringent manner – for instance, on the basis of a priori models of developmental changes (e.g., Hoppe-Graff, this volume; de Ribaupierre, Rieben, & Lautrey, 1988). In terms of content, developmental end states are defined as nonreading versus reading, and the focus is on the role of phonological awareness as the source or the result of this change; that is, the paper examines, on the basis of a number of studies, both cross-sectional and longitudinal, whether reading proceeds from phonological awareness or the reverse. It is finally concluded that transition occurs in three steps: some elementary type of pholonological awareness such as that which is used in rhyming, then reading, and finally a more elaborated phonological awareness. Because the essay is methodologically oriented, it is relatively difficult for the reader to assume what the authors' hypotheses are with respect to general underlying mechanisms of transition – that is, with respect to the reasons why at a given age the child is able to categorize words into rhymes or why, besides formal instruction, reading is at all possible.

Stattin and Magnusson's chapter focuses on the emergence of problem behavior in adolescence and on the necessity of longitudinal study for long-term predictions. Developmental end states are defined in terms of behaviors or social "habits," that is, nonproblem versus problem social behavior. Interestingly enough, the problem behavior that is examined (i.e., drinking behavior) is only a problem because of the age at which it is studied, while later on it will be defined for most individuals and within certain limits as a socially acceptable habit. Problem behavior can thus serve as evidence of a transitional state between childhood and adulthood. No transition principles or laws are defined in the essay as to the type of change involved, but a biosocial hypothesis is proposed with respect not only to broad factors such as biological changes and social influences, but to mediating factors. Specifically, the influence of three such sources on social behavior is tested – namely, biological factors, perception of self (in particular self-perceived maturity), and interpersonal relationships (in particular through peer relations). Besides focusing on individual differences, the interest being on different outcomes for different subgroups of subjects, the essay also demonstrates convincingly the need for long-term longitudinal studies. Indeed, this chapter as well as Magnusson's work in general (see also Magnusson, 1988) shows that only long-term studies can help avoid overgeneralizations and errors in prediction. If early onset of puberty, as mediated through self-perceived maturity and peer relations, does indeed seem to induce early drinking habits, the relationship does not hold later on; the late maturing girls caught up, so that at adult age no difference was found between early maturers and late maturers in terms of alcohol consumption. Adopting a long-term longitudinal design helps demonstrate that it is only within a limited period of time that early maturers can in some respect be considered socially deviant.

Harris is interested in the development of self-knowledge with respect to one's own emotional experience, specifically in the developmental decalage (what Piaget would probably call a vertical decalage) between the behavioral manifestation of emotion and its acknowledgment by the child in two domains, ambivalence and display. Development end states are thus behavioral expression of emotion (for instance, ambivalence as early as 1 year of age, or the possibility of masking emotions or disappointment by 4 years of age) versus verbal acknowledgment of the same emotions, which appear only much later. In the two domains, the developmental sequence is described as consisting of three levels: denial of the co-occurrence of two emotions, acknowledgment that two conflicting emotions can coexist but only successively or when reasons for hiding emotion are made explicit by the experimenter, and finally acknowledgment that the same situation can elicit two conflicting emotions (or that the same person can display one type of emotion while feeling another way). Incidentally, such a sequence can be compared with Siegler's sequence of Rules (e.g., Siegler, 1986) or to the system of dimensions of transformation proposed by the research group to whom the present author belongs (e.g., de Ribaupierre & Rieben, 1985; Rieben, de Ribaupierre, & Lautrey, 1983; 1986).

In Piagetian terms, the mechanism of transition responsible for the development of acknowledgment (and therefore for the vertical decalage) would probably have been that of reflexive abstraction (e.g., Piaget, 1950; 1977), allowing for a reconstruction of the behavioral system on a representational level. In contrast, Harris suggests that the decalage is due to the existence of two different modes of appraisal, "a rapidly developing and relatively exhaustive mode of appraisal that immediately translates itself into emotional behavior, and a more slowly developing system of conscious appraisal." In turn, this asks the question as to why there are two different modes and why an exhaustive search is not possible earlier. The factor responsible for the development of the second system is, according to Harris, socially marked and consists in an amplification by the environment of the child's variations in behavior.

That environment plays a role in forcing the child to carry out a more exhaustive search looks indeed like a promising hypothesis, but this hardly seems to constitute a sufficient reason or a psychological mechanism. Harris discusses individual differences in terms of speed differences, and across-task stability; longitudinal studies would then prove necessary to test whether differences of speed in development are stable. A second objective of longitudinal studies is to test the relationship between early behavior and late behavior – for instance, would securely attached children demonstrate earlier consciousness of ambivalence?

Attili's chapter represents a further elaboration of the development of the expression of ambivalence in children, by reviewing different research traditions, those of attachment theorists, of psychoanalytic theorists, and of cognitive developmentalists. In contrast with Harris's position, Attili argues that display of ambivalence relies on the same system as understanding of ambivalence, and that both develop slowly and through different stages, their main difference being that one is unconscious and the other conscious. The transition principles would consist in the construction of different internal working models and of their progressive integration. Cognitive capacities are considered to constrain the possibility to integrate constrasting information. As a consequence, although Attili does not explicitly say so, increase in cognitive capacities might represent the main mechanism of transition explaining the development of both expression and acknowledgment of ambivalence. Individual differences are dealt with in terms of vulnerability to conditions that lead to pathological development, whereas longitudinal studies are considered necessary to understand when attachment patterns change and what are the factors of change.

The objective of Hofsten's chapter is to discuss some of the problems and transitions encountered during sensorimotor development and illustrate them through research in the domain of manual development during infancy and early childhood. Developmental products are defined in terms of perception–action systems, which are analyzed from the viewpoint of the changes occurring from early coordinations already present at birth to later similar coordinations (which may be smoother, more accurate, or faster); developmental functions are also shown to undergo regressions frequently. Transition principles seemingly correspond to the well-known principles of differentiation and integration, which are considered to explain the apparent regressions in development. These principles are illustrated in particular with respect to the number of differentiations in the development of reaching and of visuoproprioceptive systems; four factors are supposed to contribute to the development of successful reaching: breaking up of the extension synergy (i.e., differentiation of the grasping and approaching systems), sensitivity to binocular disparity, uncoupling of head and arm movements, and development of postural stability of the upper trunk. More global transition mechanisms, such as the role of maturation and environment, are also discussed; with respect to the former aspect, biomechanical constraints are invoked and, although important, are not considered to be sufficient to account for development. A number of longitudinal studies conducted by Hofsten are mentioned, but seem to have been used mainly to analyze group results. Nevertheless, Hofsten discusses the importance of individual differences, seen mainly as differences of speed, and illustrates with an interesting example the relevance of longitudinal design for unraveling developmental function and rate of development. This is particularly important when U-shaped developmental functions are found: In the case of the study mentioned, reaching frequency was found to decrease and then increase after 2 months of age. When individuals develop at different rates, averaging data over the group (as is usually the case with cross-sectional data) may possibly mask this U-shaped function completely; through the longitudinal data, Hofsten could show that a decrease followed by a dramatic increase occurred in all individuals.

Bloch's paper examines the status of early sensorimotor coordinations such as eye–head coordinations and eye–hand coordinations, asking whether they constitute precursors of later behaviors; thus developmental end states are early coordinations versus late coordinations. Several types of changes are suggested: stability (e.g., eye–hand coordinations), increasing accuracy, and regressions. An interesting transition factor that is hypothesized is that of different maturational levels of the different components; that is, the more mature component (for instance, vision in eye–hand coordination) would drive development of the less mature one. Broad transition mechanisms such as biomechanical constraints (considered insufficient as illustrated in her own studies of walking), postural development because it contributes to the elaboration of spatial referents, maturation, and experience are also discussed. Bloch stresses the importance of longitudinal research for studies dealing with the form of development and with the issue of continuity–discontinuity, while seeing its role essentially as one of hypothesis testing.

Finally Butterworth's paper represents another attempt at describing developmental transitions in early infancy. The neonatal period itself is defined as a period of transition leading from adaptation to intrauterine environment toward adaptation to extrauterine environment; the developmental end states that are being considered are prenatal coordinations versus neonatal coordinations. With respect to transition principles and transition mechanisms, which are not clearly distinguished, Butterworth proposes a combination of Changeux's and Prechtl's models, illustrated by the development of neonatal stepping, of hand–mouth coordinations, and of imitation. Specifically, the transition principles proposed are stabilization, labilization, regression, disappearance, replacement by substitution (without developmental continuity) or replacement by integration (progressive embedding of innate systems in higher-order control processes), inhibition by higher centers, connection of different motor systems, and separation of neural components. The respective role of biomechanical constraints as they interact with innate pattern generators and of cognitive changes, in that they allow an instrumentation of the motor systems, is also discussed. Longitudinal studies are essentially seen as dealing with the issue of developmental continuity.

Wanted: developmental longitudinal studies

Although longitudinal research is seemingly the most obvious if not the only method for studying developmental changes (e.g., Hoppe-Graff, this volume; Wohlwill, 1973), it is amazingly scarce in developmental research at large; this is somewhat paradoxical given the number of developmental models that have been proposed (indicative of the diverse types of developmental changes that should have been tested). The present book is no exception, even though the authors make a laudable effort to stress the relevance of a longitudinal approach. Given that the objective was to focus on a longitudinal perspective, this book can be taken as a yardstick against which the difficulty of working with longitudinal perspectives can be measured.

Difficulties of longitudinal studies are indeed large; a number of them are discussed at length in an interesting review by Schneider (in press). Three classes of problems are defined: practical problems such as cost factors, recruitment of staff, data storage and funding; conceptual problems linked with the issues of continuity–discontinuity versus stability–instability, the former dealing with the development of a function while the latter is concerned with individual differences; and methodological problems such as appropriate measures of change, models of data treatment, reliability of scores. Hoppe-Graff (this volume) adds the problem of conceptual vagueness, referring to the fact that none of the authors that he mentions can provide an a priori precise prediction of a developmental sequence. This is probably combined with a lack of focus on methods (and underdevelopment of appropriate methods) in developmental psychology, while longitudinal studies inevitably raise complex methodological problems.

I would like to add yet another reason for this scarcity of longitudinal studies; it has to do with the lack of interest on the part of most developmentalists for individual differences. Baltes and Nesselroade's rationales for longitudinal research (Baltes & Nesselroade, 1979; Hoppe-Graff, this volume) all deal with identification of individual changes, whether intraindividual or interindividual changes and whether for a descriptive or explanatory purpose. In contrast, most developmental models have been concerned with discovering universal laws, applying them either to a general theoretical subject such as Piaget's epistemic subject or to age groups data. In so doing, most models have remained fundamentally unidimensional and have confounded developmental changes with developmental differences (e.g., Schneider, in press; Wohl-will, 1973). In this case, longitudinal studies in their model-testing aspect still prove necessary to test the transitions that are hypothesized; however, the fact that they are then seen as restricted to testing the continuity–discontinuity aspect of the developmental function might not represent a strong enough incentive for overcoming all of the difficulties mentioned earlier. Further, when relying on a unidimensional model of development, results of cross-sectional studies might do the job almost as well (provided the samples examined are close enough in age) and much more easily. Inferences from the group data are then transferred to individuals – that is, age differences are translated into developmental changes.

The last statements may seem to contradict somewhat the remark at the beginning of this chapter that developmentalists had started acknowledging individual differences. However, in most cases, although considered important, individual differences are most often construed as mere differences of speed or rate of development at a surface level (e.g., Dasen & de Ribaupierre, 1987); a longitudinal study would then only serve to demonstrate that such differences of rhythm are stable, which may not prove fundamental for a test of the model under question. Only when development is considered as multi- or pluridetermined (e.g., Pascual-Leone, 1983; de Ribaupierre, in press; de Ribaupierre, Neirynck, & Spira, 1988; de Ribaupierre, Rieben, & Lautrey, 1988; Rieben et al., 1986), both by general developmental and by differential mechanisms, does it become really important to study developmental forms and their stability. Individual differences then play a fundamental and probably qualitative role in terms of processes, and it becomes crucial to test whether their influence is stable. For instance, Longeot (1978) modified the Piagetian model by assuming the existence of developmental loops, followed by different types of subjects, leading from one developmental end state to the next; if one assumes two types of loop (A and B) at two different stages, it becomes fundamental to test not only the continuity of one type of loop (i.e., to determine whether Loop A at Stage 2 is a direct continuation of Loop A at Stage 1), but also the individual stability (i.e., whether subjects following Loop A at Stage 1 will also follow Loop A at Stage 2). Similarly, Rieben et al. (1986; 1988) have recently argued that, at a given developmental level, there are at least two different modes of processing applicable to Piagetian situations, namely a digital and an analogical mode; such modes are not only assumed to be differently elicited by situations, but also to correspond to individual differences. It is then essential to conduct longitudinal studies to test whether there is a continuity between the digital mode inferred during an age period x and the digital mode at age $x + 1$, and, still more important, whether subjects qualified as preferring a digital mode at a given age still present this preference later on (de Ribaupierre et al., submitted). A final example can be taken in the field of memory. As well analyzed in Schneider and Weinert's chapter, memory development is presently conceptualized as depending on at least four sources. The relative contribution of each source may differ during different periods of development (e.g., Siegler, 1986); it may also differ across individuals of a given level. Provided each source could be empirically singled out (de Ribaupierre et al., submitted; Schneider & Weinert, this volume), it would again prove crucial to conduct longitudinal studies to test the relative impact of each source at different moments, and the stability of its influence for a given individual.

A further argument in favor of the thesis according to which longitudinal studies have been little used in developmental psychology because of the lack of interest for individual differences comes from the fields of personality and psychopathology: In these areas, researchers have been primarily concerned with interindividual or intergroup differences, whether for purposes of prevention or for explaining deviant behavioral outcomes, and longitudinal studies are flourishing. Incidentally, it has to be remarked that very often these studies have neglected the study of changes within individuals (e.g., Rutter, in press). Longitudinal studies certainly are no panacea, and have limits that have not been analyzed here; nevertheless, let us hope that, in the near future, more developmentalists will be convinced of the existence of different developmental paths for different types of subjects and will be ready to overcome practical and methodological difficulties, which, although heavy, are not insurmountable. To limit the costs, however, longitudinal studies should preferably be restricted to their model-testing aspect – that is, used to test hypotheses about developmental transitions that have been derived from cross-sectional studies.

REFERENCES

Baltes, P. B. (1987). Theoretical propositions of life-span developmental psychology: On the dynamics between gains and losses. *Developmental Psychology, 23,* 611–626.

Baltes, P. B., & Nesselroade, J. R. (1979). History and rationale of longitudinal research. In J. R. Nesselroade & P. B. Baltes (Eds.), *Longitudinal research in the study of behavior and development* (pp. 1–39). New York: Academic Press.

Campbell, R. L., & Bickhard, M. H. (1986). *Knowing levels and developmental stages.* Basel: Karger.

Campbell, R. L., & Richie, D. M. (1983). Problems in the theory of developmental sequences: Prerequisites and precursors. *Human Development, 26,* 156–172.

Case, R. (1985). *Intellectual development from birth to adulthood.* New York: Academic Press.

Case, R., Marini, Z., McKeough, A., Dennis, S., & Goldberg, J. (1986). Horizontal structure in middle childhood: Cross-domain parallels in the course of cognitive growth. In I. Levin (Ed.), *Stage and structure: Reopening the debate* (pp. 1–39). Norwood, NJ: Ablex.

Dasen, P. R., & de Ribaupierre, A. (1987). Neo-Piagetian theories: Cross-cultural and differential perspectives. *International Journal of Psychology, 22,* 793–832.

Fischer, K. W., & Pipp, S. L. (1984). Processes of cognitive development: Optimal level and skill acquisition. In R. J. Sternberg (Ed.), *Mechanisms of cognitive development* (pp. 45–80). New York: Freeman.

Fischer, K. W., & Silvern, L. (1985). Stages and individual differences in cognitive development. *Annual Review of Psychology, 36,* 613–648.

Flavell, J. H. (1977). *Cognitive development.* Englewood Cliffs, NJ: Prentice-Hall.

Flavell, J. H. (1984). Discussion. In R. J. Sternberg (Ed.), *Mechanisms of cognitive development* (pp. 187–209). New York: Freeman.

Flavell, J. H., & Wohlwill, J. F. (1969). Formal and functional aspects of cognitive development. In D. Elkind & J. H. Flavell (Eds.), *Studies in cognitive development* (pp. 67–120). London: Oxford University Press.

Lautrey, J. (1980). *Classe sociale, milieu familial, intelligence.* Paris: Presses Universitaires de France.

Lautrey, J. (1985). Stades et différences. In J. Bideaud & M. Richelle (Eds.), *Psychologie développementale* (pp. 299–316). Brussels: Mardaga.

Lautrey, J., de Ribaupierre, A., & Rieben, L. (1986). Les différences dans la forme du développement cognitif évalué avec des épreuves piagétiennes: Une application de l'analyse des correspondances. *Cahiers de Psychologie Cognitive, 6,* 575–613.

Longeot, F. (1978). *Les stades opératoires de Piaget et les facteurs de l'intelligence.* Grenoble: Presses Universitaires de Grenoble.

Magnusson, D. (1988). *Individual development from an interactional perspective: A longitudinal study.* Hillsdale, NJ: Erlbaum.

Neimark, E. D. (1985). Moderators of competence: Challenges to the universality of Piagetian theory. In E. D. Neimark, R. de Lisi, & J. L. Newman (Eds.), *Moderators of competence* (pp. 1–14). Hillsdale, NJ: Erlbaum.

Pascual-Leone, J. (1970). A mathematical model for the transition in Piaget's developmental stages. *Acta Psychologica, 32*, 301–345.

Pascual-Leone, J. (1983). Growing into human maturity: Toward a metasubjective theory of adulthood stages. In P. B. Baltes & O. G. Brim (Eds.), *Life-span development and behavior* (Vol. 5, pp. 117–156). New York: Academic Press.

Pascual-Leone, J. (1987). Organismic processes for neo-Piagetian theories: A dialectical causal account of cognitive development. *International Journal of Psychology, 22*, 531–570.

Piaget, J. (1950). *La construction du réel chez l'enfant* (2nd ed). Neuchatel: Delachaux & Niestlé.

Piaget, J. (1956). Les stades du développement intellectuel de l'enfant et de l'adolescent. In *Le problème des stades en psychologie de l'enfant. IIIe symposium de l'Association de Psychologie scientifique de langue française* (pp. 33–42). Paris: Presses Universitaires de France.

Piaget, J. (1977). *Recherches sur l'abstraction réfléchissante*. Paris: Presses Universitaires de France.

de Ribaupierre, A. (in press). Operational development and cognitive style: A review of French literature and a neo-Piagetian reinterpretation. In T. Globerson & T. Zelniker (Eds.), *Cognitive development and cognitive style*. Norwood, NJ: Ablex.

de Ribaupierre, A., Neirynck, I., & Spira, A. (1988). Memory development in childhood. Unpublished manuscript.

de Ribaupierre, A., & Pascual-Leone, J. (1984). Pour une intégration des méthodes en psychologie: approches expérimentale, psycho-génétique et différentielle. *L'Année Psychologique, 84*, 227–250.

de Ribaupierre, A., & Rieben, L. (1985). Etude du fonctionnement opératoire: quelques problèmes méthodologiques. *Bulletin de Psychologie, 38* (372), 841–852.

de Ribaupierre, A., Rieben, L., & Lautrey, J. (1988). Developmental change and invididual differences: A longitudinal study using Piagetian tasks. Unpublished manuscript.

Rieben, L., de Ribaupierre, A., & Lautrey, J. (1983). *Le développement opératoire de l'enfant entre 6 et 12 ans: Elaboration d'un instrument d'évaluation*. Paris: Editions du CNRS.

Rieben, L., de Ribaupierre, A., & Lautrey, J. (1986). Une définition structuraliste des formes du développement cognitif: Un projet chimérique? *Archives de Psychologie, 54* (209), 95–123.

Rieben, L., de Ribaupierre, A., & Lautrey, J. (1988). Cognitive development and individual differences: On the necessity of minimally structuralist approach for educational sciences. Unpublished manuscript.

Rutter, M. (in press). Longitudinal data in the study of causal processes: Some uses and some pitfalls. In M. Rutter (Ed.), *Risk and protective factors in psychosocial development*. Cambridge: Cambridge University Press.

Schneider, W. (in press). Problems of longitudinal studies with children: Practical, conceptual and methodological issues. In M. Brambring, F. Lösel, &

H. Skowronek (Eds.), *Children at risk: Assessment and longitudinal research*. New York: De Gruijter.

Siegler, R. S. (1983). Information-processing approaches to development. In W. Kessen (Ed.), *Handbook of child psychology: Vol. 1. History, theory, and methods* (P. Mussen, Gen. Ed.) (4th ed., pp. 129–211). New York: Wiley.

Siegler, R. S. (1986). *Children's thinking*. Englewood Cliffs, NJ: Prentice-Hall.

Strauss, S., & Stavy, R. (Eds.). (1982). *U-shaped behavioral growth*. New York: Academic Press.

Sugarman, S. (1987). The priority of description in developmental psychology. *International Journal of Behavioral Development, 10*, 391–414.

Wohlwill, J. (1973). *The study of behavioral development*. New York: Academic Press.

Name index

Subject index

abstract mappings, 44, 45, 52, 55; age of emergence of, 44, 60; and ambivalence, 221, 222, 226; and emotional vulnerabilities in adolescence, 62; spurts in, 53, 54, 54f
abstract systems, 44–45; and emotional vulnerabilities in adolescence, 62
abstractions, 36; development of, 37; and emotional vulnerabilities in adolescence, 59, 61–62, 63; levels of, 37–45, 38t
accommodation, 6, 8–11, 276, 299; defined, 9; neonate, 238
accuracy (coordination), 266, 311
action: in language acquisition, 307; and posture, 238
action system(s), 233, 237, 291
adaptation: neonatal period as time of transition between states of, 285–287
adaptive skills, 237
Adjustment Screening Test, 159, 160
adolescence: alcohol use in, 156–173; attachment patterns in, 226; cognitive and emotional transitions in, 33–67; emotional vulnerability and cognitive development in, 58–62; levels of development in, 40–41t; rebellious period in, 217, 226; social cognitive development in, 34–47; social transition in, 147–190
adolescents: emotional turmoil of, 44, 58; psychosocial functioning of, 147–148
Adult Attachment Interview, 217
adulthood: reflection on parent-child relations in, 200; risk of alcohol abuse in, 181–182; social maladaptation in, 186
affect activation, 222–223
affective components: in internal working models, 225
age: and acknowledgment of ambivalence, 194–195, 197–200; and alcohol use in adolescence, 159, 160–163, 163f; in

communicative development, 114; and emergence of mappings, 44, 60; and memory development, 70; and memory performance, 69; and memory span, 72–73; and metamemory development, 82, 83; optimal levels and, 5, 7; and problem behavior, 184; and understanding of emotions, 208–209; as variable, 13
age differences: in memory development, 70, 73–74, 85; in memory performance, 74, 75–76, 77–78, 80, 83; in memory span, 73; in recall, 78
age-graded influences: in adolescence, 147–149
agent use, 17
aggression: alcohol use and, 157
aids (memory), 54, 73, 74
alcohol abuse: risk of, 181–182, 185–186
alcohol use by adolescents, 183, 184, 185, 187, 308–309; biological maturation and, 160–174, 185; biosocial model of, 156–173; by girls, 160, 182–187
alcohol use by adults, 157, 185–186; long-term effects of biological maturation on, 179–182, 181t
alcoholics, 157
alertness, 262, 264
alliteration, 133–134, 135, 137
allometrics, 267
alphabet, 126–127; phonetic, 210
alphabetic system: learning to read in, 137, 139–140, 141–142
ambivalence, 192, 206, 210, 214–229, 309, 310; acknowledgment of, 193–200, 208, 226–227; capacity for, 214–215, 217–218, 220, 223, 226; display of, 220, 223, 225, 310; double meaning of, 219–220; expression of, 192–193, 194, 198, 215, 216–218; in insecure children, 223–224; in secure children, 223; term, 215; understanding of, 215, 218, 220, 221,